Endorsements for *I Should Be Dead, The Life of Z*

Damian Sanders

Some people make an impact on your life from the first moment you meet. We met at Donner Ski Ranch in Lake Tahoe in the late 1980s. We were rat packing at Donner hitting jumps left and right. I backflipped a big kicker, landed and stopped to watch him try it. Literally this kamikaze psycho was blazing down the hill towards the jump. To myself I thought there's no way this guy's gonna pull this off. Way too much speed. But to my surprise he did the backflip and at the last millisecond, he flipped to fakie and stuck it. He pulled up right beside me, I'm sure I gave him a high five and the rest was history. We rode together for the rest of the day and that blossomed an almost 40 year friendship.

Szabo was the personality snowboarding needed. Goofy, funny, life on the edge, push everything to the limits personality. And he had the skills to back it up. We toured the world together. Japan, Canada and all over America. Snowboarding is a better sport because of Szabo. Riding with Szabo was always a blast, always an adventure. Always pushing each other to the limits. And not just snowboarding. Motocross, filming goofy skits for Creatures and Crusty Demons, skateboarding, pretty much any extreme sport, Szabo ripped with an effortless style and grace! Rock on Brother!

Damian Sanders -
Old School Snowboard Pro

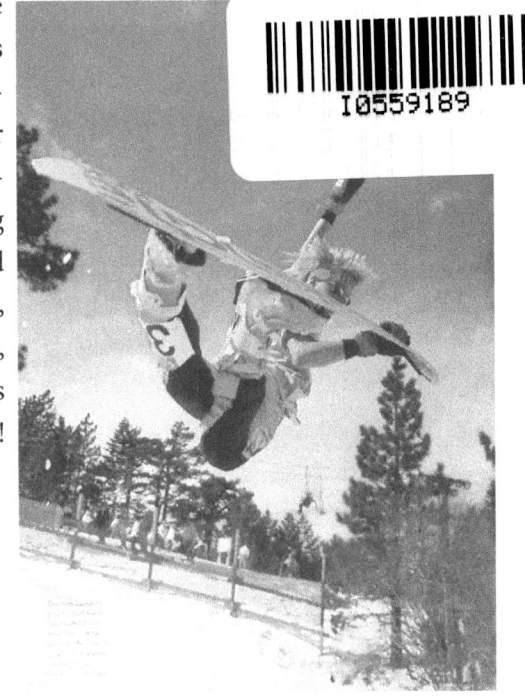

Photo: Jon Foster

Seth Enslow

Szabo was one of the first friends I made when I moved to California in 1994. I had already watched him in the Creatures of Habit Snowboarding Videos when I was in high school. Szabo always excelled at any board or 2 wheeled sport we did. He would keep a Daily Journal and I knew someday Z would write a fantastic book. Here it is. *I Should Be Dead, The Life of Z* — check it out!

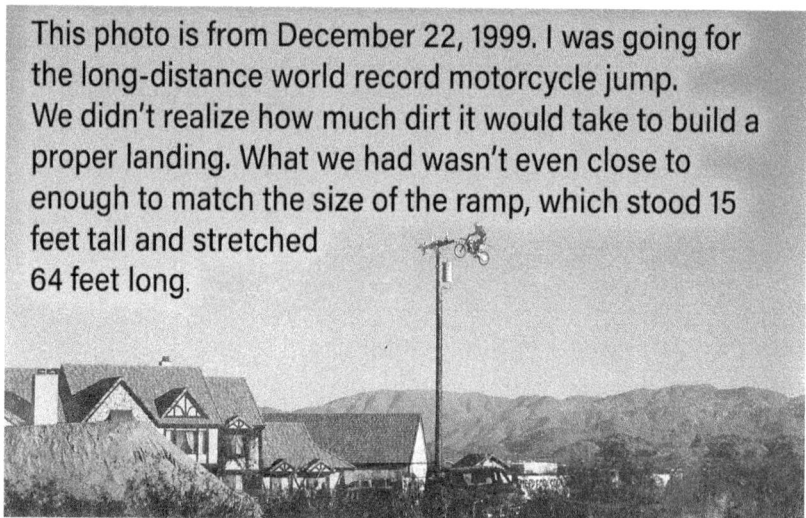

This photo is from December 22, 1999. I was going for the long-distance world record motorcycle jump. We didn't realize how much dirt it would take to build a proper landing. What we had wasn't even close to enough to match the size of the ramp, which stood 15 feet tall and stretched 64 feet long.

Needless to say, the landing wasn't nearly big enough for how high and far I jumped — but I hit it anyway and it almost killed me. I smashed my forehead on the handlebars, crushed my frontal sinus canal, and broke my right collarbone.

The doctor had to cut my head ear to ear, pull my face down out of the way, remove the crushed bone, and rebuild the sinus canal with titanium screws, plates, and mesh. Then he put my head back together with 55 staples.

Seth Enslaow - Freerider / Distance Jumper
Photo: PINEMAN

Dave England

When I was a kid back in the 80s every so often Szabo would magically appear at one of our poorly constructed backyard skate ramps. My friends and I would watch in awe as he effortlessly floated ginormous backside ollies on our barely skateable wooden death traps which featured no less than 3 feet of vert. A few years later, my first time ever seeing a snowboard magazine, I opened it up to find a stunning photo of Szabo launching off a cliff that looked to be several thousand feet high. I figured he must have died on impact. 25 years later I was floating on an inner tube at a local water-park's lazy river without a care in the world when suddenly the back of my head collided with an unyieldingly solid orb. Turns out the dense object was Szabo's hairless skull! In the years that have followed we have occasion-ally "bumped" into one another and it's always nothing short of a pleasure and an honor. Long live Double 0 Szabo!!!

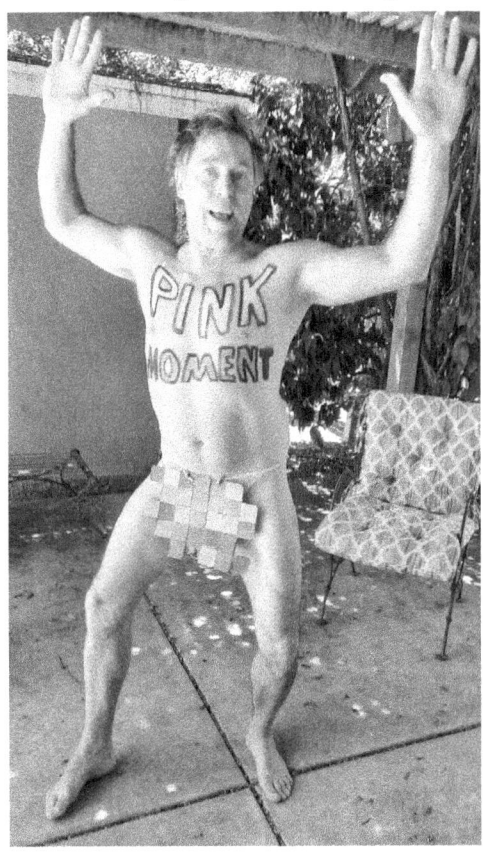

Dave England

Nathan Fletcher

I've known Don since the mid-'80s. One of my first snowboard trips was to meet up with him and his crew, and I'll never forget watching him launch massive backflips at Donner Summit. It was unreal. That moment stuck with me. Later, we became friends, and he's always been someone I looked up to. Don's energy and style pushed me to go bigger, ride harder, and keep chasing that next level.

What he's done since then, what he's been through, It's nothing short of inspiring. Most people wouldn't have made it through half of what he has, let alone come out the other side still smiling, still charging, and still lifting others up.

Don's not just a friend I value, he's a true legend, a real-life warrior, and a hero to many. His story is heavy, real, and guaranteed to hit deep.

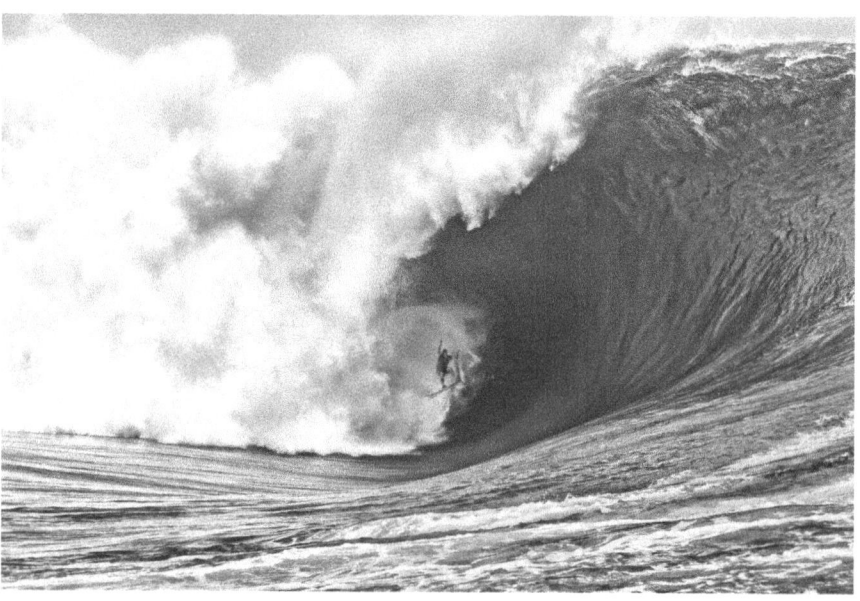

Nathan Fletcher, big wave rider / life enjoyer
Photo: Brian Beilman

Christian Hosoi

Don was one of us. He was part of the brotherhood of skateboarders that gathered at backyard ramps, pools, and ditches, where style, guts, and passion mattered most. Szabo stood out from the pack, not just for how he rode with raw power and smooth style, but for how he brought the session to life, chopping it up on the sidelines, cracking jokes, heckling, and pushing all of us like we owned the world and it owed us for shredding on it.

Don's snowboarding was next level. I saw him launch backflips off cliffs without even knowing where the landing was, just pure trust and fearless flow. It blew my mind. He ripped at moto too, and honestly, just about anything he set his mind to.

But it wasn't just talent. Don always showed respect for the culture, especially in skateboarding. He never forgot who paved the way, always honoring the tricks and riders that came before. That kind of heart and presence mattered.

There weren't many kids I knew back then who had it all, talent, guts, and the drive to push beyond the limits of what seemed possible. Don was the real deal.

Christian Hosoi,
skater at heart, son of God
and lover of life.

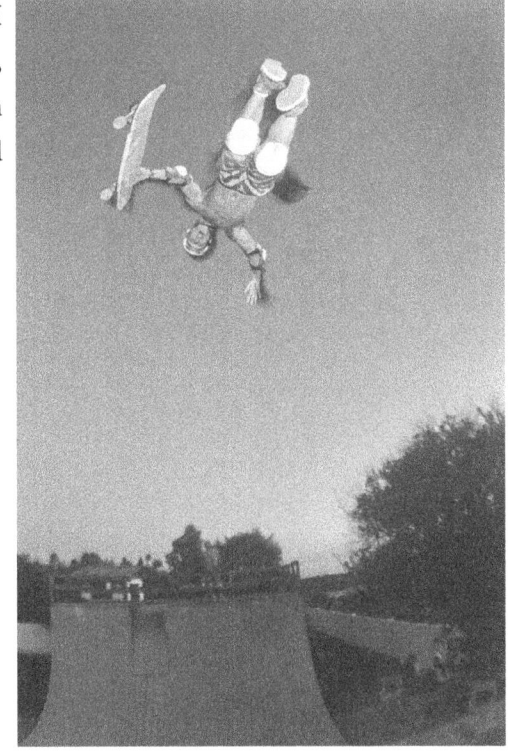

Photo: Grant Britain

Steve Caballero

If I could describe this gentleman in one fragment of a statement, I would say…"resiliently, motivated and courageous." He's lived a life full of ups and downs, literally and metaphorically, and he has the scars to prove it!

A man of many talents that I've known for decades, but it wasn't until recent years that I got to know him more on a personal level by hanging out on two wheels instead of the four wheels we both started on.

Mountain biking has been our reconnection and has given us the ability to hang together and share stories and life adventures. I'm extremely proud of him for what he's been through and admire his grit and dedication to sustain this chaotic life he's endured, never second-guessing his ability to bounce back and send it. And when I say send it, the dude flies on a MTB.

Szabo is one of the friendliest dudes I know, and it's always a pleasure to ride with him. Love you buddy, and keep charging.

Stevie Caballero
(Skate Legend,
Action Sports Icon,
Artist, Musician,
Father and more)

Trick — Caballerial

Location — Rätvik, Sweden

Year — 1981

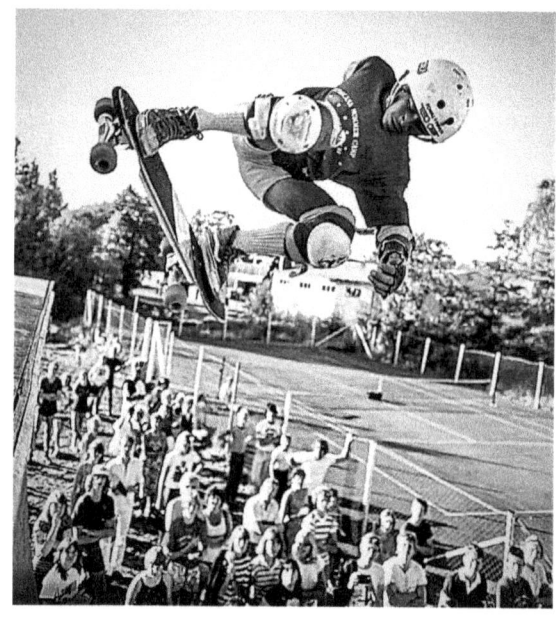

Photo: Martin Willners

Michael Bernoff

Don's journey is a powerful reminder that even in life's darkest moments, resilience is possible. In this book he lays it all out…the heartache and loss, trauma, hard truths and experiences most would never be able to speak about and through it all - he keeps showing up and fighting for healing, purpose, and meaning. The honesty he shares isn't just a testimony - this book will speak to anyone who's ever felt on the edge and needed proof that it's possible to come back stronger.

Michael Bernoff-Mindset Coach

Dusty Henricksen

Double O sZabo! I had the pleasure of growing up around a bunch of super bad-ass people, to say the least, and sZabo is one of the gnarliest. We used to rip mountain bikes all day, every day, in semi-recent years, and he was always pushing the limits. Fun to follow, that's for sure.

This photo I've chosen was shot out in Montreal this past winter of 24–25 while filming for a video project with friends called BUSTER. It's all street snowboarding, meaning we would shovel and find our own things to shred in the city. Hands down, it was some of the most fun I've had on a snowboard, just hanging with friends and pushing each other to send it harder and harder.

This specific spot is famous for skateboarding, so when we saw it, I knew I had to try to get a trick in. I mainly compete on the World Cup circuit these days in Slopestyle and Big Air, so trips like this are always refreshing and bring the style and fun back into snowboarding for me.

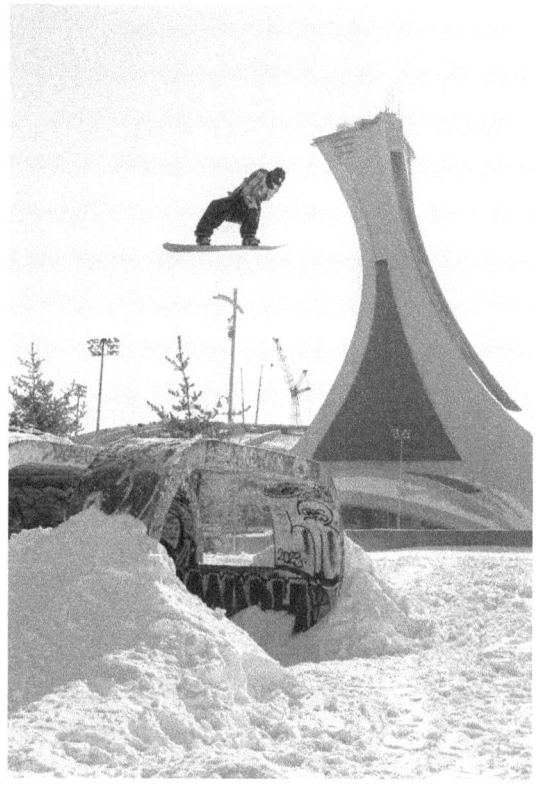

Super stoked to hear some of the crazy stories sZabo has in store for us, and I'm really honored to be a part of his book. Keep sending it, Double O — love you, bro!

Dusty Henricksen
Pro Snowboarder
– Olympian – Street &
Slopestyle Shredder

Photo: Lil John

Lance Mountain

As we were kids in the late '70s, we all grew up at different skateparks throughout California. When the parks closed, skateboarding seemed to have died. Few stuck with it, and it was recreated as a DIY backyard ramp scene. Only the die-hard few from the skateparks continued, and it lit a new fire for the next generation of skateboarders.

Skateboarding was intense and progressive, born out of desperation to show the world how great it is. This push took it far beyond where it was in the past. Don was part of that scene, and he took his aggressive ability and fearlessness from skateboarding, which would lead him into the emerging snowboarding scene.

He went on to make many lifestyle snowboarding videos that led the way in that booming industry for 10 years. He got into riding motocross and charged it in that sport, following his love for the adrenaline in moto the same way he did in snowboarding and skateboarding in the past. He has been paving the way for years in these sports that we now know as action sports.

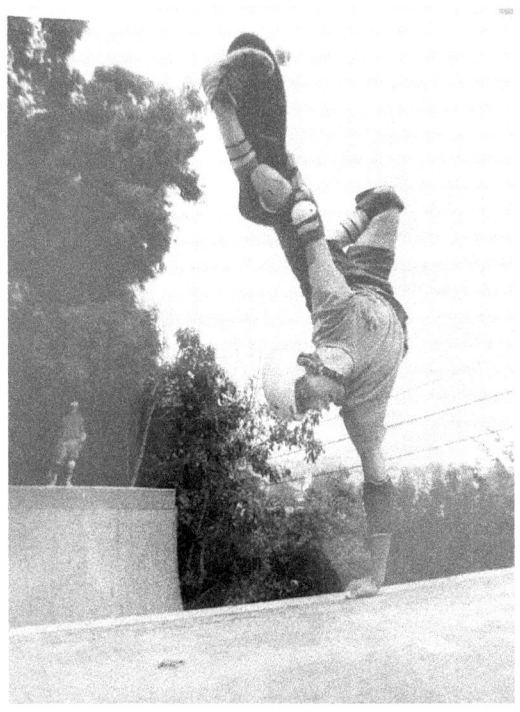

He has had the passion and drive to push through injuries and the ups and downs of life. He has continued to live in the moment rather than follow the path most people have taken in life, and it has served him well.

Lance Mountain
Skateboarder

Brett Tippie

I remember Don Szabo from the early snowboard freestyle days. He was in many different snowboard magazines and I saw him in video segments in the snowboard movies back in the day. He was able to do a bunch of different tricks and he didn't mind going big! I also saw him absolutely send it on a dirtbike in a video and I knew he had a hand in helping with Crusty Demons of Dirt, a pivotal FMX video. A very talented multi sport athlete and he is now also enjoying ebiking on a YT Industry Decoy! Check out his book, his life has been wild, inspiring, and definitely worth reading about!

Brett Tippie - Freeride MTB Pioneer
MTB Hall-of-Famer, Legendary
World Cup Snowboard Racer

Photo: Ale diLullo

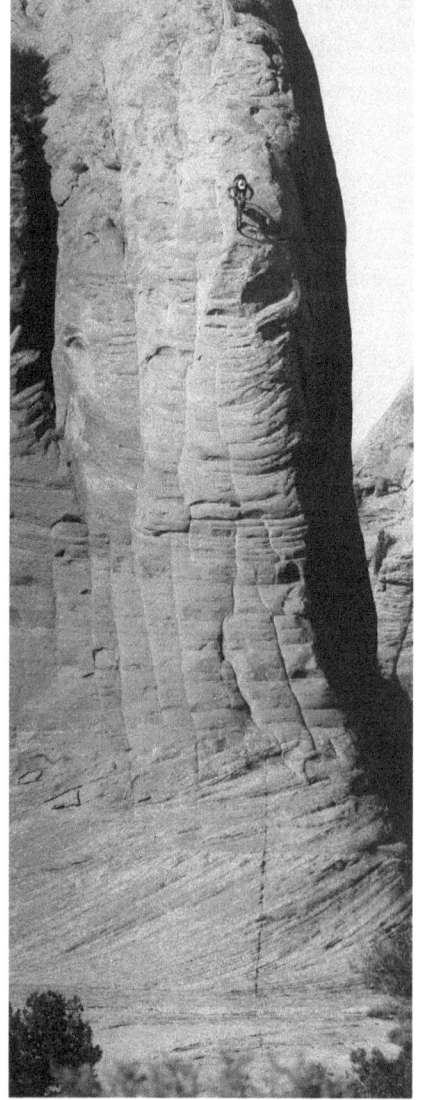

Mike Metzger

When I think of Don Szabo, the first thing that comes to mind is pure entertainment, smiles, and huge laughs. The first time I remember seeing this bald, crooked-headed maniac was in the snowboard movie Creatures of Habit. That was my introduction to the raw insanity Szabo brought to my young, growing mind, thanks to the producers behind what would soon become the mind-blowing Crusty Demons of Dirt.

Szabo, being the ridiculously creative visionary that he is, always saw things differently than most people. He brought massive amounts of energy to anything he and his friends were doing. I remember how stoked he was on moto and how he found himself at the Morrow snowboard/motocross races they promoted in Albany, Oregon. Szabo was always the guy to go for it, especially if he saw a friend do it first. He was next in line to huck himself on his number-double-zero–plated dirtbike.

A multi-talented athlete who wasn't afraid to push his limits and push others to do their best, going for it with no worries about the consequences. A true legend in the minds of many other talented athletes.

Mike Metzger — The Godfather of Freestyle Motocross, Artist / Entrepreneur

Photo: Garth Milan

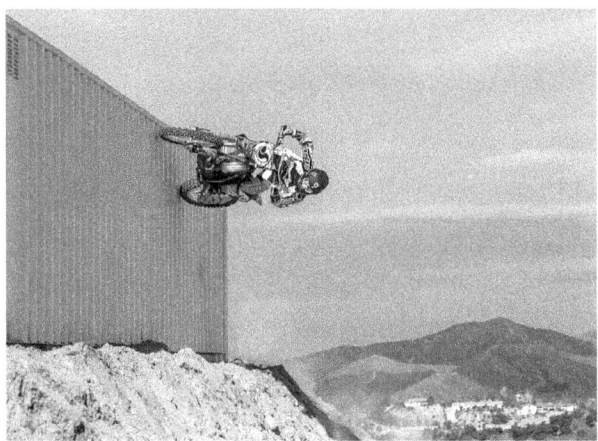

Contact The Author:

Don Szabo

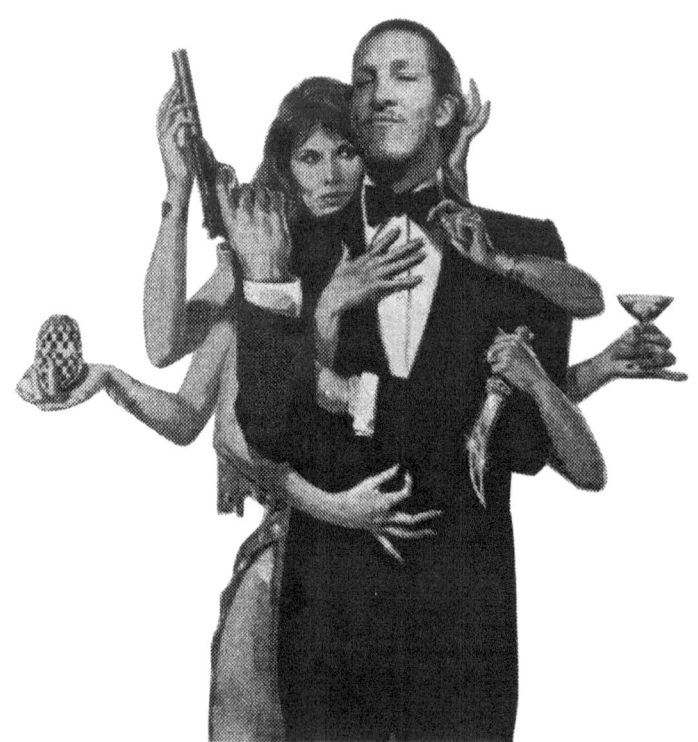

@DoubleOSzabo

IG = @DoubleOSzabo

Facebook = Don Szabo

Youtube = DonSzabo

Email = ZLifeBook@gmail.com

Website = DonSzabo.com

I SHOULD BE DEAD

The Life of Z

Don Szabo

Published in the United States by:
Blue Jay Ink, 451 A East Ojai Ave., Ojai, California 93023

"Now I understand some of the challenges that come with putting your life into words. You have to share something that feels right to you and hope the reader enjoys it, connects with it, and understands the life you've lived. Writing your story is a great experience, and I'd encourage anyone who's into it to give it a try. It's a powerful way to connect with your own life, document it for yourself, and share it with others. It was a mind-expanding journey, and I'm glad I got to experience it."

Don Szabo

open

DEAD-ICATED To:

My family on this side of the dirt. My sister, Karen, and my daughters Kaylee and Ashlyn.

My family that is no longer here. My mom, dad and my wife Heather (it's about half-and-half)

Photo: James Cassimus

Rock and roll: Don Szabo falling from Heaven's Gate, an hour from his house in L.A., while 1,300 miles to the north Masoto Ogawa floats a little closer to the ground at Whistler Mountain, B.C. Same instruments, different song.

Foreword by Vince Kitchen

Author of *Normally Unusual…Path of a Volunteer Stuntman*

"We are like books. Most people only see our cover. A few skim the introduction. Many believe the critics. But only a rare few ever read the content."

Every one of us is living a story. We spend most of our time trying to piece it together — filling in the blanks as we go. But here's the trick to keeping our sanity: stop obsessing over ourselves. As someone once said, "Humility isn't thinking less of ourselves, it's thinking about ourselves less."

Reading helps us do that. It takes us out of our own heads and into the lives of others. It's a form of therapy — a kind of time travel that brings peace, perspective, and sometimes, clarity. I've found all of that in both reading and writing.

Writing this foreword takes me back — way back — to the first time I met Don Szabo in our teens. We didn't just share the same age — we shared the same addiction: adrenaline. And our first fix was skateboarding.

My parents let us build a proper half-pipe ramp in our San Fernando Valley backyard, and it quickly became a magnet for talent. One of the most fearless riders to ever drop in was Don. Even back then, he was pushing the limits. He had raw style and next-level skills — more radical than even I could claim.

I've always been competitive, but I've also gravitated toward people who were better than me. Being around Szabo raised my game in every sport we touched. And we touched a lot of them.

Out of the four action-sport disciplines — skating, surfing, snowboarding, and motocross — Don was always a step ahead. Light on his feet, fearless on the throttle. But the higher you fly, the harder you fall. And Szabo flew high.

Z has lived through things that would've broken most people — physically and emotionally. But he always found a way to get back up. I remember him once saying, "We'll still be having adventures when we're in dentures." And damn if that's not exactly what we're doing.

Don Szabo is a huge part of my story, and now you get to read his. What you'll find is a man who's more than just skill and guts. He's a truth-seeker. He's real. Page after page, through each stage of life, you'll see it for yourself.

I thought I already knew everything there was to know about my lifelong friend. Then I read "I Should Be Dead." Watching him peel back the layers of his life, finding clarity as he wrote each chapter — it surprised me. And moved me.

That's the gift of writing your own story. You don't just tell it — you understand it. And in the end, I realized the title wasn't quite right. He should be alive. Alive to share this incredible ride with all of us.

So buckle up. Look out below. Here we go.

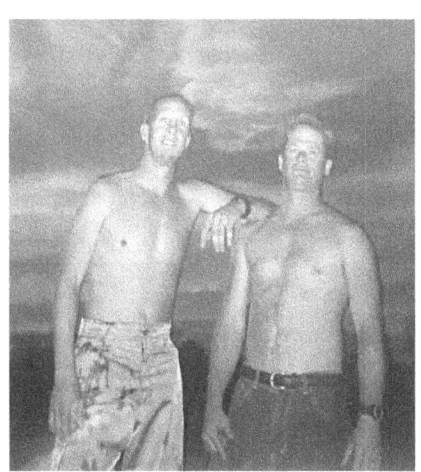 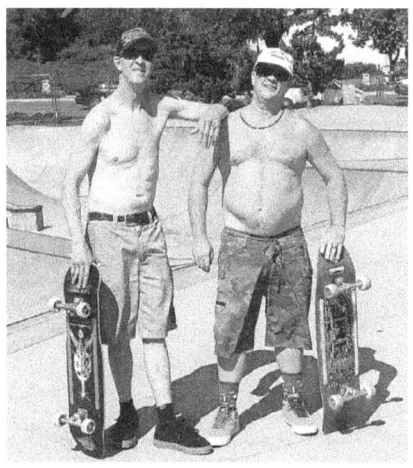

A Life on Bikes and Boards — 1999, 2021, and Beyond

Table of Contents

If you're not familiar with some of the terms in this book, there is a glossary in the back that may give you a definition of something you don't understand, or ask AI.

-Chapter 1-
Early Rollin'

The Beginning of the End of the Beginning...

My eyes crack open, and a sharp, sterile blur floods my vision as my eyes flutter open. There's the cold hum of hospital lights and steady beeps pulling me back into reality. My mind races as I try to piece together where I am and why I'm here. Faces hover in and out, people moving around like I'm some kind of emergency. They're saying my name, but it feels distant, echoing, like I'm still halfway somewhere else.

This wasn't part of the plan. I mean, I'd been through my share of hard knocks before. Snowboarding, motocross, high-speed wipeouts, and miscalculations — they've landed me under the knife ten times. Misjudged a *line* I was taking, maybe went too big off a lip, or came up short. But this? This wasn't some predictable crash with a prescribed fix.

I've always been willing to pay the price for the adrenaline rush from extreme sports. Hell, I've even had a 1,400-passenger Carnival Cruise Line ship turn around to get me the serious medical attention I needed. But this time, it was different. This time, I wasn't supposed to wake up.

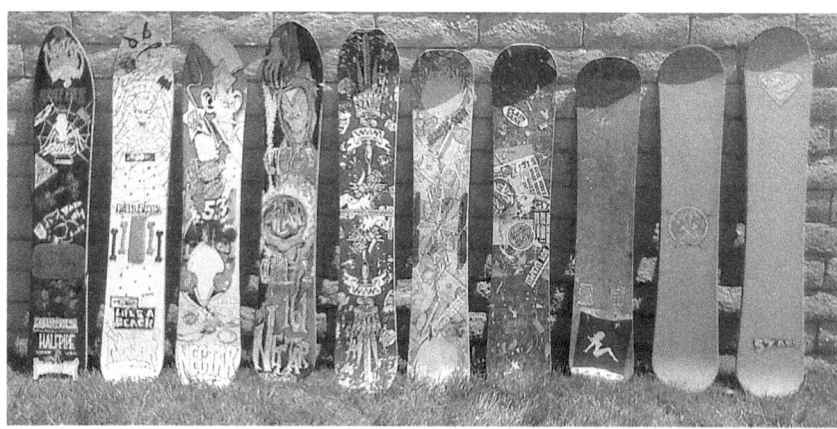

Don Szabo's 10 Signature Snowboard Models

How did it come to this? I mean, I'm the guy who lived life full throttle — ten snowboard models with my name and graphics on them splashed across dozens of magazine pages, there in the '90s as a main figure and part of the heartbeat of snowboarding's rise: spinning in videos, making waves on TV, an icon in the world I loved. Over ten years of getting paid to shred around the globe, chasing snow and adrenaline, living my passion.

After the snowboard career, I didn't just fade out. I built something — a company — and ran it strong for over 16 years. Married the woman I loved, had two incredible daughters, and put down roots in Huntington Beach, California, a paradise for our family.

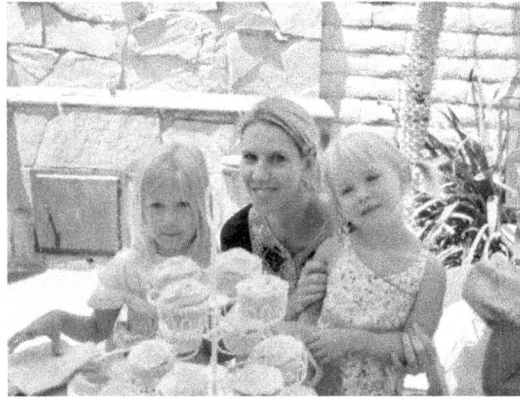

My late wife Heather with daughters Kaylee and Ashlyn

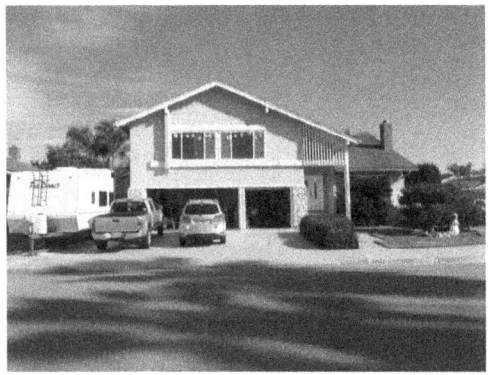

Our beautiful home we thought we'd live in forever

1988-1989
Face Spider
Nectar

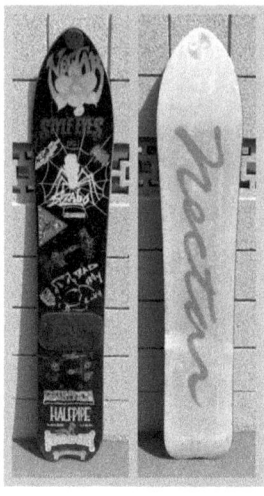

1990-1991
Sherrif Model
Nectar

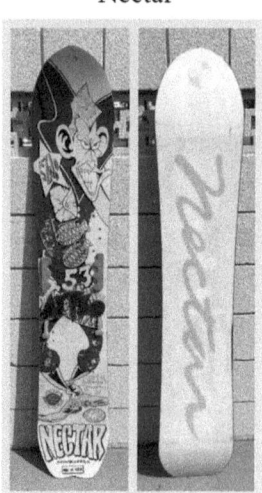

1989-1990
Skull Spider
Nectar

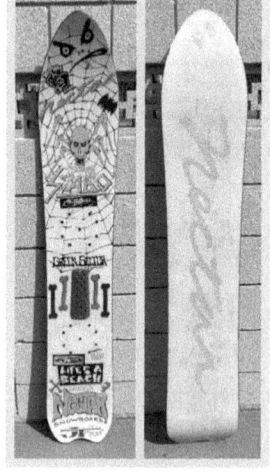

1991-1992
Nectar Wizard
Lamar

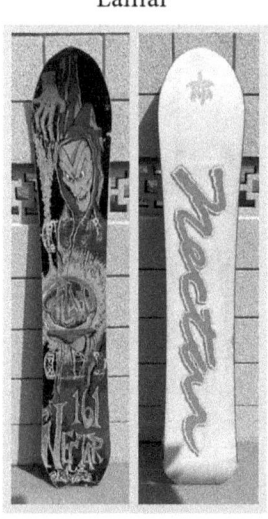

1992-1993
King Model
Lamar

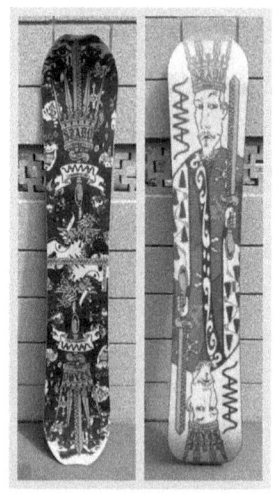

1993-1994
Money Model
Lamar

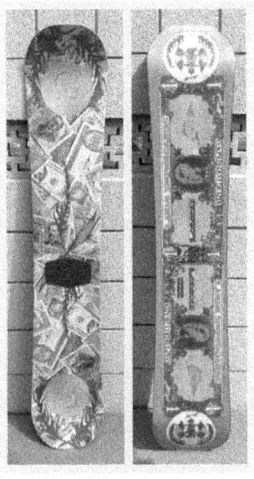

1995-1996
Trucker Model
Lamar

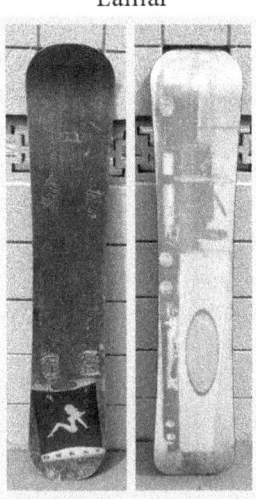

1994-1995
Shag Carpet
Lamar

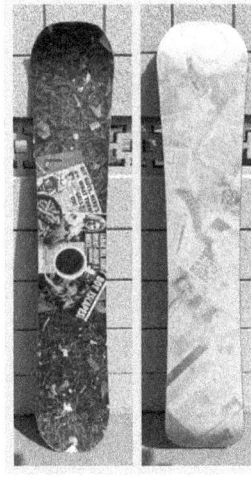

1996-1998
Super / Slayer
SZABO

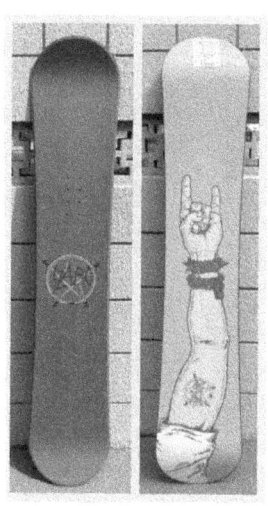

1996-1998
Super / Slayer
SZABO

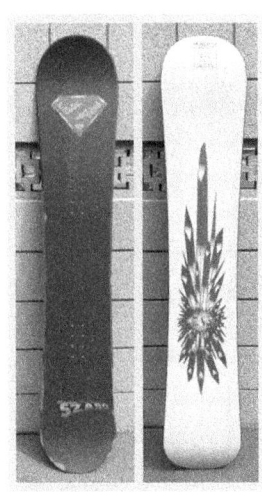

We chose the neighborhood for the schools, for our family's future, and the great life that we'd all have together.

So, how does a guy go from that — a dream, a legacy, a life built with purpose — to lying in a hospital bed because he thought leaving was the best option? Life has many twists and turns, ups and downs, and somewhere along the way, my mindset veered off course big time. I convinced myself that I'd be doing everyone else a favor. That I was the obstacle, and my absence would clear the way for everyone else's happiness.

The mind…it's a beast, especially when it's steering down a dark path. You lose traction, spin out, and before you know it, you're sinking deep, buried in a place you never thought you'd be — or able to get out of — without proper mindset.

So, who am I? How does a life that reads like an adrenaline junkie's dream morph into a decision to cut it short? To get that answer, we've got to rewind, dig back into the early chapters of life, sift through the scars, surgeries, highs, lows, wins, losses, and triumphs. Because my story is more than just the falls. It's the rise, the crash, and everything in between and after. Buckle up — you're about to see what almost took me out, and what helped me claw my way back to live life full throttle.

Family Ties and Wild Beginnings

I grew up in what you might call a middle-class family, though labels never really fit us. My dad, Lou Szabo, was a real estate agent, a title he took

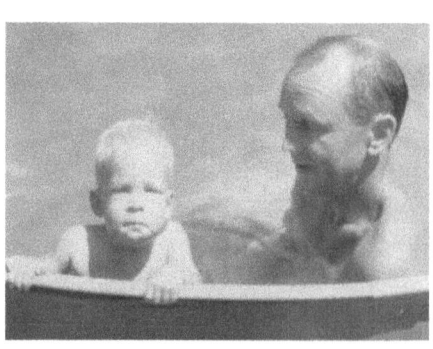

A swim with my dad when I was very young

on around my birth so he could stay home raising me while handling business in the background.

Only later did I realize the juggling act he mastered: parenting, with all its spins, flips, twists, and turns.

Before real estate, my dad's life was a series of moves in different directions. He'd been a chemist at

Shell, studied the rhythms and taught dance at Arthur Murray Dance Studio, served in the Navy in his younger years; he even pulled off one of the first "giant swings" on the gymnastics high bar, a pioneer in a move that's now a staple. The man had a taste for adventure, from rock climbing to hiking big mountain trails, all before settling down. He embraced life's waves until they naturally brought him to shore.

It was at Arthur Murray's at 46 that he met my mom, Susan, a beautiful woman 18 years his junior. Age was just a number; they connected like they'd known each other for a lifetime. Together they soon hit the road, driving from Ohio in the Midwest to many places, sharing laughs, stories, and dreams — finally ending up in Culver City, California. They knew they wanted a family. After a few years of trying and fighting through setbacks, my mom finally got pregnant, and I arrived in 1966 — the bundle of energy they'd been waiting for.

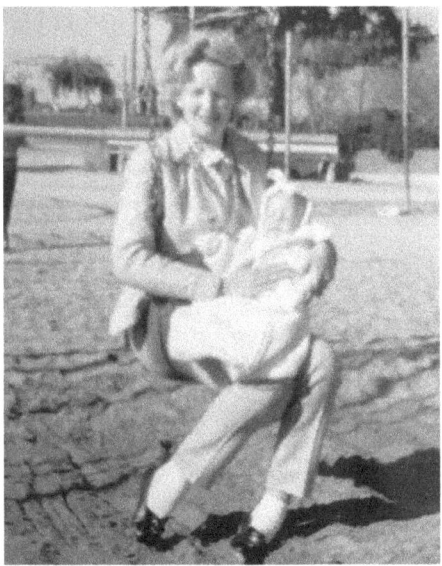

Baby me with my beautiful mom

My dad was 50, my mom 32, and I was their new adventure waiting to unfold. Mom, ever practical, went back to her career as an accountant, managing budgets and balancing numbers to keep the company's finances in check. While Dad handled both me and his real estate clients from home, he now had something new to keep track of, and that was me.

As a kid, my playground was the streets, the hills, and "the wash" near our house — a concrete riverbed that carried rainwater through Culver City to the ocean. At just three years old, I would wander down to the bridge over the wash to 'fish' with a rock tied to a string, pulling up the same soggy stone time and time again, content as could be.

I never needed a crowd to keep me busy; the world around me was my playground, and I played it solo like a seasoned pro.

Dad and I hiked the Baldwin Hills, an often daily challenge for my little legs, but a thrill I couldn't resist. On our walks, I took "extra credit" lines, scaling pipes up walls, coming down slanted walkways, always rejoining Dad with a grin, ready for the next part of the journey. At the top of Baldwin Hills, we found "tree tunnels," short, twisty paths perfect for a kid my size to run through, leaving my dad in the dust. I remember poking my eye once on a rogue branch; my eye had a red dot on it for months, but I kept on going. Nothing could keep me down.

Sometimes, we'd take on even bigger challenges, like the day we decided to walk all the way to the ocean, a six-mile journey through the wash that emptied out near Santa Monica. My dad had planned it all out, and Mom met us at the beach where we got hot dogs and snowcones as a reward for our epic trek. Those were the best bites, the ones you earn after a journey with someone who's part teacher, part teammate, and always a friend. That was my dad.

Life was simple — a mix of meat, potatoes, vegetables, spaghetti, stew, and other wholesome meals, built around family routines that worked. Fresh eggs and milk would be waiting for us on the porch at dawn since that was a thing back then.

Three years after I came along, my little sister Karen was born. I've seen pictures of us from that era — classic shots where you can tell my parents came from a different time, dressing us up like dolls for photos meant to freeze the moment forever. But no picture is truly timeless. Styles shift, trends fade, and what once felt stylish becomes a snapshot of a specific era, stamped by the fashion, the hair, and the choices that seemed so right at the time.

And just like those old family photos, I have my own throwback memories to look at. Snowboarding in the late '80s, rocking gloves that climbed halfway up my forearms, neon colors, skulls, and wild patterns everywhere. Looking back years later, it's impossible not to laugh and think, "What were we thinking?" Every era leaves its mark. My sister had her 1980s big hair, while I cycled through my own transformations — from long blonde locks in grade school to punk rock spikes and black-tipped hair in junior high. It was all part of the ride, one phase rolling into the next, each just as wild as the last.

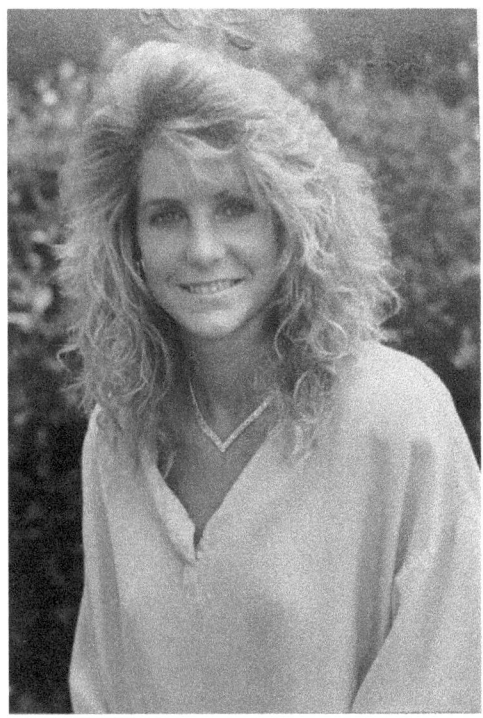

Sister Karen rockin' that classic 80's hair

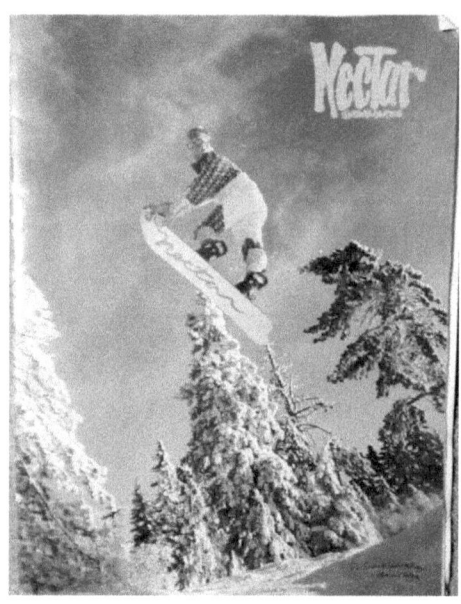

Rockin' my crazy 80's neon gear

Sibling Shenanigans and the First Taste of Danger

I loved my little sister, Karen, even if we didn't always hang out. I mean, she was three years younger than me, and, well…she was a girl. But when we did spend time together as kids, I definitely took on the role of the bratty older brother. One of my signature moves? The "open wide for a surprise" trick, where I'd tell her to close her eyes, open her mouth, and, bam — I'd give her a mouthful of dirt, or something yucky.

There was also the time I tossed a spider her way — not really on purpose, but as a split-second reaction. I had let it crawl on my hand, and the moment it scurried toward the other side, I panicked and flung it. Unfortunately, it landed right on Karen. She screamed and jumped, and before I could even process what had happened, she burst into tears. I knew if she ran to Mom and Dad, I'd be in trouble, so I had to act fast. Let's just say I quickly became an expert at pulling out all the stops with funny tricks, doing whatever it took to make her laugh and forget about my accidental — or sometimes intentional — mischief.

But payback came (unintentionally) when I hid behind a door; my new front teeth were right at doorknob height. She swung that door wide open looking for me and, bam — the doorknob snapped one of my new front teeth clean in half. I'd like to say that taught me a lesson, but it didn't, and I got her back a while later, totally by accident. Her arm was already in a cast after a wall-climbing mishap she had, and I accidentally closed a window on that arm. Thankfully, it didn't re-break her arm, but it sure spooked us both.

Our backyard was my first "training ground," dominated by a massive avocado tree, and Dad had set up a high-flying rope swing off the top of it. He showed me how to swing around the tree, and it was amazing! I learned from him, and I'd run and launch myself off the bench while holding the rope…I'd spin around the tree, stick my landing on the wall, then do it back the other way, back to the bench. I even learned how to spin myself into a 360 while swinging around the tree. It was like an early version of my own aerial tricks that I brought to board sports later on. I remember showing it off to a friend around my age who tried it himself. He didn't get the right trajectory, missing the landing entirely, crashing into the tree, and ending up in tears. Even then, I had a sense that I was built for this kind of stuff, like I had a knack for moves that other kids just couldn't pull off.

Then there was the neighbor's yard, home to Phil Frisbee, a teenage kid with a giant, shaggy dog. (And yeah, Phil Frisbee was his real name.) I'd climbed over their fence one day to get back a soccer ball Karen had kicked over. As I'm reaching for the ball, their huge dog jumped on me, knocking me straight back into a thorny rosebush. It was a rough day for backyard sports, and my mom had to pull a line of thorns from my backside. Let's just say it was the start of my lifelong beef with ball sports.

First Crush and Finding My Name

Kindergarten came with its own kind of thrill, a bit of innocence, a bit of boldness, and one unforgettable moment in the coat rack area. There was this girl, Lorraine Van Zee. Out of nowhere, she grabbed me and planted a kiss right on me. We were surrounded by other kindergartners, and of course, I had to play it cool. "Eeew, yuck! A girl kissed me, that's disgusting!" I said, scrunching my face as the kids around us laughed. But on the walk home, the truth bubbled up in my head: that was kind of neat. I think I love Lorraine Van Zee.

Looking back, it was just a silly crush, but it was my first real interaction with a girl — that first spark. And even though I had to pretend I wasn't interested, I knew then and there I was definitely into girls.

This was also around the time I insisted on going by "Don." Every time someone called me Donald, the other kids would chime in with "Donald Duck" and crack up. And if I was called "Donnie," they'd start joking around about Donnie Osmond, the TV star with the shiny teeth. The girls loved him on TV, but I couldn't stand the idea of being compared to him. So I made it clear: Call me Don. And it's been that way ever since — at least until I started saying my name was "sZabo" at nine years old, emphasizing the Z instead of the S like the traditional Hungarian way to say it. That last name nickname and "Z" have stuck till now and will continue to be nicknames I like to roll with.

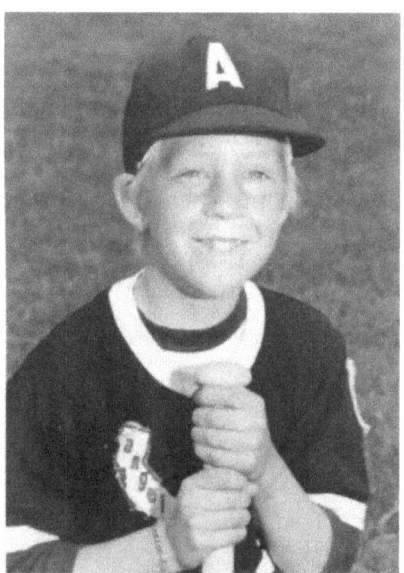

Baseball was brief — Action Sports became my world

My brief kid baseball career didn't last too long. I'd practice with Dad at times, hitting balls he'd pitch, but mostly I'd hit a baseball on one of those T-ball setups where the ball was attached to a post with a huge rubber band. I'd smack the ball around in circles, no problem. But come game day, when I was up to bat, I'd freeze. The pitches I'd crack in practice went right by me, strike after strike most of the time, my mind would freeze up for some reason, and I wouldn't even swing.

I held my own in the outfield and even ran bases pretty well, but at bat, it was like someone hit pause on me. I loved the idea of hitting home runs, but it didn't happen, and the sport just didn't spark anything real in me. Give me a different kind of action, one with a little more edge, where you've got to throw yourself into the unknown and hold on tight — that was more my style. And at nine years old, I found the kind of passion that didn't come with a ball, just the guts to go full-send into something wild.

Wheels of Fire and First Blood

When I was nine, my dad handed me a Black Knight skateboard. It had a cool graphic of a knight on a horse, but that was the coolest thing about it. Clay wheels clattered like a freight train over every crack and pebble. The trucks were flimsy, with no real bushings — nothing that absorbed the shock.

Every bump on the sidewalk felt like a mini-earthquake. But when my dad showed me how to ride it, pushing off with one foot, gliding down the driveway and turning onto the sidewalk, I was hooked. The sound, the motion — my mind was set. I was gonna ride that skateboard, learn how to do it well and enjoy it!

Every day after that, I'd take that board out, clanking and rattling down the street, having the time of my life. But it wasn't long before I realized this wasn't quite a "real" skateboard. Sure, it had the cool knight graphic, but the ride was rough, brutal even. Soon after, for my birthday, I asked for, and got a true game-changer: a skateboard with urethane wheels.

Rolling smooth as silk over the cracks, it was like going from an old clunker to a Cadillac. Suddenly, the streets and sidewalks were mine to enjoy on a whole new level. My "magic carpet ride" could actually take me around the neighborhood, smooth as could be — it was awesome!

With my new board, I started experimenting. One of my first big ideas happened when our neighbor, Phil Frisbee, was out mowing his front lawn. Phil had a skateboard too, and as he piled grass clippings on the sidewalk, I got this wild idea. "Make the pile bigger," I told him, gearing up to jump over it onto his board on the other side. Phil, always game for some chaos, kept piling the grass higher and higher and each time I'd have to jump higher to clear the bigger and bigger pile of grass.

Until, bam! One jump, I caught my toes on the top of the grass pile, I missed the board landing, and went down hard, chest and chin smacking against the sidewalk. Dazed, I looked at Phil. "Am I okay?" He just stared and said, "You've got a lot of blood on your shirt." I looked down, and sure enough, my yellow shirt had a big red stain spreading across it. I touched my chin, my fingers coming back smeared with blood.

The sight of it and the raw sting hit me all at once, and I burst into tears. I hadn't known that kind of pain yet, the kind that leaves a mark on your body and your mind.

Twelve stitches later, I had my first real lesson in the thrill and the danger that come with going all-in. There was an adrenaline rush in flying over that grass pile, in pushing for "one more" even when it was risky. But now I knew: sometimes you pay hard when you play hard. That day was just the beginning of chasing that balance, where pain and pleasure ride side-by-side. And for me, it only made the ride even better to push boundaries. This was just a part of the wild ride of life.

-Chapter 2-
Valley to Sk8 Love

The big move to the San Fernando Valley happened because my mom landed a job in the accounting department at Dunlop Corporation, a big opportunity that meant leaving Culver City and settling into Reseda, California. My parents bought a house this time instead of renting, which felt like a permanent step forward. During the moving process, we found ourselves eating roast beef sandwiches from Arby's almost every night. Mom had newspaper coupons, and it was easy while our kitchen was still in boxes. At first, they tasted great, but after a few days, I was already craving something different. This was just the start of adjusting to our new life.

Once we settled in, I met the Portaro brothers down the street, Joey, who was my age, and his younger brother Eden. Joey and I clicked right away, and he introduced me to his family's wild sense of humor and a bit of the Valley's edge. I remember his dad pulling me aside once with a marijuana joint in hand saying, If you tell anyone I smoke this stuff, I'll kill you, with a half-crazy laugh that seemed to be out of the crazy professor's mouth from a sci-fi movie. It was wild. For an eleven-year-old who'd never been exposed to drugs or anything close to it, it was a bit shocking, but also oddly thrilling to see new things.

One unforgettable night, Joey's dad took us to see KISS perform live at Magic Mountain, in front of the Colossus roller coaster. There was fire blasting onstage with loud heavy rock 'n' roll music, and all the band members were wearing crazy leather-spiked outfits. Gene Simmons blowing fire out of his mouth was an awesome sight to see! Watching KISS was a rush in itself, and it felt like this new world — the Valley, rock concerts, bigger-than-life energy — it was all opening up a whole new side of life for me.

We moved to the Valley in the beginning of the summer, just after school let out. I was a graduated fifth grader from Culver City looking for my next step in life and now planted in Reseda in the San Fernando Valley. Around that time, I heard about a skatepark called SkaterCross just a mile and a half from our house. It didn't take long before I was skating there every day. I'd ride my skateboard a mile and a half to the park, spend the entire day skating there, and then skate all the way back home in the evening. Soon, SkaterCross became my world. It was where I got my adrenaline and flow at that time in my life, and I loved it!

At SkaterCross, I quickly figured out how to game the entry system and how to ride for free. There were daily color-coded tags they'd staple to our shirts that you would buy to skate for the day. Each day had a different color, and I'd collect tags in every color. On blue tag days, I'd staple a blue one on; for red tag days, a red one, etc. With this little trick, I was able to skate more without constantly paying to skate all the time since I couldn't afford it. This allowed me to have fun at SkaterCross almost daily, and my skills were improving all the time. It was a win-win situation for me.

One of the biggest influences I met there was Shreddi Repas. He was sixteen, a local pro with talent I could only dream of at eleven. He quickly became my skateboarding mentor, showing me the ropes not only at SkaterCross but also in other iconic skate places around the Valley, Los Angeles, and other spots in Southern California. Sometimes, he'd take me to empty backyard pools hidden in tough neighborhoods, like one called the Mulatto Cage. This was deep in L.A., surrounded by graffiti-covered walls and shady characters lingering around the edges. We were just there to skate, so they left us alone.

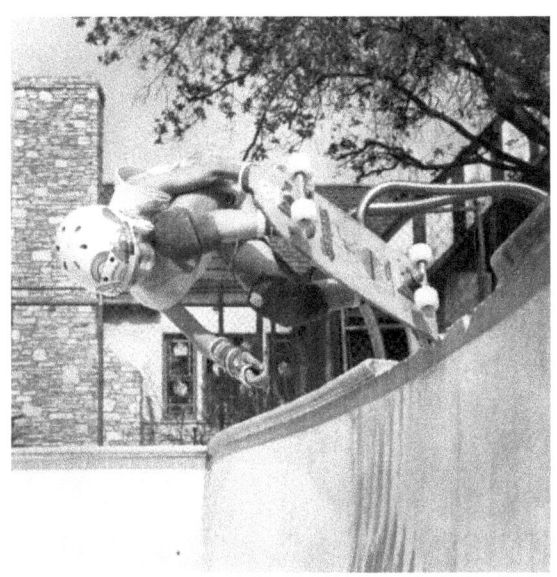

Tail Tap at the Mulatto Cage pool, deep in LA

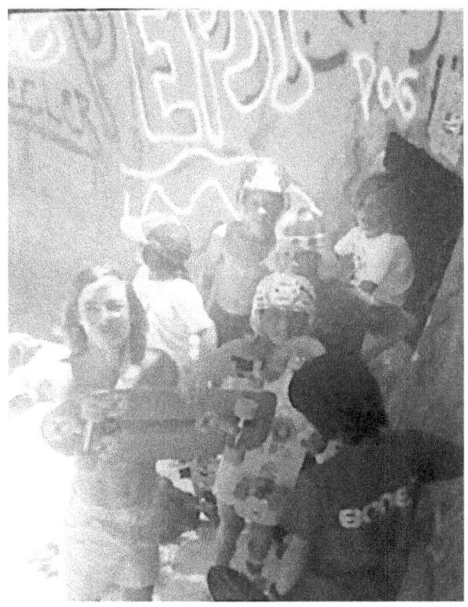

Shreddi in the front, me in back, graffiti everywhere

Shreddi was a local legend with some magazine recognition, including a cover of Skateboard World Magazine, and he would take me skating everywhere when we got the chance. Since he could drive, we sometimes ventured down to Del Mar Skate Ranch in San Diego, Marina del Rey Skatepark, The Concrete Wave, Big-O, Skatopia, Upland Skatepark, and other spots all up and down Southern California. Out of all of them, Marina del Rey became my favorite skatepark to visit when we weren't *shredding* our local park, SkaterCross, back home in the Valley.

SkaterCross had become a hub for talent, and the owner, Lou Peralta, knew it. He let a handful of us skate for free — not just me and Shreddi, but also up-and-coming pros like Bert LaMar, Jay Smith, and Eric Grisham. Lou understood that having strong riders at the park on a regular basis created a buzz and brought in more skaters eager to ride where the best were hanging out. All three of those guys made names for themselves in different ways from that era, and they were close friends of ours as we lived and loved our skate life back then.

Shreddi and I would skate every possible line at SkaterCross, especially in the snake run — where creativity ruled. The snake run was a series of vertical bowls and banks that you could carve through in countless ways. You could even skate in the opposite direction when no one was in the way. You could weave back and forth in many untraditional ways — forward, backward, and sideways over rollers — creating some truly unique lines and gaps. There's really no easy way to describe it. If you know, you know.

In case you're wondering, a "line" refers to the path you take — connecting tricks and transitions in your own way and direction — ideally with a smooth, flowing rhythm and style. We explored every possibility — carving unexpected routes, doing aerials in untraditional spots, gapping and carving through different sections, and squeezing the most out of every transition. That's how we learned the ins and outs of the park — by constantly pushing what was possible and sharing it with each other.

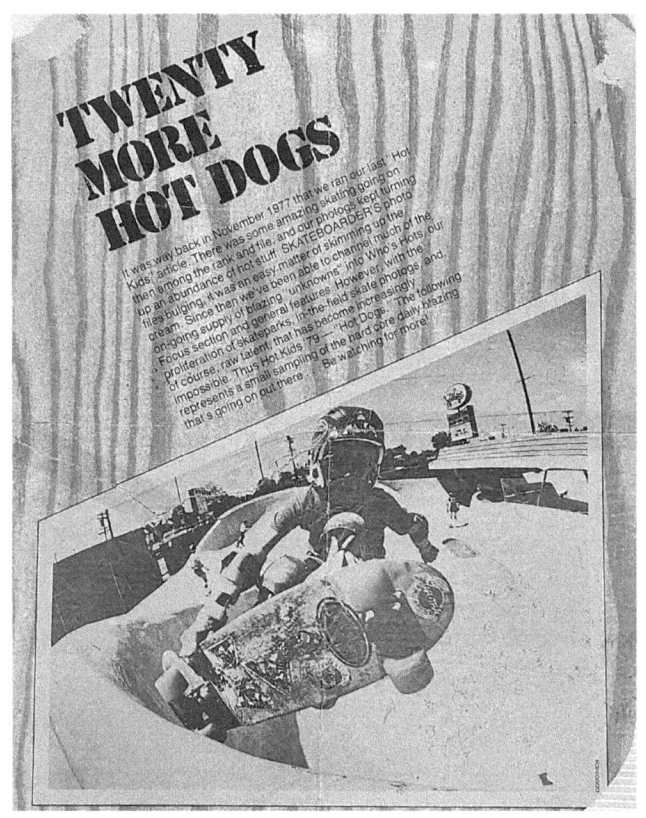

TWENTY MORE HOT DOGS

It was way back in November 1977 that we ran our last "Hot Kids" article. There was some amazing skating going on then among the rank and file, and our photogs kept turning up an abundance of hot stuff. SKATEBOARDER'S photo files bulging, it was an easy matter of skimming up the cream. Since then we've been able to channel much of the on-going supply of blazing "unknowns" into Who's Hots our Focus section and general features. However, with the proliferation of skateparks, in-the-field skate photos and, of course, raw talent that has become increasingly impossible. Thus "Hot Kids 79 — Hot Dogs." The following represents a small sampling of the hard core daily blazing that's going on out there... Be watching for more!

First magazine shot - 12 years old at SkaterCross

Even now, I can replay every line in my head — every angle I carved, every boardslide, tail tap, and air like I'm still there. Those sessions with Shreddi were the building blocks of my skate life, and he wasn't just a friend — he was a mentor, always pushing me to see new possibilities.

His house was like a second home for me at times. It had that lived-in, dog-smell feel from his mom's dog, but it didn't matter. We spent the night there so we could get up early and go on whatever adventure we had planned.

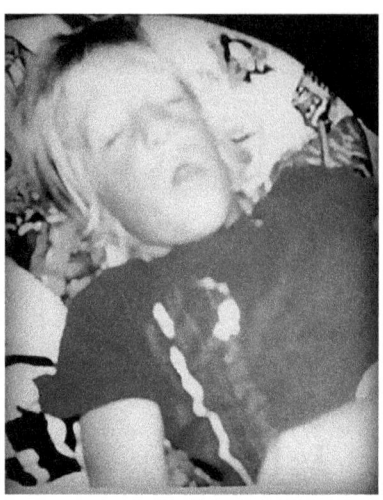

Catching Z's at Shreddi's house

We would skate and hit the parks and pools as much as possible — it was the skate life that we loved to live.

Now traveling up, down, and around Southern California with Shreddi and the crew was like a dream for a 13-year-old, although it exposed me to some "adult" things too. Some of the older skaters drank and smoked pot, and they let me try both, but neither one impressed me much. For me, skateboarding was the true high. I didn't want anything messing with my mind or slowing me down. I'd found something pure in skating, an adrenaline rush that felt unbeatable, and I didn't want it to end, so I just kept taking that ride.

As we kept rollin', we'd go hit Marina del Rey Skatepark quite a bit. We loved it, and it was just over the hill from the Valley where we lived. I'd sometimes spot a young 12-year-old skater named Christian Hosoi, ripping it up in the small clay six-foot bowls known as the brown bowls. He was good, but at the time, I thought of him as just a young skater in the warm-up bowls and didn't think much of it. I was now a 13-year-old ripper that was there with Shreddi Repas, and we were skating and ripping the big pools, including the "Dog Bowl," that was a replica of a legendary backyard skateboard pool before

Marina Skatepark was built. We would skate with some local skate legends at times like Tony Alva, Shogo Kubo, Brad Bowman, Jay Adams (RIP 🙏), and other rockstar skaters from way back then in the early vert skatepark days.

One evening, Shreddi and I got to Marina Skatepark and saw a full-blown photo shoot happening at the main back pool called the "Back Keyhole." We looked closer, and there was Christian Hosoi, only twelve, skating with the kind of style and skill that blew me away! He tore through that pool like he owned it, flying high across the seven-foot-wide drop-in gap of the keyhole, and shredding the pool better than I could imagine. I'd thought I was one of the best young skaters coming from SkaterCross, where I rode really well, but seeing Christian that evening at Marina humbled me. It was one of those moments when you realize that there's always someone out there pushing even harder, going even bigger, and taking things to the next level; it was quite a show and quite a blow to my ego, you know?

I kept skating at SkaterCross and meeting new riders who'd become part of my world. We even formed our own "color gang," with everyone in the skate crew representing a different primary color. My color was yellow. I dyed all my T-shirts and socks yellow, rode yellow Tracker magnesium trucks, had yellow Sunspots wheels, and rocked my yellow "Mad Rat" shorts. We had a great group of guys in the color gang and shared some amazing times. It was one of the ways I stood out and claimed my place in the local skate scene. Later on, when I chased my motocross adrenaline fix, I'd "ride red" with my Honda dirt bikes. But that's a story for another chapter.

For now, life was all about the skateparks, the thrill of learning new tricks, finding new lines, and the deep satisfaction of carving out my place in a skate world that I loved. Those early years at SkaterCross gave me everything I needed to feel alive, to push limits, and to define who I was.

It was an incredible time where the pursuit of air and style was sacred ground. Every new trick that was learned and landed was a hard-earned badge of honor. The lines we created and shared with each other were amazing, and the unique worlds that these skateparks created were truly life-changing, and I know it set my own life onto a different trajectory. For that, I'll always be grateful to Shreddi, and Lou Peralta from SkaterCross, for having the vision to create such an amazing skatepark just a mile and a half from my house in Reseda that changed my life.

It's amazing to think that these skatepark entrepreneurs had the vision to create places where skaters could express their creativity, bond with others, and thrive in a positive environment. Each park had its own unique vibe and community and things you'd never forget. From the food and arcade area where skaters would hang out, meet, talk and then say, "Let's go take some runs in the park," the memories were as rich as the skating itself.

Then there were the unforgettable characters, like Gyro George. He was a very fit, Italian-looking young man with curly brown hair, probably around 20 years old. He always wore dolphin shorts, always had his knee pads on, and spoke with uncontainable excitement, shouting, "Gyro, Gyro, Gyro wheels are the best!"

Gyro wheels had a CNC metal insert with the urethane wheel itself molded around the metal where the bearings were placed. Every other wheel was just made of urethane, and you had to press the bearings into them, which was no big deal. George loved Gyro wheels, but that era faded out with the end of the Gyro metal insert wheels a few years later..

George had Tourette's syndrome, which made him shake and talk uncontrollably, but he was harmless to others — just a wildly enthusiastic, quirky guy that no one who met him could ever forget.

Looking back, I see those days as the foundation of everything that came next. It was the spark that led me into a life fueled by *action sports* adrenaline and an endless pursuit of the next big thrill.

Skateboarding, snowboarding, motocross, surfing sprinkled across them, and most recently, mountain biking. These five sports have been the sport loves of my life. They've given me joy, challenge, and purpose.

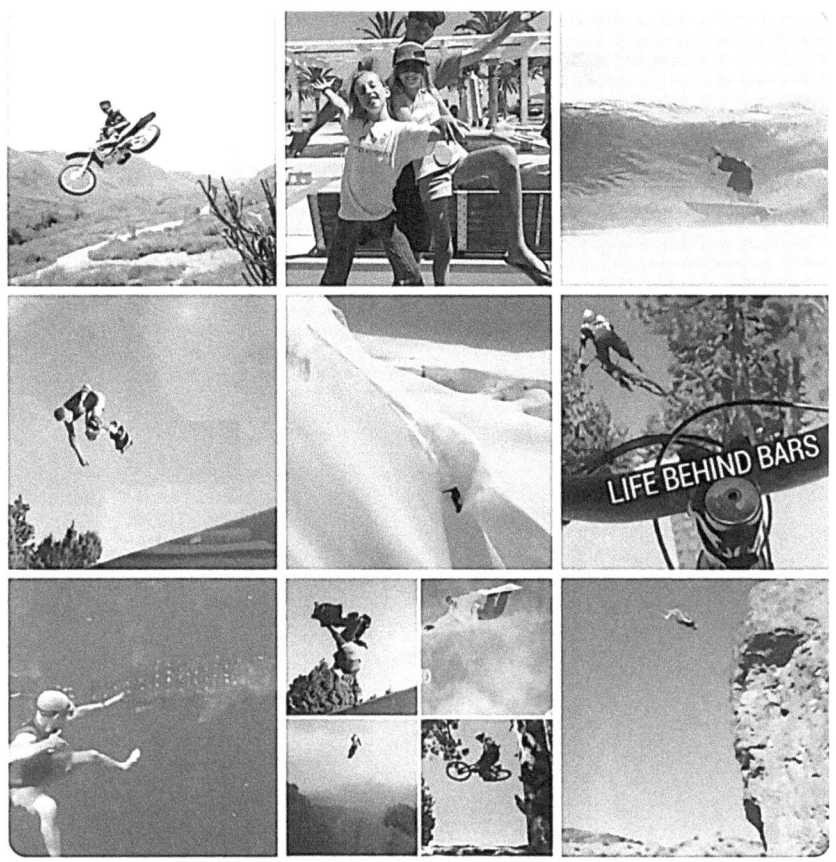

Some of my sports life, and my kids, but not my wife

I've poured into them with all the passion and drive anyone can have for something they truly love. They've been my fuel, my escape, and my identity, and I wouldn't trade those experiences for anything. Even now, they still bring a warm feeling to my heart and remind me that, for the most part, I've lived a life that I've truly loved.

Chapter 3

Next PhaZe of
My Sk8 CraZe

By my mid-teens, the San Fernando Valley — and all of Southern California — had become an endless playground of *ramps*, *halfpipes*, and backyard pools waiting to be shredded.

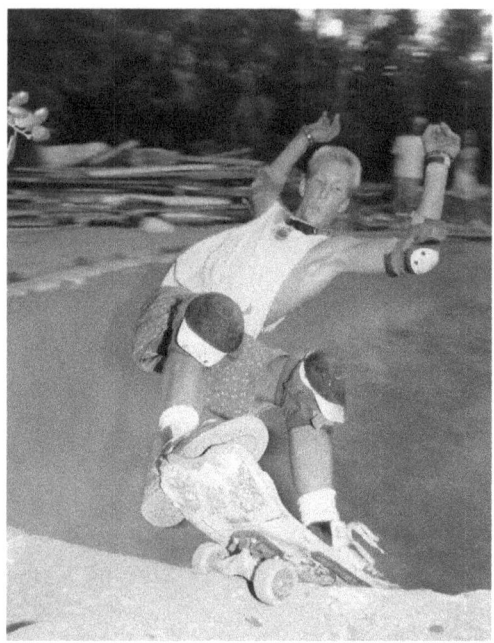

Back to the grind

But something was missing. Most of the legendary skateboard parks were gone, closed under the weight of lawsuits from parents who would sue the skateparks. They couldn't accept that skating came with its own risks. Back then, the court system hadn't caught up, and if a kid got hurt, it was the park's fault. That kind of system and thinking drained the life out of skateparks. Skyrocketing insurance costs forced them to shut down, killing off the very spaces that fueled the skateboarding scene.

It's wild when I think about it now. Today, public skate and bike parks are everywhere, and the courts finally understand — and have rules in place — that if you get hurt, that's on you.

That's how it should've been all along.

When SkaterCross finally closed its gates, it didn't feel real. That place wasn't just a skatepark — it was home for many of us latch-key kids. For a little while after it shut down, we still managed to sneak in and skate our favorite local park. We were like ghosts in a place that had been alive just weeks before. Sometimes the cops would show up, but we had our escape routes dialed in. If they came through the front, we'd bail out the back. If they rolled up the alley, we'd hop the opposite fence. It was a cat-and-mouse game, and for a while, we always won.

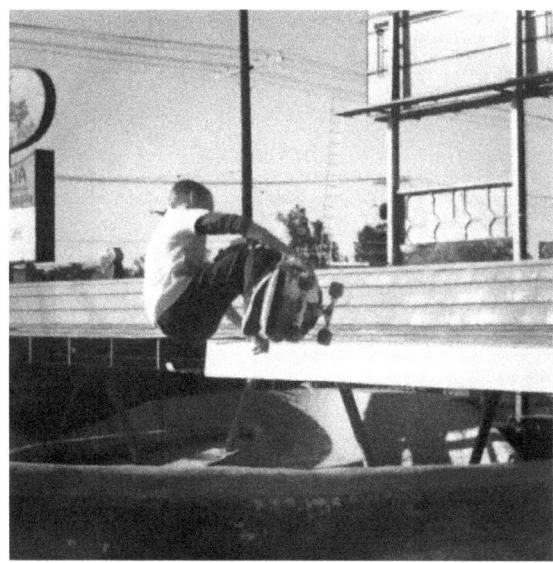

Frontside Air after SkaterCross closed down

But that didn't last. One day, the cops weren't messing around. They rolled up from every direction, boxing us in like we were pulling off a heist. No matter which way we ran, there was a squad car or cop waiting to take us into custody. A handful of us law-breaking skate rats got hauled off to the police station for trespassing.

I'll never forget sitting there in the station, all of us handcuffed to a bench, laughing and joking like the kids we were. We started singing some chain gang song, cracking up at the fact that we were "locked up" for the crime of loving our skatepark too much. It was ridiculous and perfect at the same time — a fitting end to our time spent at SkaterCross.

Our parents were called to come pick us up, and that was it. SkaterCross was bulldozed, flattened into nothing more than a memory. For us and the hundreds of kids who skated there during those great years, it was more than just a park. It was a piece of who we were — a second home and a community of our peers. But now it was gone.

We weren't alone in that loss. Parks across California and the rest of the country suffered the same fate, crushed by insane insurance costs and lawsuits. Skateboarders everywhere suddenly had no place to go, no park to call home.

But skateboarders are built different. You can tear down the parks, but you can't kill the passion that was in all of us.

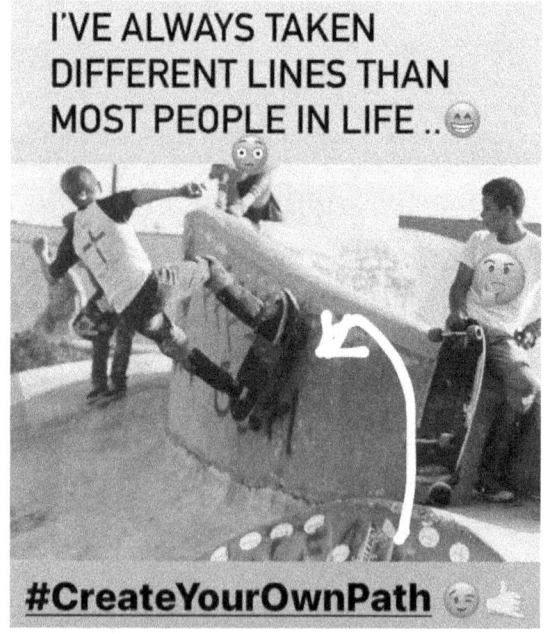

Built different, still rolling different

With the parks gone, a new era was born.

Every ramp and every backyard pool we could find became our new playground. Each spot had its own story, its own quirks, and its own crew of misfits pushing limits without a care in the world. We weren't following rules anymore — because there were none. We skated like there was no tomorrow, living in the moment, skating whatever concrete, wood, and *masonite* transition we could find or create — and it was great!

Masonite is a smooth, hardboard sheet, used as the 4' x 8' sheet size it comes in or cut to size for wherever it's needed. It's thin, fast, and grippy — great for ramp surfaces and it bends well over the transitions of the ramps.

The skateparks were gone, but skateboarding wasn't. It just got more raw, more real, and more alive than ever.

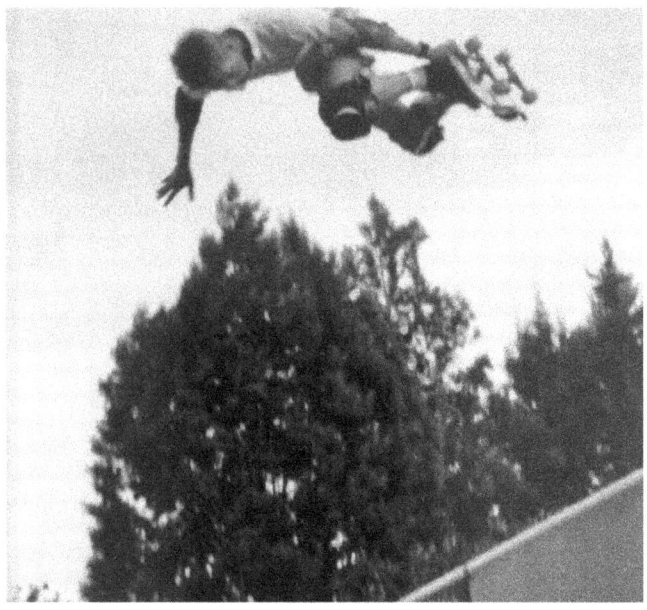

Backside air when I had hair

Randy's ramp became a staple and a second home. After school let out, we'd roll over to his backyard, our boards and bodies primed to launch airs and tricks with each other and have a blast!

Randy Wild, the owner of the ramp, was a man of few words and many laughs. He had this dry, sarcastic humor that could throw you off balance more than any trick. Once, he introduced me to a kid on the ramp as Sam. Weeks went by before Sam burst out with a frustrated confession that his name wasn't Sam — it was John Swope! Good on him for speaking up. He went on to make a name for himself, and even a decade later, he was still ripping in the 1995 Crown Jewels and 1996 15 Pool Punishers skate videos.

One memorable trip, Randy and I headed out to Ridgecrest, driving deep into the desert. There stood a ramp bigger than most — it was a 32-foot-wide beast of a ramp. Ten feet high, with extensions reaching twelve feet, and a four-foot-wide drop-in channel. It was the kind of ramp where you could draw cool lines all over the entire thing, doing tricks on different features during each session. It felt like sacred ground.

On the drive home, Randy had his usual six-pack at his feet in the passenger seat. A cop pulled us over and was suspicious of the beers. He grilled me with multiple tests: saying the alphabet backward, balancing on one leg, then closing my eyes, leaning my head back, and touching my nose — all while still on one leg. At the time, I didn't know I was just being tested for my reaction. I just felt like I was failing everything. Finally, I told the cop, "Do you think I could do this if I was drunk?" I put up a solid ten-second handstand right there on the highway shoulder. After I came down smoothly, the cop took Randy's beer and let us go. I'd saved us from a ticket and stacked another story from this ride home — one that would last a lifetime as a classic memory from those days.

There was another ramp that became a key part of our scene — rebuilt by Billy Spann — and it had a little Hollywood history behind it. This was the same ramp from the skateboarding movie Thrashin'. In the film, they show it going up in flames, but that was just for the cameras — a quick mockup made from 2x4s to look like the real deal. The actual ramp was properly dismantled after filming, and Billy brought it back to life near CSUN College in the San

Fernando Valley. We ended up skating that ramp for well over a year, and it became a solid fixture in the early '80s.

All the ramps we were hitting back then — Billy's, Randy's, Arnold's, Charlie King's — they were all scattered throughout the Valley. At different times, certain ramps would become more of a home base, depending on what was happening and who was around. We rotated through them naturally, always chasing the next good session. And when we had the time, we'd branch out — go hit ramps outside the Valley, meet new locals, and ride with different crews. Those longer missions were always worth it when we could make them happen.

We weren't skating to film or shoot photos — we were just living it. It was about the freedom, the feeling, the flow. I'm glad Chris Fithian happened to snap a few photos of us at Billy's ramp back then. Without those, it'd all just be another great memory slowly fading away like so many others from those golden days.

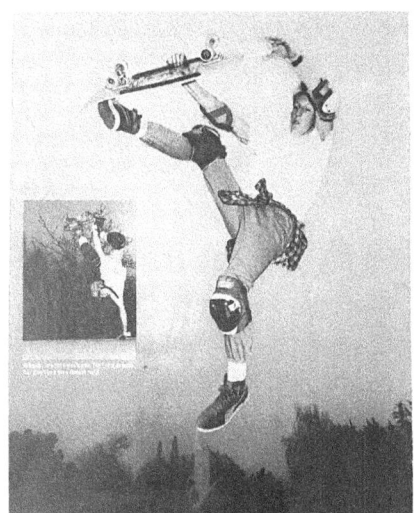 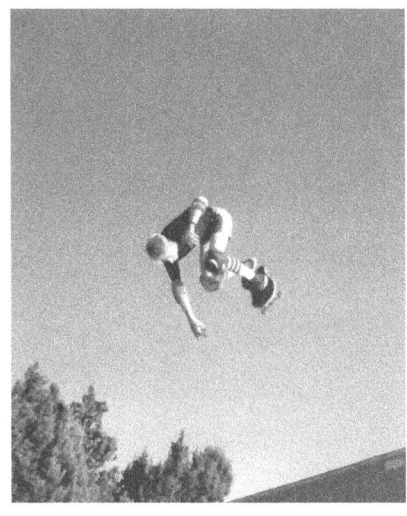

Biliy's ramp flair, glad Chris Fithian was there 📷

Pro's, Bro's and Contest Flows

Reflecting on that era, I sometimes crossed paths with skateboarding legends like Lance Mountain. Even now, at 60, Lance remains an amazing presence in the skateboarding world. He turned pro in the early '80s and joined the Bones Brigade Skate Team. He was featured in iconic videos, including The Search for Animal Chin — a film etched in skaters' minds forever. Over the years, he's founded several skate companies and continues to produce artwork cherished by passionate skateboarders and collectors alike.

He also participates in expression sessions, which aren't contests. There are no rules — just skaters throwing down their style, their tricks, and their soul for whoever's watching. No judges, just raw, creative energy. It's you, your board, and the chance to show the world how you do it. Lance still rips in legend skate competitions too, showcasing his enduring talent and commitment to the sport.

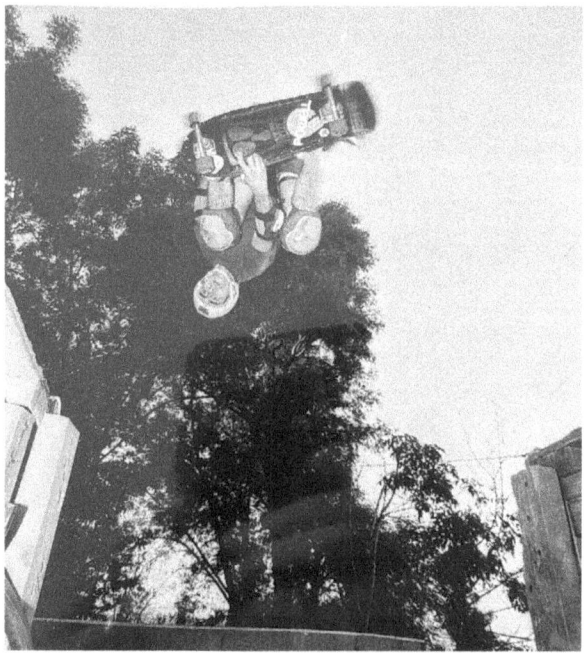

Lance Mountain — Indy Air over his channel, backyard magic

Lance's ramp in Alhambra was legendary — a magnet for professional skaters seeking a prime session spot. Nestled up winding roads in the Alhambra hills, his property was surrounded by towering oak trees. The ramp itself was situated on a lower level, separate from his home, creating a dedicated zone for skateboarding. While the happenings inside Lance's house remained private, the ramp area buzzed with energy and camaraderie for the skaters lucky enough to experience this little piece of skateboard heaven.

To escape the Valley heat and dodge traffic, I'd sometimes show up late at night or very early in the morning and camp out in front of Lance's place, sleeping in the back of my truck. In 1985, Lance welcomed his son, also named Lance. At that time, thoughts of family or settling down hadn't even crossed my mind — skateboarding was my baby.

Mornings would find me waking up outside Lance's house, sometimes joining sessions alongside some of the best skaters in the world. Lance's larger ramp transitions opened the door to bigger airs, and it was incredible! Along with my regular arsenal of tricks — handplants, footplants, ollies, smith grinds, and a solid lineup of aerials — I picked up a few new moves there, including Christ Airs.

This game-changing, *no-footed trick* was pioneered by (the now-famous at the time) Christian Hosoi. It involved doing a big backside air, then, as you left the top of the ramp, you would hold your board out away from your feet in one hand while striking the pose of Christ on the cross — high above the transition — then bringing the board back under your feet before landing. I learned my own smaller version of this trick, but no one did them like Christian himself. His style and air height were beyond belief — a true master of his craft.

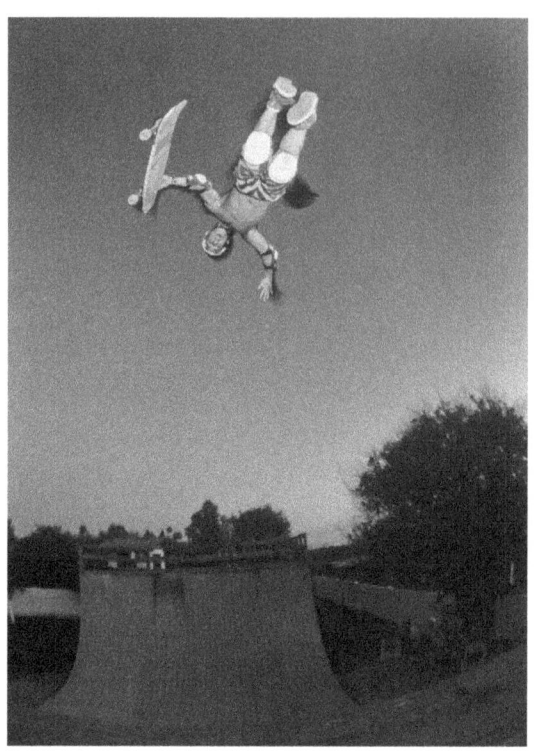

Hosoi, blasting the Christ Air that he invented

Christian is still ripping on a skateboard over 40 years later — a true legend in the skateboard industry. His skating and life have been well documented, ensuring he'll never be forgotten. His documentary film The Rising Son shows his incredible rise in skateboarding, his struggles with addiction and incarceration, and his inspiring comeback. Beyond thriving again in the skate world, Christian is now also a pastor — spreading God's word, positivity, and creating good vibes everywhere he goes. His story is truly remarkable.

At the time, I had my own skate style — bold and creative — skating at a level that rivaled the pros at times. But competitions? They just weren't my thing. For me, it was all about the ride. Getting free skateboards and having a network of underground spots scattered across Southern California was all I wanted.

It was raw, unfiltered, and fueled by word of mouth — each scene offering something fresh and unique. We'd catch wind of a new spot, roll out, meet the locals, and shred with them. Those days were nothing short of epic and will be etched in my mind forever as great times.

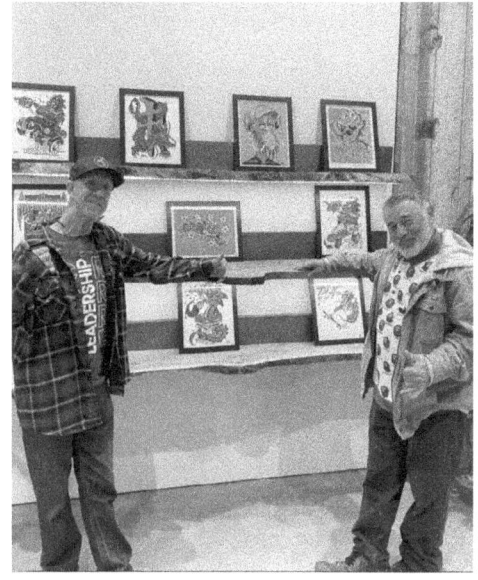

Cab and I at his art display in LA

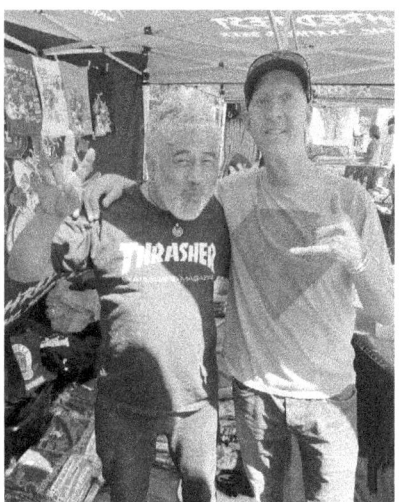

Cab's Urethane band rocked the Pink Motel Skate Jam

One of many MTB rides with Cab

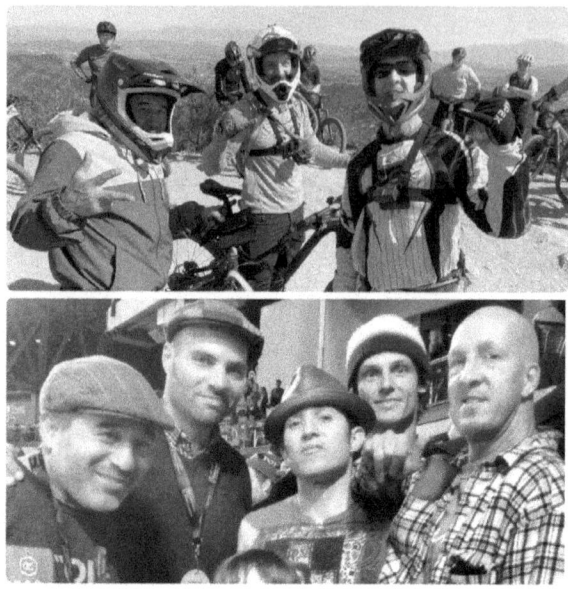

Steve Caballero, Salman Agah, Christian Hosoi, Terry Cook, Don Szabo

Steve Caballero was another skateboard icon — skating since 1979 for Powell Peralta — and he still skates for Powell now, over 45 years later. He's a legend in the skate world. We crossed paths at Lance's and other skate spots in the '80s and early '90s. Then again in the early 2000s on dirt bikes. And more recently, from a few years ago till now, on mountain bikes. We've ridden together many times. We share a passion for the freedom and expression that two wheels can give you.

He's still a force in the skateboarding industry, still skating strong at 60 years old, and over three decades in with a Vans signature shoe. He's also an artist and creates work that ties into his dragon skate graphic legacy, along with many other very cool and unique styles. On top of that, he plays guitar in a semi-new band he rocks with called Urethane, which has a great vibe and energy!

Caballero's creativity runs deep — a true legend with multiple talents and a longtime friend of mine that I have the utmost respect for. He is still truly rockin' life to the max!

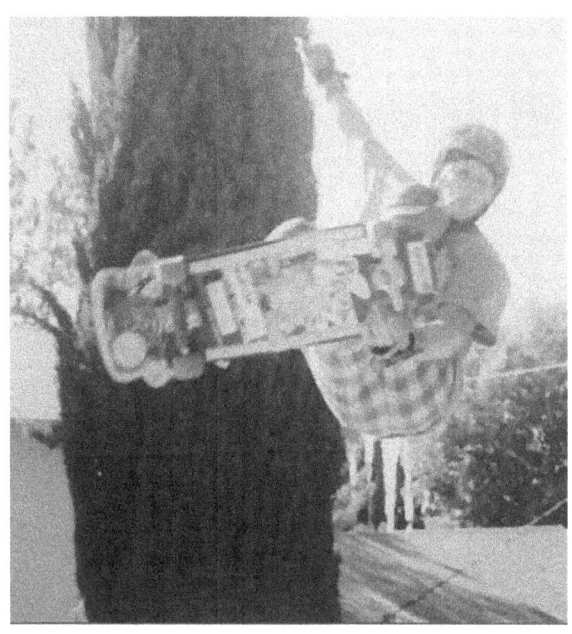

Vince doing a LIEN when we were both 16

But one of the most memorable ramps for me was Vince Kitchen's. It was a modest setup: 12 feet wide, 6 feet high, with a 4-foot-wide, 7-foot-high extension, and the skating surface was beat-up masonite. But what made it stand out was Vince himself — a character straight out of Fast Times at Ridgemont High. He was like Jeff Spicoli in the flesh. We were both 16, and we bonded over our shared passion for skating and good vibes — we quickly clicked as friends.

Vince not only had a very unique style of tricks but also a surreal way of thinking and speaking — twisted phrases and out-of-this-world thoughts that made him unforgettable. He once had a dog named "Stay" that caused some confusion and laughter. Our friendship stuck, and even now, all these years later, Vince is still one of my closest friends — even though he lives so far away in the Philippines with his wife, Yolly, who's from there. How they met over ten years ago and are still going strong is a story for another time, but it's definitely another one of his "Normally Unusual" tales. Vince comes back to the US at least once a year for a month or two to see family and friends and catch up with a bit of his previous life from when he lived in the States.

His book, Normally Unusual, shares stories of his life, his battle with alcohol and drugs, and some of the unusual thoughts, words, and phrases that have kept me entertained for over 40 years. His "Pre-Ramble" to his book (usually called a preamble) is a classic — "20 years in 2 minutes" rap-style message that I've heard him say many times. He always comes up with classic stuff that doesn't come from normal thought patterns. A Normally Unusual entertaining guy for sure.

It's packed with interesting stories of skate, surf, snow, dirt, travel, and his journey to becoming clean and sober more than 14 years ago. I was honored to endorse it on the back cover of his book as a fellow rider, and I found it very entertaining and inspirational to read.

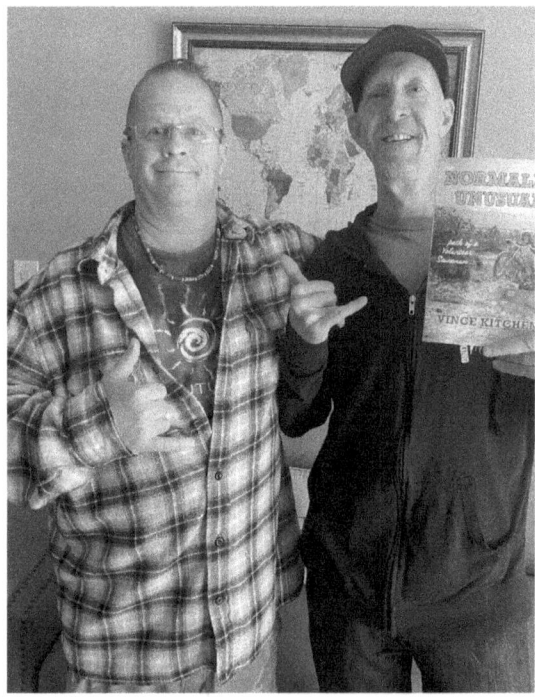

Hey look, I'm holding Vince's book

Now, as a fellow autobiography writer, I understand some of the challenges that come with putting your life into words. You have to share something that feels right to you and hope the reader enjoys it, connects with it, and understands the life you've lived. Writing your story is a great experience, and I'd encourage anyone who's into it to give it a try. It's a powerful way to connect with your own life, document it for yourself, and share it with others. It was a mind-expanding journey, and I'm glad I got to experience it.

After high school, I kept skating hard and signed up for community college, choosing business as my major. But my heart was still set on the thrill of skateboarding.

I was now twenty and restless as I found myself at a crossroads. A couple of years ago, when I graduated high school, my dad said, "You know you'll need a real job, son." He had that parental logic that I couldn't argue with, so I tried the responsible route. I did two years in junior college studying business, and then made an attempt at studying the then-new field of lasers. I remember those drives to Simi Valley College, dreading the commute, trigonometry, calculus, and everything that made my eyes glaze over. Passion was absent from this part of my life, and I felt every minute of it.

Eventually, I couldn't ignore my calling. I told myself — and then my dad — "I'm going to be a pro skateboarder." When I broke the news to my dad, I was surprised at his lack of pushback. It was like he could see that this wasn't just a phase — it was what made me feel alive. With that, I dropped the textbooks and made a plan to try to keep following my passions.

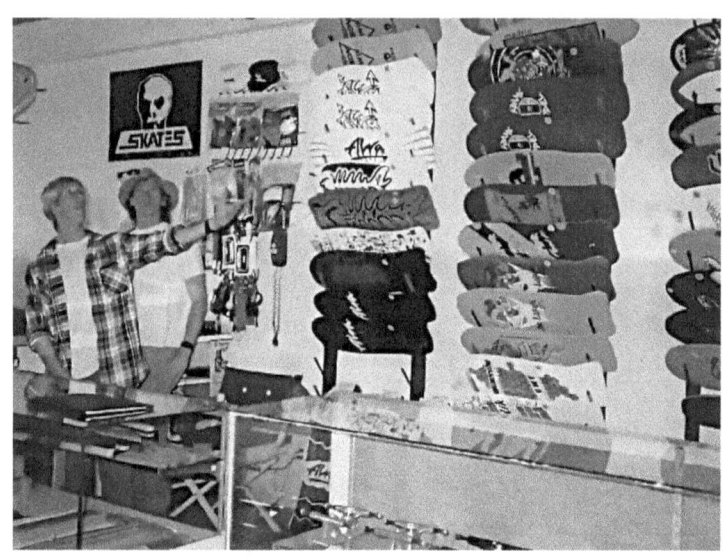

Throwin' it back to 1985, me and Don Jayne at Green Sector

My skate shop sponsor, Green Sector, and Don Jayne, who owned it, were my gateway into the Life's a Beach Hell Week skate contest in 1987. They covered my entry fee, and Don even filmed some footage of me warming up on the contest vert ramp. Back in the '80s, capturing skateboarding on video was rare for me. I still have access to that footage on YouTube — one of the few clips I have from a life chapter spent on four wheels. Like I said, in those days, we were living in the here and now, not thinking about preserving it for the future. It was just pure, raw skating for the love of it — and just loving the skate life that we were living daily.

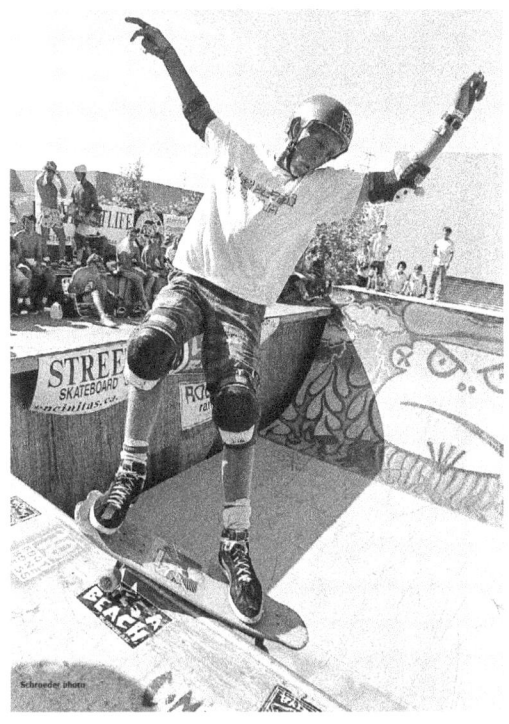

Smith grind at the 1987 L.A.B. Hell Week Contest

In that contest, I entered the amateur division as a warm-up — and won. That was just the beginning. I took a shot in the pro division. This wasn't a main pro competition circuit contest, but I was facing off against legends like Danny Way, Gator, and other well-known pros. I was an unknown, a wildcard — and I came out swinging. I ended up beating them and many other well-established riders and landed on the podium. I'm sure people were wondering who this random kid from the Valley was that was shredding with the heavyweights and beating most of them. I knew I could skate with the best of them. I had now arrived, and there was no going back to college, calculus, and the kind of suffering and lost-life-direction feeling I had at that time. I was back to where I was supposed to be — with a purpose, drive, and love for what I was doing — which felt completely right at that time in my life.

A podium position at the Life's a Beach contest opened doors. New sponsors came on board: Life's a Beach, Airwalk, and JT Eyewear instantly sponsored me after my results shined out of nowhere. Skateboarding was evolving into a career. Soon, I was doing demos, photoshoots, and starting to see a future in skateboarding.

Along the way, I met Sonny Miller — a professional photographer with a reputation in the surf, skate, and snowboarding industries. Sonny, who left us too soon in 2014 at 53 years old from a heart attack, became a huge influence. He saw my potential not just in skateboarding, but in something else — the then-niche sport of snowboarding.

I'd been into snowboarding during the winter for a couple of years, thanks to Don Jayne's suggestion and bringing me up to the mountains initially. It had that same rush as skateboarding, just with fresh, unlimited terrain and many new possibilities. Sonny and I hit the slopes together, and he was blown away by my skate-style approach — backflips and all — which were a rare trick back then.

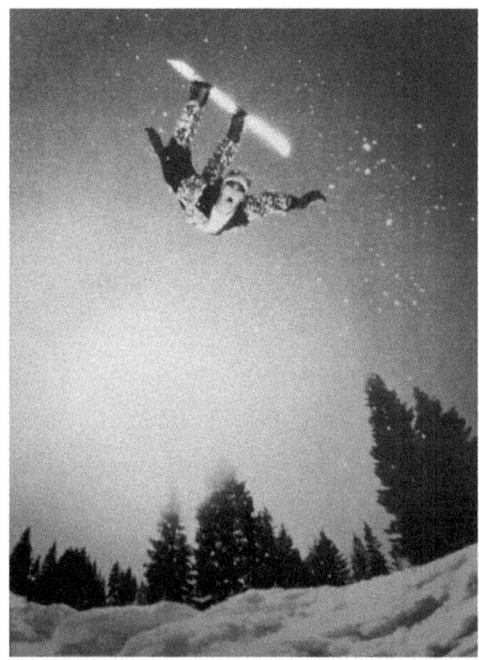

Backflip Shot captured by Sonny Miller (RIP 🙏)

Those days, barely anyone was going that big on a snowboard or riding one with a full skateboard style — but for me, it was just natural. Sonny spoke to Jamie Mosberg, my team manager at Life's a Beach, and they got the word about my snowboarding skills to my other skate sponsors, Airwalk and JT Eyewear. These companies were also investing in this new sport of snowboarding, and they saw me as a part of that vision. They already had enough pro skaters, so they wanted me to be their pro snowboarder and would start to pay me for representing their brands in this new sport.

I was into it — since I loved the sport of snowboarding — so I was in. And it was on!

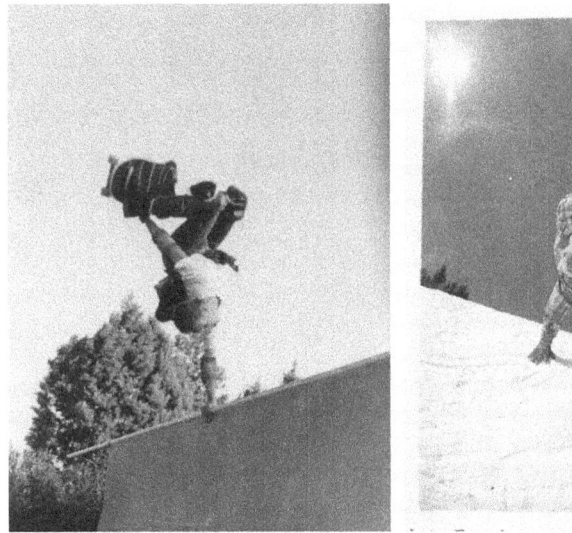

From skate handplants to snowboard handplants

It was a big pivot, going from a rising pro skateboarder to becoming a pro snowboarder. It was a wild ride — so let's check out the highs and lows and where it all goes.

-Chapter 4-
CraZy Teen TimeZ

I loved skateboarding, but when I went snowboarding, it was like a whole new level of adrenaline. Skateboarding was incredible, especially as a vert skater, where you're defying gravity and executing precision tricks at the highest level you can. But snowboarding? It was like skateboarding on steroids! Flying down a mountain at full speed, catching air off anything you could find or create — it was pure freedom. The mountain became a canvas, and we were painting flowing lines on it like an artist.

In the early days, in 1985, Mountain High was one of the only resorts with chairlifts in Southern California allowing snowboarding. Back then, snowboarders were seen as second-class citizens, and ski patrol wasn't thrilled about us riding — especially when it came to jumping. They'd patrol the mountain like watchdogs, making sure we weren't catching air anywhere. But for every hard-headed ski patroller who wanted us gone, there were way more curious skiers and staff who saw our style and fluidity of snowboarding and couldn't help but be impressed. Every time we'd wait in a lift line, people would ask how these snowboard things worked. We'd explain as best we could, trying to be cool to people and represent snowboarding in a positive light.

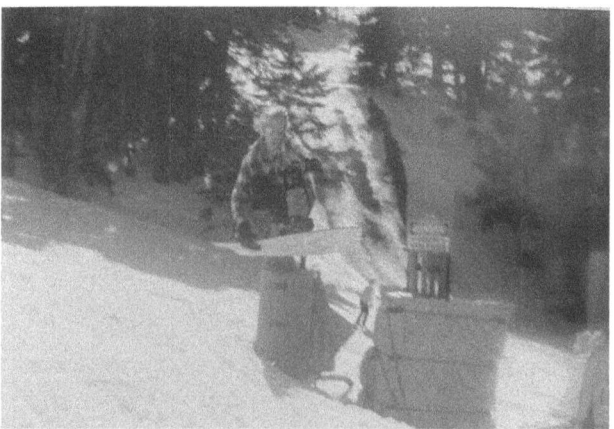

1985 Mountain High days on a Sims Swallowtail

I would say it was like a blend of surfing and skateboarding on snow. It's a great sport that is always improving, and it gives us a whole new way to express ourselves and enjoy the mountains in a different way than skiing. You should get on a board and try it — it's awesome!

Despite the occasional ski patrol hassle, we always managed to have fun. We'd carve up the runs, slashing snow everywhere and surfing across the mountain with speed and style. We'd hunt for jumps — whether it was a natural feature, a mound near a ski pole, or a snow-covered stump or rock. If there was a way to take off and land smoothly, we were hitting it. This was before they made *jump lines* — we had to get creative to make jumps happen on the mountain and not get caught by ski patrol. If you got caught jumping by a grumpy ski patrol, he would pull your lift ticket for the day. That would suck, but then we'd be back another day, or another way, to play the game again.

When I say "we," I'm mostly talking about my longtime friend at the time, Victor. He and I went way back to junior high school. He was my bad-influence, good friend — the guy who'd sometimes push bad boundaries, and I'd usually roll with it. On the slopes, we'd feed off each other's energy, trying to one-up each other with tricks and antics like slashing a bit of snow at people as we flew by. We'd rip down runs, dodging ski patrol and laughing the whole time. But Victor's rule-breaking influence extended far beyond the mountains in the years before snowboarding.

Trouble and Teenage Antics

Victor was the kind of friend who always had a scheme. One Christmas in junior high, we both got remote-controlled cars that needed six D-size batteries each. Batteries weren't cheap, and we didn't exactly have a steady income. Victor's solution? Wear big coats, head to the store, and steal battery packs. With our heavy down jackets, we'd stuff multiple battery packs into hidden pockets, casually buy a small item to throw off suspicion, and walk out with enough batteries to keep our RC cars running strong until the next time we needed power.

He also taught me how to cheat arcade games. We'd tape a quarter to a piece of thread, feed the quarter right down to the money counter clicker, and rack up dozens of free games. We'd play Asteroids and Defender for hours at the local store, restaurant, or arcade. Just another way we were gaming the system.

Canyon Drives and Reckless Adventures

By high school, our antics escalated. My first car was a beat-up 1972 Opel station wagon that I bought for $200 from Steve Fransman with my paper route money. That car became a rolling prank machine. I discovered that turning off the engine key while driving, then switching it back on, would cause a loud backfire — sounding like a gunshot. We'd click the key off while rolling toward someone and then click it back on near the unsuspecting victim. BOOM! People would jump in shock as we rolled by, laughing our heads off.

I also rigged the windshield washer squirters to spray sideways toward the passenger side instead of up onto the windshield. Victor loved this. We'd roll up to friends — usually — and while he distracted them with conversation from the passenger seat, he or I would twist the washer handle and spray them in the face while they talked through the window. One time, at Zuma Beach, Victor pulled this trick on a surfer we didn't know. We pulled up, Victor asked how the waves were, then sprayed the guy in the face mid-sentence. We pulled away laughing, parked, and paddled out into the surf.

When we came back in from the water, my car seats and floor were filled with sand. The guy had gotten his revenge, and my seats looked like sand dunes. We scooped it off, and I ended up laughing it off. After all, it gave my car a permanent beach vibe, and now I always had my toes in the sand, I actually liked it. I even put more sand at my feet on the floorboards, confirming my new "sand floor interior" style. It was a wise-guy blessing in disguise.

Victor had a VW Bug with big fiberglass fenders. One day, I was standing along a two-way road saving him a parallel parking spot at a surf break called Drainpipes. I thought he'd stop. He thought I'd move. At the last second, I dove into the sand, but his fender grazed my arm and sliced it open. I still have the scar from that day — a permanent reminder of our wild teenage surfing years.

Our drives through Malibu Canyon to Zuma Beach were just as eventful as our beach days. Victor would stockpile baseball-sized rocks at his feet in the passenger seat. As we'd drive past roadside vendors selling fruit and nuts, he'd launch a rock at their signs, knocking them over as we sped by — laughing while the vendors yelled and shook their fists.

I remember one time, driving away from Victor's house, he was holding and scraping a six-foot stick along the ground out the passenger window. As we passed a cyclist on the main road, he lifted the stick and whacked the guy across the back. The guy grabbed his back and yelled at us as we kept driving. It was reckless and wrong, but back then, it was just another reckless stunt we'd laugh about as we tore through the streets. Crazy young days.

Toward the end of that summer, my 1972 Opel station wagon met its end in Malibu Canyon. Driving back to the Valley after another epic beach day, me, Victor, and Dave Troy (RIP 🙏) were navigating the winding canyon road. It included a tunnel — a sudden burst of darkness after the bright California sunshine.

As fate would have it, an elderly driver two cars ahead panicked when entering the tunnel and slammed on her brakes. That triggered a chain reaction. One car rear-ended hers, I hit the car in front of me, and another car slammed into the back of mine. Once we got through the tunnel and back into daylight, all four cars pulled over to the shoulder.

Victor and I stepped out, jokingly yelling, "Ouch, my neck! Ouch, my back!" as we laughed, trying to ease the tension — typical jokers that we were. After the initial humor wore off, we exchanged insurance info with the other drivers and went our separate ways.

Fortunately, since I wasn't the last car in the chain, the driver who hit me covered the damage. My trusty Opel was totaled, but the payout was $800 — a solid return on a $200 car. That wagon had given me a summer full of memories, and in the end, I'd quadrupled my investment. With the settlement, I upgraded to a 1978 Toyota Celica — a newer, better ride that marked the start of my next adventure.

That crash in Malibu Canyon taught me a lesson that stuck: life is full of twists and turns, and sometimes a hit comes out of nowhere and changes everything. The best thing you can do is roll with it, stay alert, and keep moving forward — because the next curve or tunnel might hold a surprise you didn't see coming.

Sideways in the Celica

Getting behind the wheel of my new — well, new-to-me — 1978 Toyota Celica stick shift changed everything. The road wasn't just a path to wherever I was heading, it now became a playground. Compared to my old Opel station wagon, which was basically a beach cruiser on wheels, the Celica was a bit of adrenaline on asphalt. The Opel's days had ended in the Malibu Canyon pileup, but this Celica was alive, waiting for me to push it to its limits — and so I did.

On rain-slick or misty streets, the Celica became even more fun, and I was the artist learning how to paint with speed and control. A quick shift, a clutch dump, and the rear wheels would break loose and slide, letting me drift through corners like I was in some backlot rally. It wasn't just driving anymore — it was an adventure.

Every street offered a new kind of thrill, every turn a chance to feel the tires hug the pavement — or break them loose if I wanted to. This car wasn't just about getting from one place to another; it was about finding excitement along the way.

Of course, pushing limits has its price. And I was about to learn that lesson the hard way.

I didn't drink or get stoned much, but there was the infamous night I told Victor, "I drive great when I'm drunk and stoned!" I'd had a few drinks, smoked some pot with him and some friends, and thought I was invincible. Driving to another party we were trying to find that night, shortly after I said that, Victor shouted, "Turn here!" I tried to turn right down the street I was nearly passing and went up the far-side curb with my car, wrecking my radiator, wheels, and front end. I backed up my steaming car and parked it. We then did the walk of shame back to his house that night.

The next day, I lied to my parents, saying that another driver forced me off the main road and up the curb of that side street. My dad and I later bonded by finding another Celica body with a blown motor for cheap. We rented a Cherry Picker, which was an engine hoist. We took the good motor out of my crashed Celica and put it into the good Toyota frame, giving me a second chance with another Toyota Celica — ready to roll again. Those were the good old days when you could just bolt things together. Now, I think you need an engineering and electronics degree to do an engine swap like that.

Clipping Tickets and Chasing Dreams

When it came to snowboarding, Victor and I were resourceful. We didn't have money for lift tickets, so we'd show up to the mountain after lunch and "clip tickets" at Mountain High. We'd wait in the parking lot, find someone wrapping up their day, and ask if they were done and if we could have their ticket. Using wire cutters, we'd remove the person's ticket and reattach it to our belts, making it look brand new. This trick let us ride for free, honing our skills on the mountain without breaking the bank.

No Ticket for Us, We Win

Once Mammoth Mountain opened its slopes to snowboarders, it felt like a game-changer. The mountain was massive compared to Mountain High and Big Bear, and snowboarding there was a big deal for anyone who loved the sport. But it hadn't always been that way. For a couple of years before this, June Mountain — Mammoth's smaller sister mountain — had cautiously allowed snowboarders as a sort of trial run. They wanted to see if we could coexist with skiers, follow the rules, and ride safely. When they realized snowboarders weren't just a bunch of reckless kids but a valuable source of revenue, the

McCoy family, who owned both resorts, gave snowboarding the green light at Mammoth Mountain.

It wasn't just about money either — snowboarding brought a fresh, exciting vibe to the mountains, drawing in curious skiers and inspiring new riders to try something different.

Times were simpler back then. This was before one of the corporate giants, Alterra Mountain Company, took ownership of Mammoth and June Mountain, turning them into part of their corporate wheelhouse of resorts to play by their rules.

Alterra also now owns resorts in Colorado, Utah, Tahoe, and back East. Between Alterra and Vail Resorts — which owns resorts in all of those areas as well as Whistler and Blackcomb in Canada — it feels like everything is getting bought up and centralized, swallowed by massive institutions in every industry.

The charm of family-owned operations is fading, but I guess that's just how business goes. You have to adapt with the changes. Back then, though, Mammoth felt like an untamed playground for us as snowboarders, and Victor and I had figured out how to ride there for free as well.

Another trick we learned was simple: sneak onto the bottom lift and avoid going all the way to the base of the mountain once you were up. The lift operators at the higher chairs didn't bother checking tickets, and as long as you stayed away from the lower lifts, you could ride all day without paying a dime. It was a perfect system — until the day it wasn't.

Victor and I had made it to the top of the mountain in the morning, as usual, and were carving through some fresh powder when we got back in an upper lift line. When a lift operator asked us for our lift tickets, he wasn't buying our excuse that we'd left them at the bottom. He wanted ski patrol to escort us down the hill to confirm our story. We weren't about to let that happen. As soon as we could, we strapped into our boards and bolted, racing down toward the bottom of the mountain as fast as we could. For a brief moment, we thought we'd pulled it off.

But the lift operator had called the bottom of the mountain, and by the time we reached the base, a police car was already waiting for us in the main lodge parking lot. They nabbed us on the spot and hauled us off to the local police station, where we were slapped with tickets for riding without lift passes. It wasn't the way we wanted our day to end, but we weren't about to let it ruin our trip.

After making it back to town, we regrouped with friends and shared the story of our not-so-slick escape. A couple of buddies who had been riding that day gave us their tickets, and before long, we were back on the mountain, ripping down some different runs since we now had lift tickets for the day.

The trip ended on a high note, but the tickets from the cops still hung over our heads. We'd have to go back to court weeks later to face the charges.

When the court date rolled around, Victor and I had a plan. We took the lift tickets we'd gotten from our friends and put them onto our jackets, making it look like we'd had lift tickets from that day the whole time.

Standing in front of the judge, we explained that we'd been snowboarding hard that day and had taken off our jackets because we got too warm. That's why we didn't have our lift tickets on us when the lift operator stopped us. We made sure the story sounded airtight.

The judge bought it. He looked at the tickets we presented and dismissed the case. Just like that, we were off the hook. If we'd been found guilty, we could've been hit with fines totaling around $1,000, but instead, we walked away without paying a cent. It wasn't just a victory — it was a testament to our tricky thinking and a little bit of luck. And it gave us one more wild story to add to our collection.

After this entire court fiasco, Victor and I had six hours to kill on the drive back to the San Fernando Valley, where we were based at the time. Naturally, we used that time to channel the adrenaline and excitement into something creative. By the time we got home, we'd come up with a rap song that perfectly captured the chaos, humor, and triumph of our escapade. It wasn't just a joke between us either — our rap and the story of what we pulled off ended up being published in Transworld Snowboarding magazine, complete with a cartoon illustration of Victor and me taking on the cops and the judge.

Seeing that rap immortalized in print, along with the cartoon, felt like the ultimate win. It wasn't just about getting away with it — it was about doing it in a way that was pure us: breaking the rules, making our own, and walking away with a legendary story to tell.

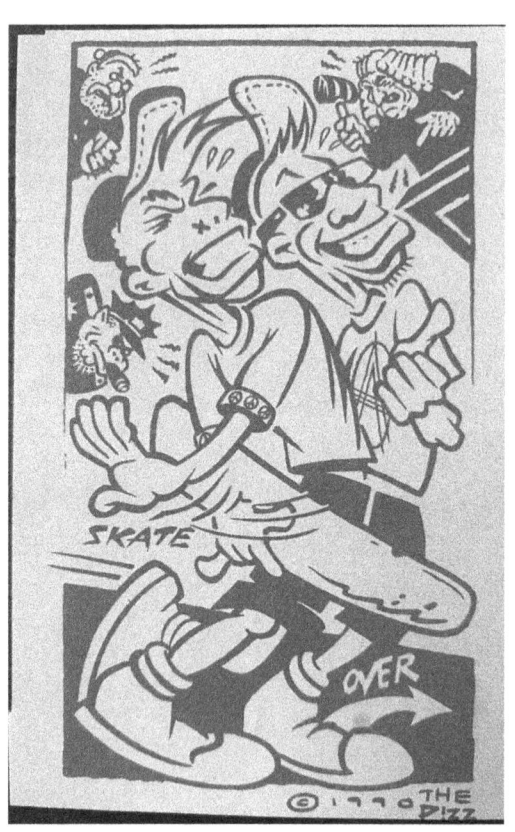

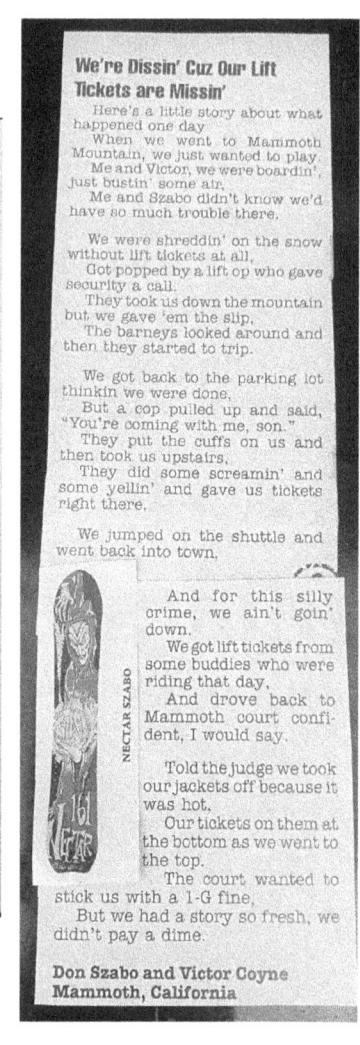

We're Dissin' Cuz Our Lift Tickets are Missin'

Here's a little story about what happened one day

When we went to Mammoth Mountain, we just wanted to play.

Me and Victor, we were boardin', just bustin' some air,

Me and Szabo didn't know we'd have so much trouble there.

We were shreddin' on the snow without lift tickets at all,

Got popped by a lift op who gave security a call.

They took us down the mountain but we gave 'em the slip.

The barneys looked around and then they started to trip.

We got back to the parking lot thinkin we were done,

But a cop pulled up and said, "You're coming with me, son."

They put the cuffs on us and then took us upstairs,

They did some screamin' and some yellin' and gave us tickets right there.

We jumped on the shuttle and went back into town.

And for this silly crime, we ain't goin' down.

We got lift tickets from some buddies who were riding that day,

And drove back to Mammoth court confident, I would say.

Told the judge we took our jackets off because it was hot,

Our tickets on them at the bottom as we went to the top.

The court wanted to stick us with a 1-G fine,

But we had a story so fresh, we didn't pay a dime.

**Don Szabo and Victor Coyne
Mammoth, California**

Our rap got published in TransWorld SNOWboarding mag

-Chapter 5-
Sk8 to Snow Pro

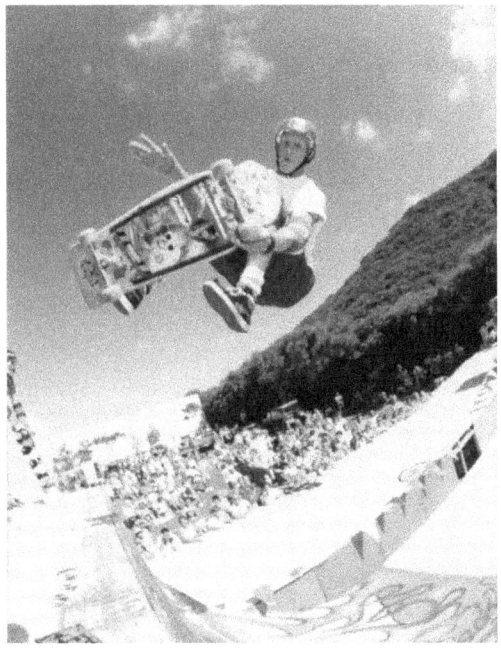

Life's a Beach skate contest shot

In 1987, the Life's a Beach skate contest turned into a game-changer. That contest led straight into a paid snowboarding gig that winter. Victor wasn't so lucky. He didn't have sponsors backing him or the right breaks to keep traveling or cover the costs, so his road got a lot tougher.

Nonetheless, we continued to hang out and ride together. I introduced him to my sponsors and connections, securing product support for him. We remained a team, moving forward together. Our photo shoots with Sonny Miller gained Victor recognition in magazines and within the snowboard community. We were even featured in a few ads together — riding and hanging out as always. Victor, being resourceful, did what he could to join the missions, which was great!

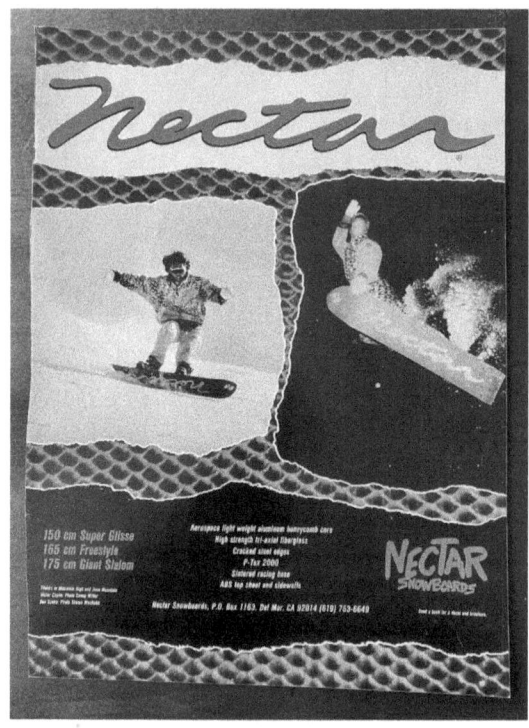

Me and Victor in a Nectar Snowboards ad

Working closely with Sonny Miller, we traveled to different mountains to capture great snowboarding shots and promote the products we endorsed. Companies and magazines also compensated Sonny for his outstanding photography, making it a win-win situation.

Sonny Miller and I shared countless crazy snowboarding missions, but one that always comes to mind is the time we were sprinting through the airport after a late-afternoon photo shoot on Mount Hood's summer snowfields in Oregon. We checked in and were told at the ticket counter that we might make the flight if we got to the gate on time. We then ran like O.J. Simpson in those old airport commercials, dodging other travelers and pushing our limits to make it to the gate. Despite our frantic effort, we could only watch helplessly as the plane pulled away from the terminal without us on it. It was one of many chaotic, adrenaline-filled moments with Sonny, who was just as passionate about getting the shot as I was about nailing the trick. At least we got some great shots that afternoon at Mount Hood, even though we had to get a later flight to make it back home from that trip.

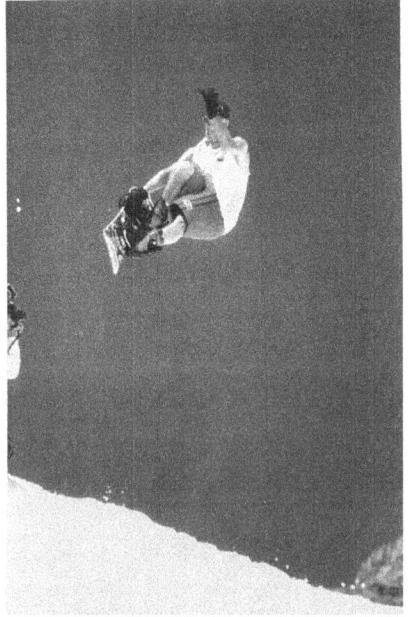

Mt. Hood, frontside air in shorts

Our partnership wasn't limited to just photo shoots. Sonny and I were friends, and we hung out and went on a string of snow missions together — sometimes waking up at 3 a.m. to head to different mountains for magazine shoots or sponsors' product features. I was based out of my parents' house in the San Fernando Valley at the time, but I spent way more nights sleeping at other places than at home. I'd also go surfing in San Diego at times when I was down there for our missions or to visit my sponsors.

We frequented places like Mountain High, Big Bear, Mammoth, and Tahoe, which became our easy-access playgrounds. Sonny's camera captured the essence of our snowboarding sessions. He had connections with Nectar Surfboards and Snowboards in Cardiff, which quickly became my snowboard sponsor. He and the owner, Gary McNabb, recognized snowboarding's potential long before it became an Olympic sport or the massive industry it is today.

For me, that area near North County San Diego became a second home, but I'd always return to the Valley to repack and regroup for the next big mission when I needed to.

Canada Camaraderie, Eh

In 1989, Sonny and I traveled to Canada for a photo shoot and competition. I remember the antics as much as the riding — like wearing a big hair wig and adopting a terrible British accent while meeting other snowboarders. By then, people recognized me from magazines, often decked out in neon Life's a Beach gear with bats, skull-and-crossbones patterns, neon panels, or other wild outfits they made at the time.

Snowboarding was still new, and standing out was part of the game. I loved being the crazy, fun guy with a shaved head and bold attitude, doing wild things with this emerging sport.

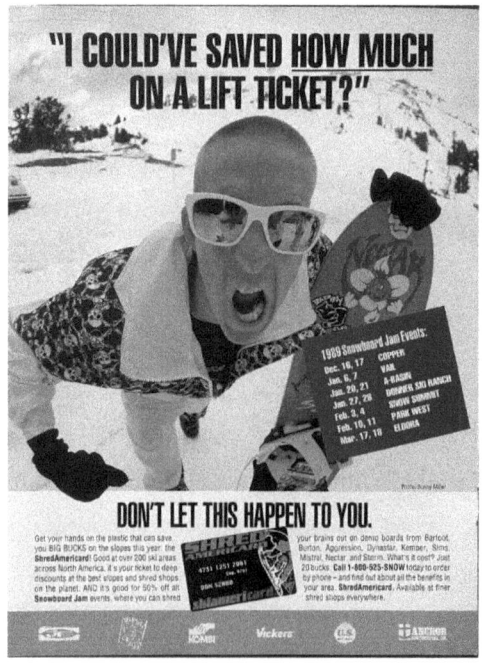

High volume, higher fashion crimes

This Canada trip was also where I competed against Damian Sanders, one of the most influential snowboarders in the sport's early days. He was a huge inspiration to me and many others. I first saw him in ISM Snowboard Magazine, produced by Tom Hsieh, which was like the Bible for snowboarders in the mid-'80s. This was before Transworld Snowboard Magazine even existed. We'd eagerly wait for each new issue to see the latest tricks, *cliff jumps*, and powder shots featuring legends like Keith Kimmel, Terry Kidwell, Tom Burt, Sean Palmer, and of course, Damian Sanders.

Damian had a rockstar image like no other. He was married to Brandy, a Penthouse Playmate, and his unique look and lifestyle turned heads everywhere. With shaved sides and the rest of his hair up in a Gothic, spiked style, he embodied the badass snowboarder vibe. But it wasn't just his image that got him noticed — Damian had the skills to back it up. He was larger than life, but when I finally met him, he turned out to be just as genuine and down-to-earth as he came across in his interviews.

Damian's brother, Chris Sanders, owned Avalanche Snowboards, one of the early snowboard companies. The two of them experimented with ways to make snowboards work better in those early development days of the sport. Damian was a natural at snowboarding, and that simple twist of fate changed the course of his life. It's crazy to think how one little thing in all of our lives can set us on a completely different path.

Flashback: Meeting Damian Sanders

Back in 1986, snowboarding still wasn't welcome at most ski resorts. But Donner Ski Ranch in Tahoe was one of the few places that allowed it, and that was all we needed to know. Compared to the bigger resorts in the area, Donner was small, but to us, it was perfect. They let us ride, so we were going.

Don Jayne, who owned Green Sector — my skateboard shop sponsor — wanted to get up to the mountains for some fresh NorCal snow. Road trip adventure and new terrain to snowboard? I was all in. Let's go!

Along with his brother Mike and our friend Adam, the four of us hit the road, ready for a good time in Tahoe.

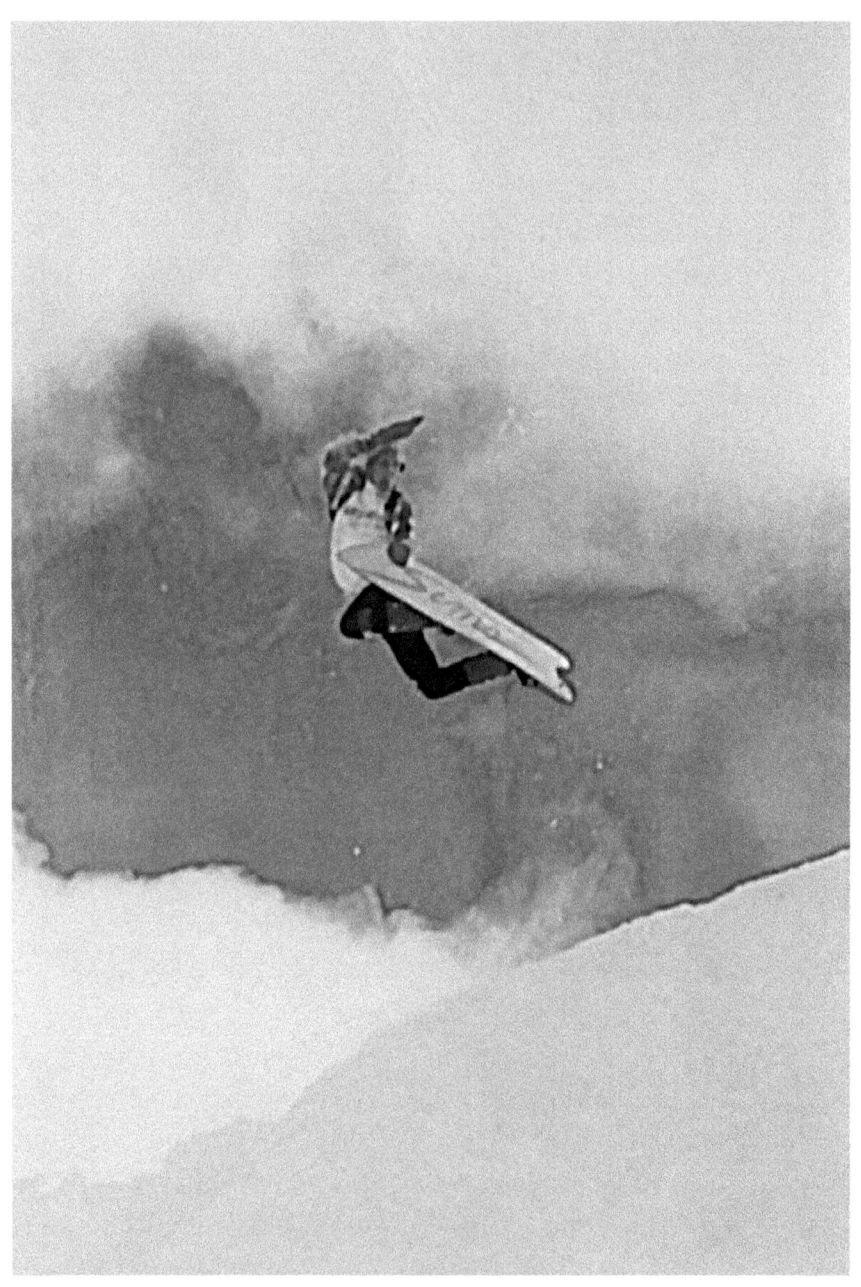
My first backflip wasn't much to look at, but this Method Air at Donner in '86 was a blast

We got to Donner and were having a blast — fresh snow, good friends, and a new mountain to ride. It was great! Then, out of nowhere, we ran into Damian Sanders. That was unreal. I had been following him in ISM magazine, as I mentioned, so I felt like I already knew something about him. And now, here he was, right in front of us.

Turns out, he was a local at Donner and knew the mountain inside and out. He offered to show us around, and just like that, we were riding with one of the most well-known snowboarders of the time. It was surreal.

Riding with Damian was next level. We carved through fresh powder wherever we could find it, and even the tracked-out runs were fun with him leading the way. He had such a smooth style — always in control — making everything look effortless as we carved down the mountain together, all of us having a great time ripping it up.

At one point, on the backside of Donner, Damian pointed out a jump and said, "This is the perfect spot to learn a backflip." He made it sound so easy, like it was no big deal. I had never done a backflip on a snowboard before, but I knew I had the motion down from other things.

I'd thrown backflips into pools, off cliffs into water, and even off stages at punk rock shows into crowds.

Still, I knew I could do it.

Standing near Damian as he took off, I watched as he effortlessly threw down a perfect backflip, landing smoothly in the fresh snow beyond the jump. Seeing him do it with such ease and style was all the motivation I needed.

When it was my turn to *drop* in, I pointed my board toward the jump, locked in, and as I hit the lip, I threw myself backward, tucking my knees as I always did when doing backflips. But this was snow, not water, and my rotation wasn't exactly how snowboarders usually did a backflip. At the last second, I adjusted my board and my landing weight, realizing I was going to come down backward. I landed backwards — also known as riding fakie — then my board rotated back to forward and I rode down to where Damian was after his awesome backflip that he showed us on this jump. I couldn't believe it worked out so well.

Damian was *stoked*. "Dude! That was sick!"

That moment meant a lot — pushing past something I hadn't done before and pulling it off. It was a good day in the mountains, riding with friends and learning something new. A personal milestone. One of those days that stands out as a turning point, an accomplishment I'll never forget.

In 1988, a year before my wig antics in Canada and a couple of years after first meeting Damian, I competed in a halfpipe contest against other pros, including Damian and some talented Canadian locals like Ken Achenbach and Don Schwartz. I pulled off a solid run, combining skateboard-inspired tricks with my smooth, high-flying style. At the end of the pipe, there was a lip I turned into a jump, and I did a backflip off it. The crowd went wild, but the judges disqualified me, citing *inverted aerials* as illegal in competition. I was shocked — Canada was usually more lenient about those kinds of tricks, but I guess not in competitions.

Damian ended up winning, but during the awards ceremony, he did something incredible. In front of everyone, he said, "Szabo, I think you won this contest. That wasn't fair." He gave me credit in front of my fellow riders, which was amazing, and then split his prize money with me — a gesture that amplified my respect for him. That was Damian. More than just a snowboarding icon, he was a class act, and he still is to this day. Definitely an amazing guy that I've had many great times with — on snow, dirt bikes, traveling, parties, and just hanging out over the years.

Crack Creates Chaos

Back in SoCal, I reconnected with Victor. As I mentioned, he hadn't quite had the same opportunities I had, but we were still a team as friends and on the snow. He just had to keep performing to get more help from sponsors that were warming up to him becoming a pro snowboarder in the near future.

Victor was talented, no doubt about it, but there was always that edgy, devious side to him. One night, that edge got razor-sharp, and the devil stepped in.

We met at this little hole-in-the-wall Mexican spot in Northridge, the kind of place where you order food at a window and eat outside at cheap plastic tables. While we waited for our food, this shady dude sitting nearby caught Victor's attention.

"Pssst! If you can guess which cup the bottle cap is under, I'll pay you some money," he said.

Victor was instantly intrigued. The guy had three cups flipped over and was sliding them around like a magician, daring us to guess which cup the bottle cap was under. His sleight of hand was wild, and I had to admit, it was fascinating for a minute, but I could tell this guy was bad news. But Victor was hooked. He leaned in, letting this guy egg him on. Soon, he was betting money, convinced he could win if he just figured out the trick to this guy's scheme.

My burrito finally came up, and I told Victor, "I'm taking this home and eating it where it's warm. I'll catch you later, bro."

But I could see it in his eyes; he wasn't leaving anytime soon. That devilish spark was alive and well, and it burned brighter when later, the guy asked Victor to go smoke crack with him. That night, everything changed for Victor.

Meanwhile, I kept pushing forward, snowboarding every chance I got, photo shoots, events, chasing the adrenaline fix that I had and loved. But Victor started slipping away. At first, he was just harder to pin down to go ride. Then I heard through the grapevine he was couch-surfing and doing whatever it took to score his next hit. The Devil had him.

Fast-forward a bit, and our once-solid friendship and partnership on the mountain was completely gone. Victor had become a ghost of who he was, caught in the grip of something much darker than any snowstorm we'd ever faced. Drugs had him, and they weren't letting go.

My addiction has always been action sports — the rush of speed, the thrill of danger, the feeling of flying. Sure, it's cost me more injuries than I can count, but I've always known it was worth it for that rush that I loved.

Watching Victor spiral down a different road, one lined with shadows and regrets, was devastating. He could've been right there with me, pushing limits and breaking boundaries. Instead, he let the wrong kind of rush take him out.

I also remember back in these early days of snowboarding when I had a bit of a head start over Victor. I remember him telling me, "I'm never going to be as good as others at snowboarding". Looking back, I realize now that his words reflected more than just doubt; they revealed a mindset that also held him back. He didn't believe he could reach that next level, and that belief became part of his barrier. It's another tough lesson he had to learn, and for me, it's a reminder of how powerful mindset truly is.

At that time, I wasn't even thinking about mindset. For me, it came naturally through pushing limits in action sports by just doing what I loved. But when it came to facing real-life challenges, I didn't recognize how important it was to actively focus on my thoughts and perspective. It wasn't until much later that I understood how crucial it is to be intentional about mindset — not just to overcome obstacles but to truly appreciate the good things in life. Staying grateful, staying present, and keeping your mind focused on where you want to go makes all the difference. You have to think about it daily, make it part of who you are, and enjoy every step of the journey. Because success isn't just about reaching your goals; it's about how you show up every day on the way to getting there.

It's another hard lesson that I learned from him: sometimes, no matter how much talent or potential someone has, the wrong choices can shred it all to pieces.

-Chapter 6-
CraZy Snow DayZ

First trip to Japan

My love affair with Asia began in 1988, when I was the only pro snowboarder representing Nectar Snowboards in Japan. This journey wasn't just about promoting my first pro model snowboard — it was an introduction to a whole new world. At the center of it all was Sohn, the representative who distributed Nectar Snowboards in Japan.

Sohn was a cool, down-to-earth guy. I had met him in the States before our big promotional trip. I remember our first meeting down in San Diego near Nectar Surfboards and Snowboards' headquarters, and later, he even visited me in the San Fernando Valley, where he met my dad and had a cool talk and interaction with him.

Traveling to Japan in 1988 felt like stepping into another universe. From the moment I landed, Sohn and I hit the ground running — literally. Our journey began right from the airport, driving to a hotel for our first night. The next day, the whirlwind truly began as we visited shops where fans eagerly awaited our arrival. They wanted autographs, pictures, and a chance to meet, even though we couldn't speak the same language. The energy in those shops was electrifying. Seeing people excitedly purchase my pro model board and getting to interact with them one-on-one was a surreal and humbling experience.

After the events, shop owners often took us out to dinner. Communication wasn't always easy since many of them didn't speak English, but Sohn stepped in as a translator, and we also relied on hand gestures, eye contact, and mutual enthusiasm. Quite often, we stayed at the shop owners' homes, where I got a taste of authentic Japanese living. Sometimes they would set up a makeshift room with folding bamboo screens and lay down a futon, blankets, and a pillow, creating a cozy area to sleep in. It was such a unique experience — living Japanese, even for a short time.

The food, of course, was another adventure. Sometimes I'd find food staring back at me from my plate or bowl. I drew the line at eating heads but embraced each meal as part of the cultural experience. I figured, if they can eat it, so could I.

Sohn had also arranged on-snow demonstrations for me, and even Japanese TV appearances with us both demonstrating this new sport of snowboarding to TV audiences. At resorts, I performed tricks for crowds of people and rode with Japanese snowboarders and shop owners. Sometimes there'd be a big enough jump for me to throw a backflip — a trick that was still considered special at the time. I'd chuckle when kids asked me to do a "back-frip," loving their enthusiasm and knowing their pronunciation of English was far better than my attempts at Japanese. I picked up a few basics like "I am hungry," "I am full," "Please give me water," "How much does this cost?" and, of course, "Thank you." It was simple, but it made the experience even more meaningful.

That first trip lasted a month, and by the next year, I stayed closer to two months. The warmth and honesty of the Japanese people left a lasting impression. At resorts, we'd leave our snowboards unattended in front of the lodge without giving it a second thought, knowing they'd still be there after lunch. That level of trust was rare and deeply refreshing in comparison to other places.

I continued to visit Japan for years during a good part of the '90s, but those early trips with Sohn were something special — just the two of us, immersing ourselves in the culture, living Japanese, and building connections with shop owners and fans. It was pure and authentic.

My time with Sohn gave me an incredible appreciation for Japan. I'll never forget those early days — eating authentic meals in family homes, signing autographs for passionate fans one-on-one, and experiencing life through a completely different lens. It was an extraordinary chapter of life, one that set the stage for many more adventures in the Land of the Rising Sun.

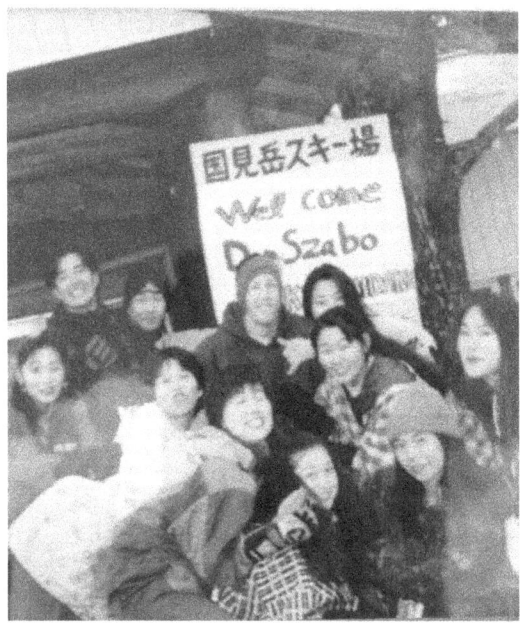

Japanese ladies were great in the 80's

A Cross-Country Ride into the Unknown

A road trip that we took from the West Coast to the East Coast was more than just another snowboarding tour — it was an all-out, unpredictable adventure packed with wild moments, unexpected disasters, and the kind of reckless camaraderie that defined our fearless youth. It was 1991, the start of the Professional Snowboard Tour of America. This was a two-month series of snowboard competitions peppered across the United States, mostly on the East Coast, happening each week at a different mountain resort. Shawn Frederick, a surf photographer aspiring to expand his horizons into snowboarding, approached me and a few local pro snowboarders with an idea.

He pitched the idea of taking a crew of California snowboarders on a cross-country motorhome trip to compete in the PSTA series, ride some fun mountains, and see and do some cool stuff along the way. He had talked with Transworld Snowboarding Magazine about coverage of our epic adventure, and he said they were interested. It sounded like a fun trip — let's do it!

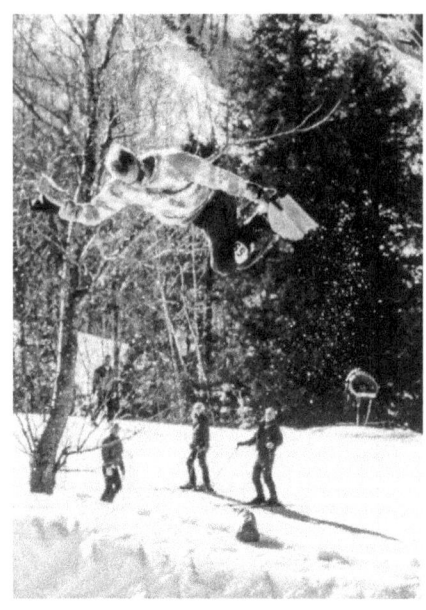

Backside Method Air, Hunter Mountain NY. Photo: Shawn Frederick

Joining the crew were Derek Swinfard, Todd Messick, and Monty Roach. The five of us were set for a two-month journey, hitting competitions and also exploring some great snow mountains across the country along the way. Pulling up to the meeting spot for this trip of a lifetime, we were expecting a decent motorhome. Instead, what was lined up was a four-cylinder Toyota pickup converted into a makeshift motorhome-style camper. It barely slept four, yet there were five of us. Instead of dwelling on the obvious problem, we tossed our bags into a side closet in the rig and embraced the unknown. Bags were packed, high-fives were exchanged, and we hit the road — full of optimism and ready for whatever came next on our journey into the great unknown.

Our first ride was at Brighton Resort in Utah, where a foot of fresh snow greeted us. Shawn talked to the resort's marketing department and scored us all free lift tickets. We wasted no time, charging through steep chutes and deep powder. It was the perfect way to start the trip — except for one minor issue. Shawn was a solid surf photographer, but he wasn't much of a snowboarder yet. He couldn't keep up and lacked the skills to get to some steeps and chutes, missing some of the best shots of the day that the rest of us rode. This problem we weren't aware of was a bit of a bummer for all of us, including him. We gave him some light-hearted grief, but in the back of our minds, we wondered how this was going to play out for the rest of the trip.

Not long after leaving Utah, the real chaos began. A sudden bang from the back of the motorhome sent a jolt through us all. The gas hose had come loose at the metal gas receptor (essential for the modified fuel system) and got sucked under the rear tire, causing a blowout. To make matters worse, the stock bottle jack wasn't designed to lift the weight of the modified camper. We had to get creative, stacking two skateboards in a crisscross pattern as a base to stabilize the jack. It worked — barely. We were able to change the tire and reconnect the gas receptor to the hose and screw it into a position that wouldn't fall apart again, but it was just the first of many situations that we'd have to improvise our way out of.

As we continued east, we ran headfirst into a monster thunderstorm. Sheets of rain hammered down, lightning cracked across the sky, and visibility was near zero. But that wasn't even the worst part. Because of the earlier gas hose and flat tire incident, a hole had been torn through the closet floor where our gear bags were stored. Water from the road sprayed directly into that hole, soaking everything inside. By the time we made it out of the storm, a lot of our clothes and gear were soaked. Luckily, the next day, some East Coast locals near Dover, Delaware took us in after a day of snowboarding. They let us wash and dry our gear, which was awesome. We had fun hanging out with them that evening, and a few of us slept inside their pad — a luxury we didn't often have on this trip.

The next day we drove north into New York. There was a brutal climb on the way to Hunter Mountain Ski Resort in the Catskill Mountains. The winding mountain roads were too steep for the little four-cylinder motorhome, and at one point, a few of us had to jump out and push the rig up sections of the road just to keep it moving uphill.

At the competitions, standing out was tough. But that didn't take away from the experience. We were out there riding hard, chasing the moments that made it all worth it, and doing our best and enjoying the ride. Reality hit us hard when we realized the magazine coverage we were expecting wasn't going to happen. Every competition was packed with pro riders, and the photographers were all capturing the same halfpipe shots. We weren't the strongest halfpipe riders, and contests weren't really our thing. We were more about riding the natural terrain, making magic happen on the mountain — but on this trip, we weren't getting much magic on film.

Next day was Stowe Mountain Resort. Conditions weren't great — hard-packed and icy, with no fresh snow. We spent most of the day riding *bulletproof terrain*, just looking for something decent to ride. Toward the end of the day, we finally found a fun run full of moguls that had softened up nicely in the sun. A few of us started having fun on that section — turning those *bumps into doubles*, *slashing turns*, and flowing down the mountain, making the best of what we had to work with. After everything we'd gone through to get there, and after searching all day for decent snow and terrain, finding that one stretch of sunny, soft snow that was actually fun to ride felt like a small win.

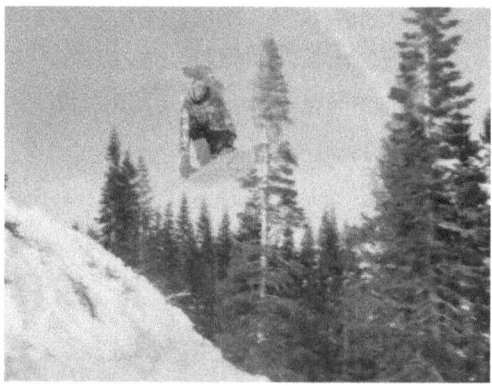

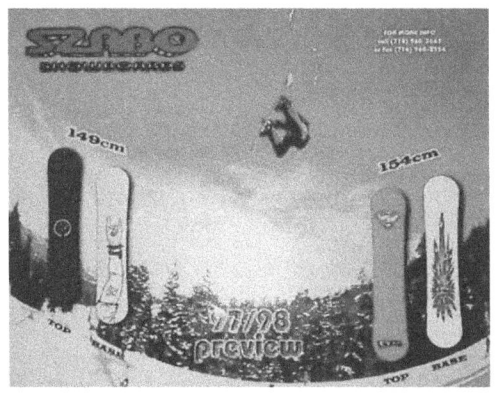

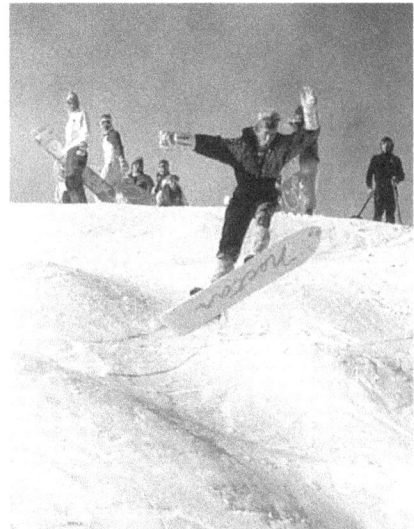

Making jumps out of bumps

Niagara Falls nearly cost me my life. We got there in the early morning hours, and the guys who were awake went out to see it while I was still sleeping in the rig. I woke up to the sound of rushing water and cold air blasting in from the open door. Still groggy, but instantly energized by the moment, I jumped out of the motorhome and ran up to the edge of the Falls, eager to take in the view. Without thinking, I jumped up onto a metal pole barrier to get a closer look in a tricky way. My feet slipped on the dew-covered surface, and suddenly, I was sliding feet-first over the railing. In a split second, I managed to hook my arm around the pole, stopping myself just in time. If I hadn't caught myself, I would have gone straight into the river and over the falls — a 160-foot drop to death. Sketchy doesn't even cover it — I could've been dead.

Looking out at it afterward, I took in how powerful the scene really was. Over one million gallons of water rush over the edge of Niagara Falls every minute — and standing that close, you feel it. It's not just a tourist spot; it's one of the largest hydroelectric power sources in North America, supplying energy to both the U.S. and Canada, while putting on one of the most intense natural shows you'll ever witness. After soaking it in for a few minutes, I jumped back into the rig with everyone, and we kept on moving to our next destination.

Besides snowboarding, close calls, random mishaps, and mayhem, we also saw some iconic landmarks like the Statue of Liberty when we were in New York, and Mount Rushmore in South Dakota as we made our way back toward California. At the time, they felt like just another couple of tourist attractions to check off the list. But looking back now, I realize how incredible they really were — the Statue of Liberty standing as a symbol of freedom and opportunity, and Mount Rushmore as a tribute to vision, artistry, and sheer determination.

As we were nearing the end of our journey, we hit Bridger Bowl Resort in Montana. We found some great out-of-bounds runs, dropping cliffs and *charging chutes* — but with no cameras rolling, those moments existed only for us. And honestly, looking back, it's okay. The trip had been less about press coverage and more about the pure thrill of the adventure and making memories that would last a lifetime.

But the trip wasn't over yet. On our way back, disaster nearly struck again. It was my turn to drive a late-night shift, and I was running on fumes. Derek sat shotgun, but despite my warnings that I couldn't keep my eyes open, he dozed off. I nodded off too — and the next thing I knew, a caution post crumpled under the front bumper with a loud bang. We all woke up, and suddenly, we were barreling off the highway into the desert, bouncing through bushes and dirt. The chaos jolted everyone awake.

"What the hell is going on?!" they yelled, as I held the right line through the desert, avoided high-siding the rig on the downsloping shoulder, and steered us back onto the road at the right time. The front of the motorhome was dented from the caution post, but we were alive. If we had drifted off in a different section — one where the road dropped off — we wouldn't have been so lucky.

Looking back, the PSTA trip was pure madness. It wasn't the polished media spectacle we had all envisioned, but it was something even better — an unforgettable, reckless, and completely raw adventure. It was about pushing limits, embracing chaos, and riding the highs and lows of the journey. We were five young guns chasing a dream, jumping off a cliff just to see where we'd land — and somehow, we survived it all. Long live adventures, friendships, and lifelong memories created from this wild motorhome trip of a lifetime.

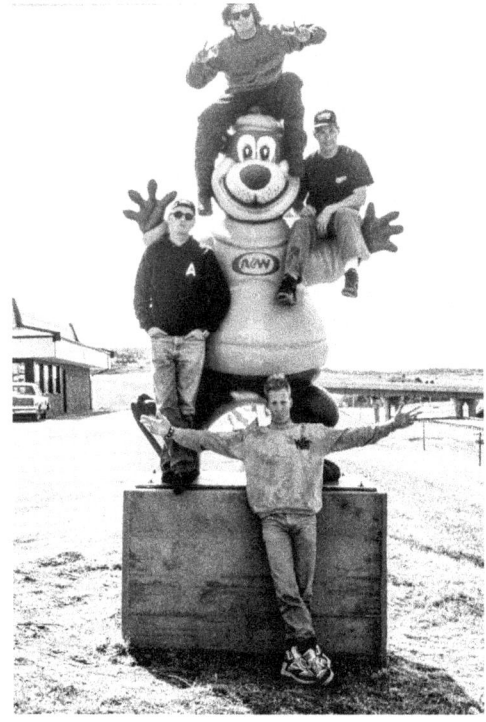

PSTA Crew on A&W Mascott — Photo: Shawn Frederick

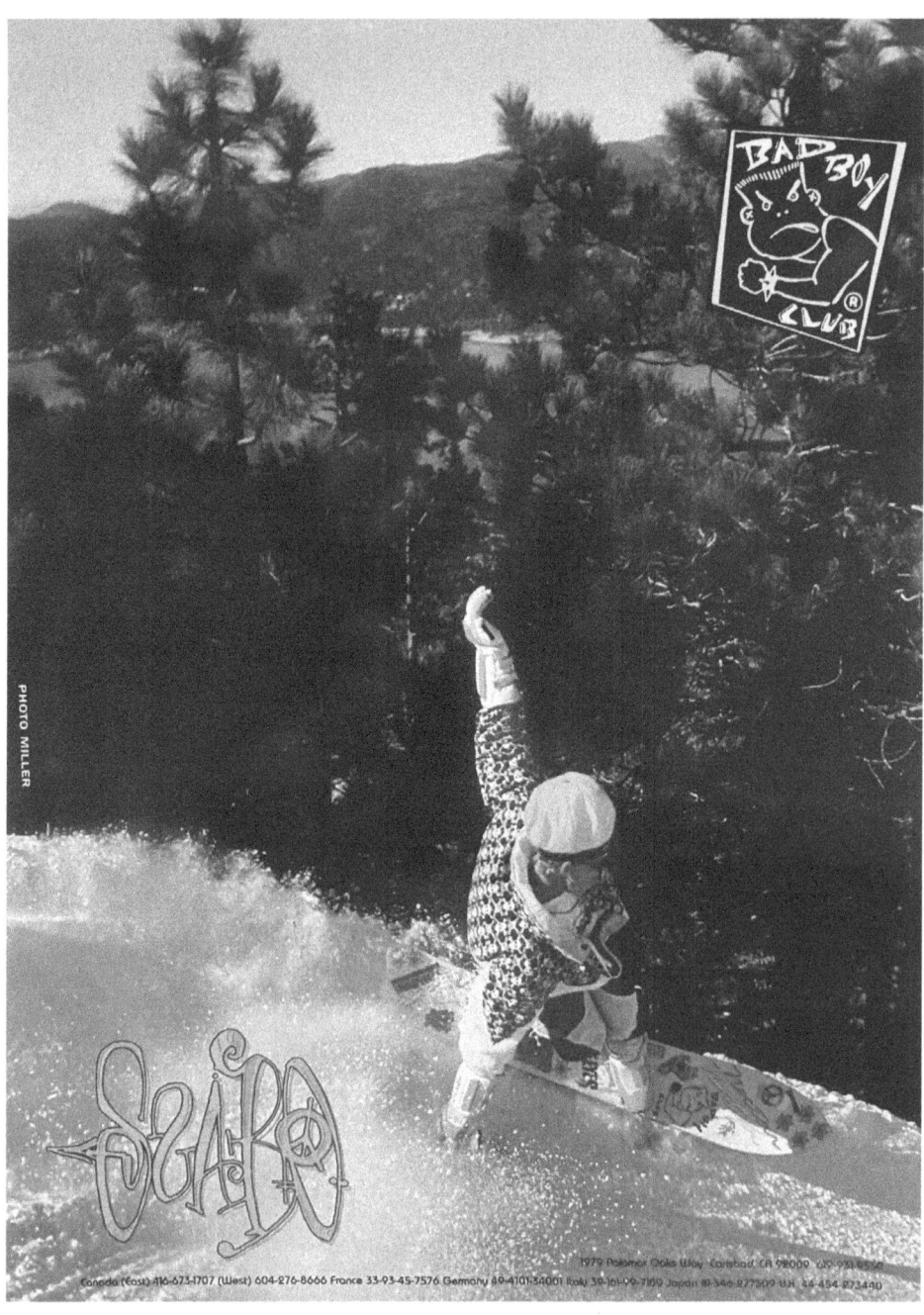

PHOTO MILLER

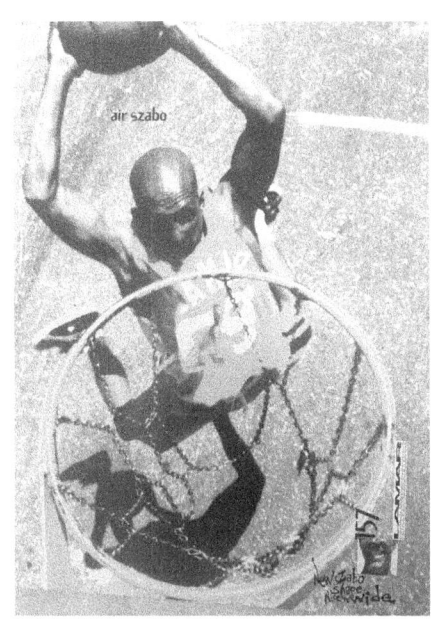

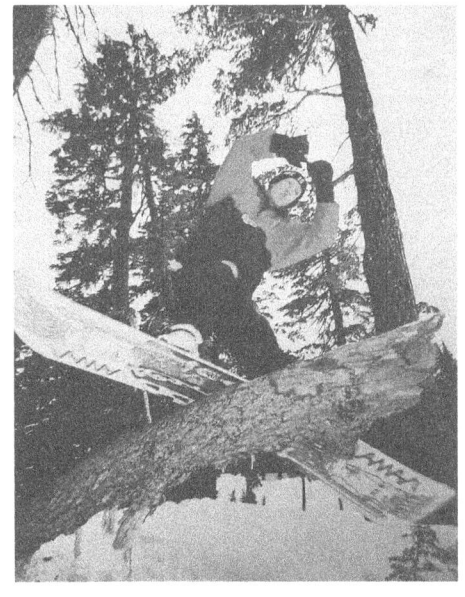

Cruise Ship Calamity

I was heading down to San Diego a lot back then. Some of my sponsors were based there, and I was seeing a girl down that way, which made the trips south even sweeter. One day, she asked if I wanted to go on a cruise to Cancun, Cozumel, and Jamaica. With a few weeks to kill before my annual trip to Japan, I figured, why not? Let's do it.

We boarded a Carnival cruise ship with 1,400 passengers. It was my first time on a cruise, and I couldn't believe it — it felt more like a floating hotel than a boat. There was a pool, hot tubs, lounges, a gym, and food everywhere. Buffets, restaurants, late-night snacks — whatever you wanted, whenever you wanted it. Days could be spent by the pool, playing games, or soaking in the ocean views. Nights brought live music, bars, dancing, and a packed casino. Whether you wanted to socialize or just chill, the ship had it all — great food, plenty to do, and a new adventure waiting at the next stop.

When we hit Cancun, scuba diving caught my eye, and she was all in. Back then they didn't care much about formal certifications there. The guys advice? "Just don't come up faster than your air bubbles, and you'll be fine." That was good enough for me. We went for it.

The moment I dropped beneath the surface, it was like stepping into another world. The water off Cozumel was crystal clear, and the reef below was alive, bursting with color and movement. Schools of fish darted past in flashes of blue, yellow, and orange, like something out of a dream. A sea turtle cruised by effortlessly, and for a second, I felt like I was gliding alongside it — just two creatures flowing with the current in this surreal, weightless world.

Beside me, she reached out, eyes wide with excitement. We kicked forward, weaving through stunning coral heads and sponges. A big manta ray glided beneath us, smooth and controlled — like a perfect powder turn in the backcountry. That's when it hit me — this was another kind of ride. No board, no wheels, just pure freedom.

When we surfaced, we pulled off our masks, laughing, the warm ocean air hitting our faces. She looked at me, still buzzing from the rush. I got it. This wasn't just a dive. It was an experience we shared, and it was a damn good one.

Afterward, we grabbed some food on the island, and soon it was back to the ship and off to our next stop, Cozumel.

Once in Cozumel, I rented us a Jeep. We were determined to find a private beach for just the two of us. A ways out from town, I spotted a dirt road that looked promising, but as we got closer to the water, the Jeep sank deep into the sand. No problem, I thought — I'd throw it into four-wheel drive. Except…there was no four-wheel drive. The system had been disconnected. Guess they didn't want people actually off-roading, but I didn't get the memo. Now we were stuck.

Instead of enjoying our own private beach, I was on my hands and knees, digging the Jeep out. I scavenged tree branches and leaves for traction, sweating like crazy in the sun. After over an hour of frustration and effort, I finally got the Jeep back to where it had enough grip to get us moving again. We headed back to the roads that would take us into town. I was hot, exhausted, and in a terrible mood — but that changed fast once we got there.

We found a bar that was absolutely raging. Back then, Long Island iced teas were my go-to if I was drinking, and I knocked back a few like they were water. After all that digging, I was wiped out and thirsty, and those drinks hit fast. Before long, "Evil Z," my drunken alter ego, made his appearance.

Next thing I knew, I was on stage in a beer-chugging contest. Three of us lined up with one-foot-tall, skinny glasses of beer, ready to go.

3–2–1, go!

I threw it back faster than the others, slammed my tall empty glass on the table, and threw my arms up in victory as the crowd cheered. Just like that, the whole Jeep fiasco faded into a hazy memory. We were having a blast, raging in town, and living it up.

Before long, the cruise ship blasted its horn — a signal to start loading up onto the boat from the shore. Time to start moving towards our next destination: Jamaica.

Back on board, my girl handed me a drink with a pineapple and a little umbrella. One drink led to another, and somehow, I found myself in a hula hoop contest. Let's just say I didn't win. Later that night, we took a romantic walk to the front of the ship. It was straight out of Titanic — except without Leonardo DiCaprio. We kissed under the stars, the ocean breeze, views and our interactions were all making it feel surreal.

Then my adrenaline kicked in.

I spotted a handrail leading from one deck to the next level down where we were headed. Naturally, I decided to sit-slide down it. Problem was, I was at a 0.22% blood alcohol level. I lost my balance and flipped backward over the rail, falling 15 feet, headfirst, onto the deck below.

I don't remember much after that. What I do know, I pieced together later from what she told me. I hit the lower deck so hard my head made a splat sound, leaving a blood pool bigger than a trash can lid.

The impact broke my nose, fractured my cheekbone and cracked the skull beneath my forehead. Blood was everywhere. We were an hour and a half out to sea, and the crew turned the entire 1,400-passenger ship around back to Cozumel, delaying its journey to Jamaica. A Learjet flew in from Texas to pick us up and get me to a hospital with the tech needed to check my condition properly.

In Cozumel, they couldn't confirm if my skull's brain sac was ruptured without advanced imaging, so I had to undergo a full scan with the higher-tech equipment in Texas. Miraculously, I survived — unlike my younger snowboard teammate Jeff Anderson (RIP 🙏), who tragically lost his life at just 23 from a similar handrail fall 10 years later. Jeff was more than a teammate — he was family to many of us in snowboarding, with a style and energy that inspired everyone around him. His brother Billy created the JLA Banked Slalom at Mammoth in Jeff's honor, a tradition that still runs strong, keeping his spirit alive on the mountain. My girl never left my side, filling in the blanks of everything that happened that I couldn't remember.

We never made it to Jamaica, but somehow, I walked away from something that should've killed me.

Two weeks after the cruise ship disaster, I was back in Japan doing snowboard jump demonstrations for Japanese audiences and snowboard fans. Every time I landed a trick, I could feel the cracks in my skull shift. The pain was intense, but I was in my early 20s and I thought I was invincible. I just kept riding and pushed through the pain, not even thinking about the potentially bad consequences that could have happened.

Japanese kids pointed at my black-and-blue eyes.

"What happened, Szabo?"

Depending on how much English they knew — or how much time I had — I'd either give them some of the story or just say:

"I went boom."

Or —

"I went splat before I got here."

Either way, I was lucky. Lucky to ride again. Lucky to heal. Lucky to still be here.

Other Times in Japan

In the early 1990s, traveling with some of the Lamar Snowboards teammates in Japan was always a mix of cultural discoveries and wild memories. If the name Lamar sounds familiar, that's because Bert Lamar — an old skateboard friend from SkaterCross and the skatepark days back in the late '70s and early '80s — had launched his own line of snowboards after a few years as a pro snowboarder himself. That connection made it extra cool when I started riding for Lamar. It wasn't just another brand — it was a friend offering me a deal that was too good to pass up. So I joined the Lamar team and had a great time riding for them for a few years.

One of the standout memories was from a trip to Japan with a few of the Lamar riders. John Cardiel was with us — one of the most radical skateboarders of the time and also a solid snowboarder. He was pure fire — raw energy and fearless. On our first day in the city of Tokyo, we were getting ready to cross a street, and Cardiel stepped off the curb, still thinking like he was back in the States. In Japan, cars drive on the opposite side, so instead of looking right, he looked left. All of a sudden — boom — a car clipped him from the right. He flew over the hood, launched off the back, and his shoes literally flew off mid-cartwheel as he flipped over the car.

Miraculously, he got up laughing, totally fine. Once we saw he wasn't hurt, we all lost it — cracking up with him. That was Cardiel for you — unstoppable.

Another hilarious memory was riding Japan's train system. Their trains are next-level — quiet, clean, and incredibly efficient. But us? We were a different story. A few of us had picked up these realistic-looking BB guns from a shop we came across earlier. They were solid black, looked totally legit, and fired little plastic pellets. Naturally, we turned the train into our battlefield.

We were ducking behind seats, popping up and firing across aisles, laughing like little kids with way too much energy. BB pellets were flying back and forth as we staged these mock gunfights, completely oblivious to how insane we must've looked. The Japanese passengers, calm and composed as always, sat quietly in their seats — wide-eyed but totally silent — probably stunned that a crew of foreign snowboarders had just turned their peaceful train ride into a low-budget action movie.

Looking back, it was ridiculous, totally inappropriate, but it still cracks me up. That was us — young, wild, and in Japan, making memories the only way we knew how.

A Night Out in Tokyo: Sliding Into Chaos

I remember one epic night in Tokyo with my friend and Pro Snowboarder teammate, Sean Johnson.

One evening, we ventured out, bar hopping in Roppongi, a lively district in Tokyo, when we unexpectedly crossed paths with Pat Ngoho, an old pro skateboarder I used to skate with occasionally during my skateboarding days in the 1980s. We decided to raise the stakes of the night by taking a shot of absinthe — the notorious liquor known for its hallucinogenic edge. Already a few drinks in, the absinthe kicked our buzz into overdrive, setting the tone for the chaos that followed.

Sean, known for his wild side, later made a series of videos in the 1990s called *Whiskey*. A running theme was trying to break beer bottles over your own head — Sean did it, and plenty of drunk friends tried too. Sometimes the bottles shattered, other times they just bounced with a loud clunk, leaving a pounding headache and leaving the viewers with some laughs. Fights and stunts kept the chaos rolling, and one wild moment had Sean riding a motorcycle through two grocery stores in a clown suit as Boozy The Clown — pure chaos and entertainment at its finest. The *Whiskey* videos captured it all — like *Jackass* before *Jackass* — and maybe even sparked ideas for my friend Dave England. After all, he's the man who threw himself into the Fire Hose Rodeo in *Jackass #2* in 2006, more than 10 years later, classic friends of mine...

As we spilled onto the bustling streets, the energy around us felt electric. That's when inspiration hit: The Dukes of Hazzard. The crowded streets and stationary cars stuck in traffic became our playground. Like Bo and Luke Duke, we slid across car hoods, shouting "Yeehaw!" and laughing hysterically. The cars we slid across were stuck bumper to bumper. Some drivers were fuming — honking their horns, shaking their fists, and yelling things in Japanese that we didn't understand. But we didn't care. We were having an absolute blast.

Later that night, we casually walked into a liquor store, grabbed six-packs of beer, and strolled out without paying. The store attendant just watched us, and whether he called the police or not, we'll never know. Back at the hotel, we shared the stolen beers and swapped stories with the rest of the team, recounting our car-sliding antics and laughing until we went to sleep for the night.

I know some of these stories involve drinking. The truth is, I've never been a heavy drinker — but somehow, the times I should remember the least ended up being the most impactful and memorable. They still pop into my mind to this day, and I've told them so many times over the years that they're easy to recall.

Riding Forbidden Powder in Hokkaido: Breaking the Rules for the Perfect Run

Japan's northernmost island of Hokkaido is home to some of the best snow on the planet. The weather patterns there create an unreal snow quality that rivals anything in the world.

The mountains of Hokkaido are more than just a playground — they're deep with culture, natural beauty, and a touch of mystery. Resorts carefully rope off areas, citing avalanche dangers or the challenges of patrolling the forests where skiers can easily lose their way. But beyond the practical reasons, there's also a deeper, more spiritual belief at play. Local superstition suggests these closures honor the tree spirits, allowing them to dance undisturbed among the snow-covered branches. It's a beautiful sentiment — but for us snowboarding Americans, those untouched lines of pristine powder were impossible to resist, boundaries or not.

Those roped-off areas were like treasure chests waiting to be opened.

While most riders in Japan played by the rules, my crew and I were the complete opposite. Perfect, untouched powder lay just beyond the ropes, and there was no way we were leaving it untracked. We ducked ropes, explored tree lines, and floated through pristine snow pillows in what we called "the magic forest." These runs were legendary — even if they were technically illegal.

Sometimes we'd find ourselves riding a powder line right below a bunch of chairlifts filled with mostly Japanese skiers and very few snowboarders. In the U.S., riders on chairlifts would cheer loudly for anyone throwing down an epic powder run under the lift. But in Japan, the silence was deafening. The skiers looked down at us with what I assumed was disapproval — though maybe, just maybe, a few of them were silently stoked for us.

Despite the lack of audible encouragement, we were ecstatic. The snow was flawless, the turns perfect, and the stoke undeniable. We yelled out in excitement, breaking the silence with our energy. These runs weren't captured on film — this was the pre-smartphone era, and we were just out riding for the pure fun of it. No footage. No followers. Just perfect powder and lifelong memories. Japan and Hokkaido hit different — and it still does to this day.

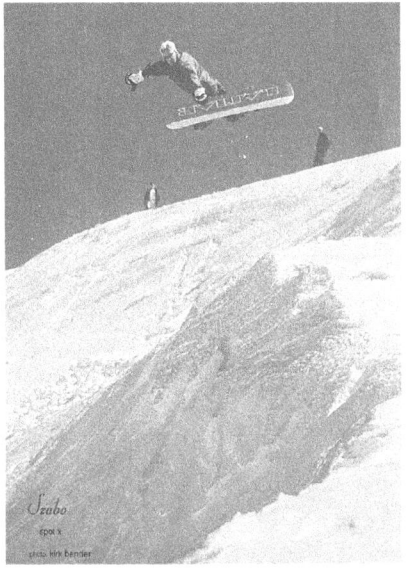

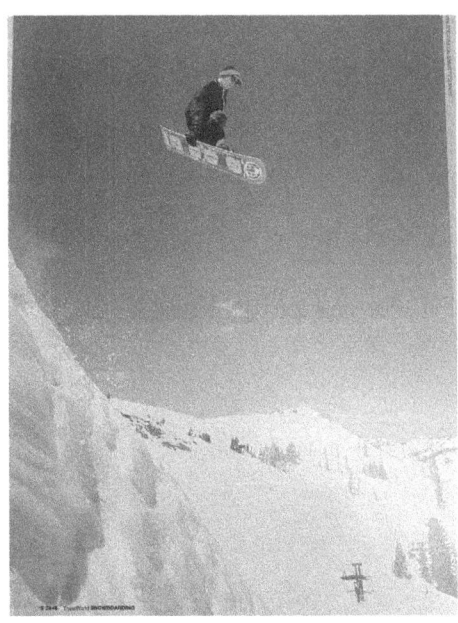

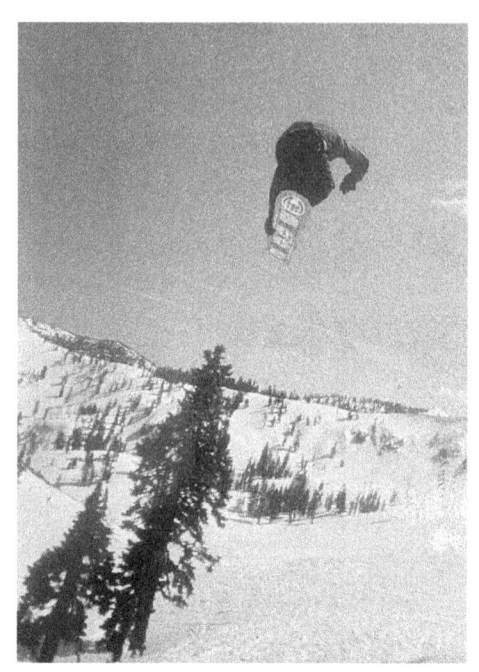

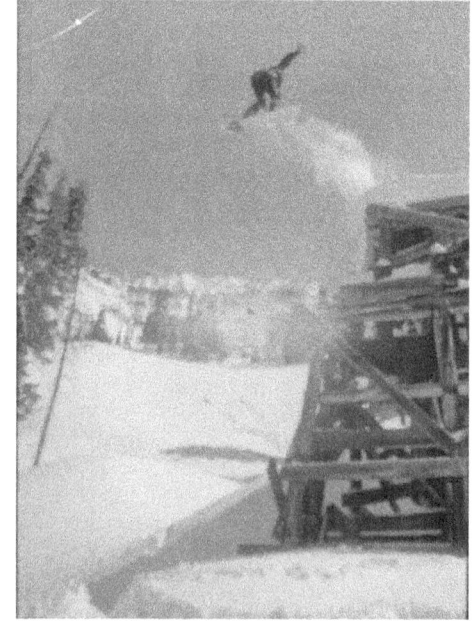

Chapter 7

Creatures of Habit

When you're pushing your limits — whether it's a massive jump, a technical line, or a feature just beyond your comfort zone — your mindset is everything. You need confidence, vision, and the ability to commit fully. That was the case on a helicopter trip with Wasatch Powder Guides in Utah, where I faced a cliff drop that would become a proud moment in snowboarding.

On this particular run, I was riding with Dana Nicholson and Martin Gallant. We were fired up — riding fresh, untouched snow, getting footage, grabbing photos, and just having a killer day in the mountains. We were filming with Jon Freeman for Creatures of Habit 5, stacking clips and pushing ourselves all the way down the mountain.

Eventually, we reached the lower part of the run where a cliff feature stood out. The elevation had dropped, and with the slightly higher temps, conditions were getting sketchy. Long icicles were hanging from the cliffside, and the snow wasn't as good as it had been at the higher elevation of the run. The other guys started eyeing it as a *double step-down* — thinking they could land on a lower shelf first, then drop the rest of the way to the base of the cliff.

Dana went first. He sent it off the cliff to that lower shelf — but it was solid ice. It threw him off balance and made him land on his back in the soft snow at the bottom.

Then Martin gave it a shot. He kind of made the double step-down work, but it didn't go that smooth. That shelf was a trap, and the line just wasn't working very well.

After watching both of them, I knew it was time for a different approach. I scoped the cliff from a new angle and saw another option — skip the lower shelf completely and send the entire thing in one shot. It was a big drop, and the landing wouldn't be easy, but if I committed to it properly, I knew I could make it happen.

I hiked back up above the cliff drop. From that higher vantage point, you couldn't see the landing — just the edge of the cliff. It was a *blind drop* like most cliffs are, but the line was crystal clear in my mind, and the visualization was locked in.

I yelled to the crew, "Outta the way, boys! Let me show you how it's done."

With full commitment, I launched off the edge, soaring about 50 feet down and out, straight to the bottom. Landed solid, rode it out, and that was it. No hesitation. No second thoughts. Just a confident send.

Photographer John Kelly got a killer shot of the cliff drop. Jon Freeman captured the whole thing on 16mm film, and the footage ended up in Creatures 5 — good music, high energy, and the drop edited in with other solid clips, just the way those Creatures of Habit videos always hit.

That moment reminded me how crucial mindset is in action sports. Without confidence — the ability to see new lines and push past the fear — it just doesn't happen. But when you've got the skill, the vision, and the will to make it happen, you can turn something that seems impossible into another proud moment in sports. Good snow on a helicopter-access day, pushing limits with your crew, and making memories that last a lifetime, this was one of those days.

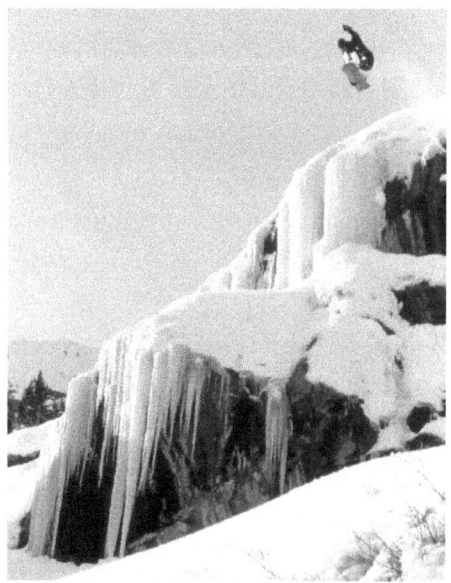

Proud moment in sports — photo by John Kelly

Double O Szabo Origins

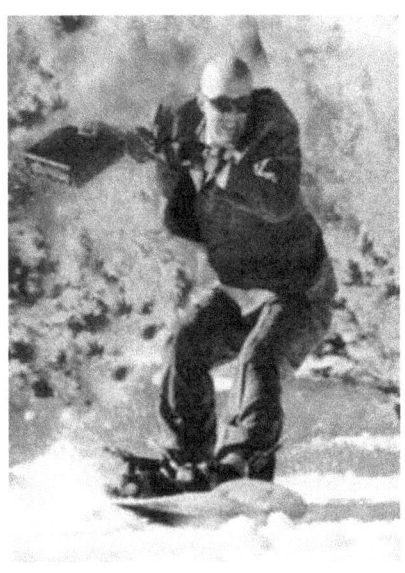

Double O going through fire

For a handful of years in the early '90s, I spent a lot of time filming with Jon Freeman. He had already released Creatures of Habit 1, the first in his six-part snowboarding video series — a wild mix of action, humor, cutting-edge music, and great riding. After seeing it, I was all-in when he invited me to film for Creatures of Habit 2 the following season.

Those next few years were packed with incredible times and trips, riding alongside close pro snowboard friends like Damian Sanders, Dana Nicholson, Steve Graham, and meeting up with legendary riders like Mike and Tina Basich, Andy Hetzel, Matty Goodman, Brett Johnson, Tom Burt, Shawn Farmer, Nick Perata, and countless others. We traveled across states and sometimes countries, stacking footage, pushing limits, and throwing in ridiculous skits just for laughs.

By the time we got to Creatures 3: Demented Chowder Pilots and Creatures 4: Plastic Soldiers, we were going *full send* on the entertainment side, on top of high-performance snowboarding in epic locations. Both films ended with eight-minute mini-movies called Double O Szabo.

They were James Bond-style, over-the-top, low-budget action skits mixed with snowboarding chaos and classic humor. I played a slick secret agent — Double O Szabo — armed with a snowboard rigged with gadgets while effortlessly pulling off wild stunts on the mission.

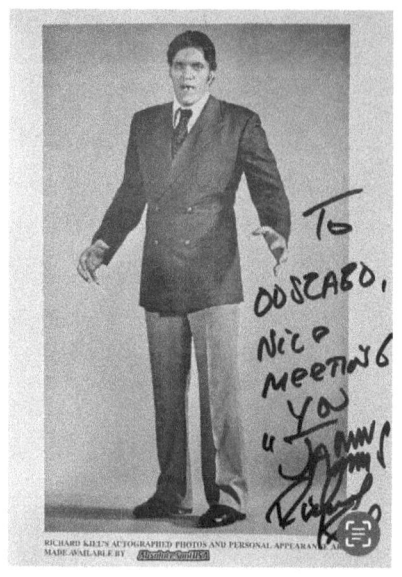

OG Bond villain Jaws, signed to Double O Szabo

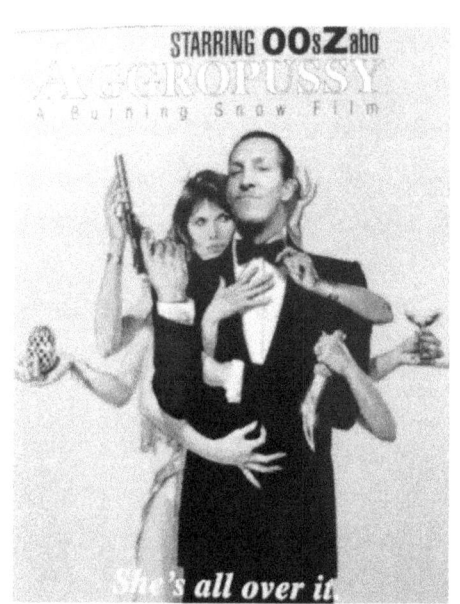

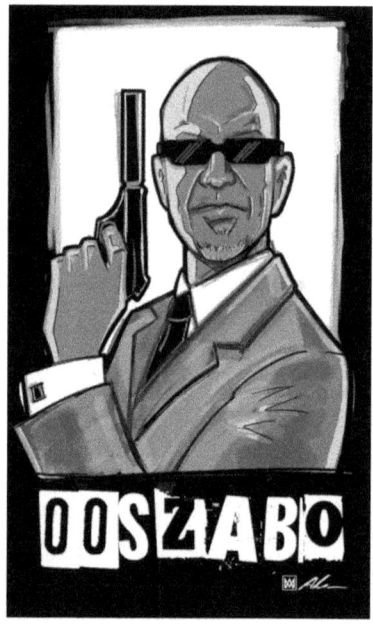

Double O ad (L) and logo (R) drawn by Adam Mock

Brett Johnson played Q, the mad scientist behind all the absurd spy tech in the laboratory. He hooked me up with everything from a snowboard with rockets and a smokescreen to hand grenades, throwing stars, and a few other gadgets. It was pure entertainment value, with some legit action built into these classic, ridiculous skits.

In one scene in the lab, Q introduced the "proctological decimator" — a modified toilet with 30,000 pounds of anal thrust — that he explained with full dramatic flair. We put on goofy eyewear protection and demonstrated how it blew up a dummy sitting on it. "A bit more abrupt than your standard enema," I would say. Then we moved through the lab to the next gadget demo for items that would help with the Double O Szabo outdoor snow action mission that was coming up.

He also debuted the Hookah Bazooka — a "deadly" device demonstrated by a lab worker taking a bong hit, then putting the modified bong weapon over his shoulder and blasting a dummy's head clean off from across the lab. It was a classic scene.

Brett absolutely deserved an action sports acting Emmy for his performance. He transformed into Q with hilarious commitment and delivered every line like a pro. I didn't know he had those acting skills in him, and it still cracks me up to this day.

Another classic scene in the lab was when I walked by and reached for what looked like a bowl of breath mints. Brett stopped me — straight-faced, completely in character — and said, "This little apre' meal sweet is an oral intake, internally processed nitro-combustible gastrointestinal propellant. In laymen's terms, a fart pellet." Then he added casually, "Take a couple, Double O — they might come in handy." And they did. Later, I popped one of these so-called "breath mints," and flames shot out of my butt, giving me extra speed on my snow-sliding device while dealing with the bad guys. It was a classic scene...

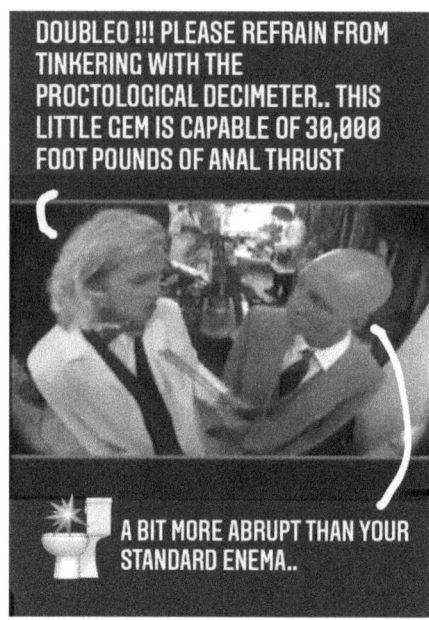

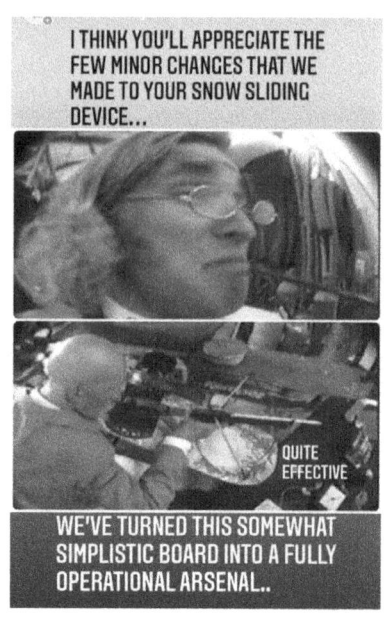

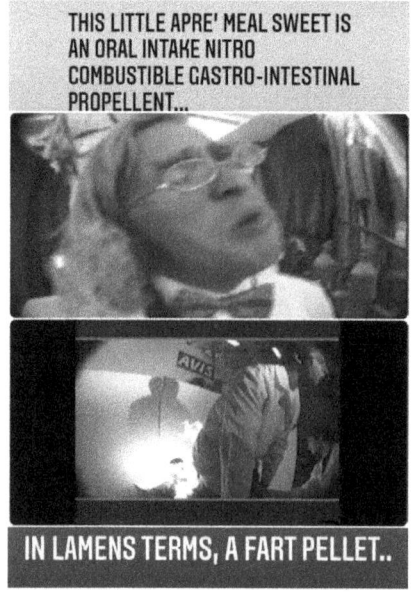

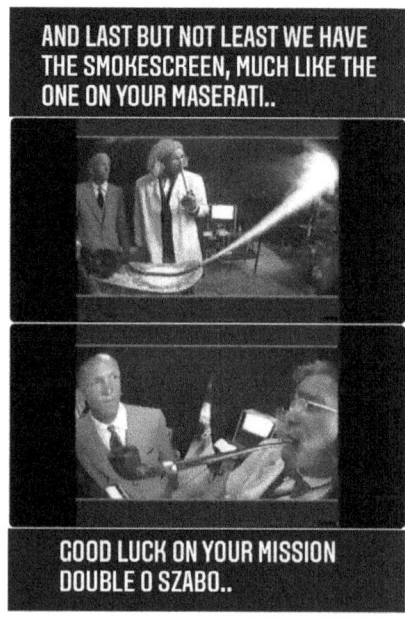

Freeman and I actually came up with the idea for Double O Szabo on a flight back from a snowboard trip to Alaska. We had just started talking about some basic skit ideas when the plane began its evening descent into Los Angeles. As we looked out the window, we saw multiple fires burning across the city. The Rodney King riots had erupted while we were gone, and L.A. was in full-blown chaos. The civil unrest had exploded after the shocking decision to let the four LAPD officers go free — even though they had been caught on video brutally beating Rodney King.

That verdict lit a fuse. The protests escalated into six straight days of riots — more than 60 people were killed, thousands were injured, and large sections of the city were overwhelmed with looting, fires, and clashes with police. Damages were estimated at over $1 billion.

Seeing those flames from the plane window was surreal. It felt like we were flying into a war zone. But thankfully, we made it home safely. Freeman didn't waste any time. He ran with the Double O concept we'd talked about on the flight, brought in Brett Johnson for his classic role as Q, lined up snowmobiles with our friend Bronco for chase scenes and backcountry access, and hired a special effects crew for explosions, gunfire, blood squibs, and bullet-hit effects in the snow.

We filmed most of the snow scenes late-season in the Mammoth back-country — one of our favorite zones where we could get away with that kind of mayhem, blow stuff up, and catch things on fire.. Snowmobiles and modified ATVs on snow became chase vehicles for the bad guys. We had a solid cast of villains, including Dana as the main bad guy, and even Freeman himself got in front of the camera, showing up as a nun-chuck warrior that I shot in the head with a bow and arrow — one of the weapons Q had modified onto my Snow Sliding Device.

The explosions and antics got even more ridiculous the next year in Double O Szabo #2. In one chase scene, Dana — totally in character — was stealing a snowmobile to continue chasing me. In the process, he accidentally cracked our friend Chris Drake in the head with the butt of his rifle. Knocked him silly for a minute. Total accident, but the commitment was real.

One of the wildest stunts Freeman came up with was in Double O Szabo #2. In a bar scene, after the action kicked off, tensions escalated and heavy bad-guy gunfire broke out. Q and I took cover behind the bar as all the alcohol bottles above and behind us got blasted. We quickly went over the next part of my mission — now that I had the blueprints showing the location of plutonium transport and production in North Korea — plans I had to get to the commander to help save the world. No big deal.

Then, Q pulled a hidden lever, triggering a secret dartboard exit for me to get out of the bar and move forward with the snow part of the mission. I returned fire, dropped a couple of bad guys, ran across the pool table, and dove headfirst through the dartboard escape route.

It cut to a shot of me sliding through a McDonald's kids' playground tube as the getaway tunnel. From there, it cut to me flipping off a wall at Zuma Beach — like I was launching out of the tunnel — then landing straight into my snowboard bindings in Mammoth. The bindings snapped shut around my feet in futuristic style, and I was off into the next part of the mission.

Freeman's vision and editing made it feel like one seamless escape — but the real magic was stitching together four totally different locations into one fast-paced, impossible getaway. It came together like a full-throttle spy chase movie that somehow made total sense.

Helicopter Crash

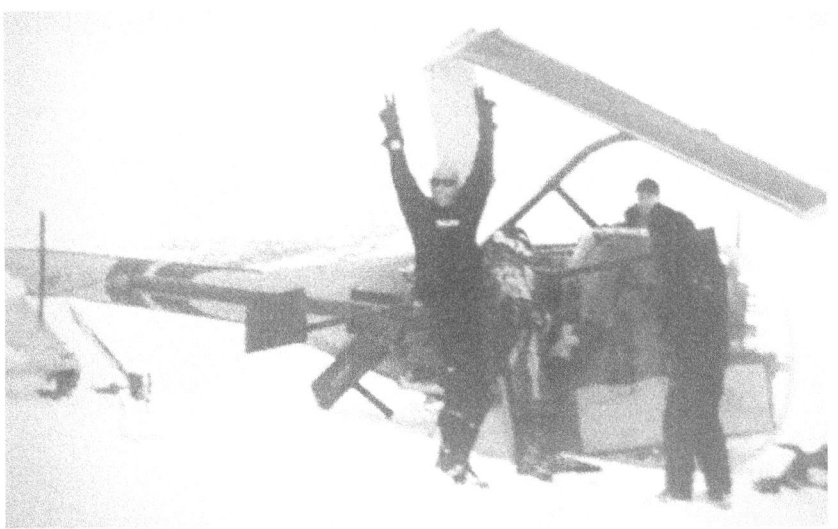

Not the landing they planned

Filming Double O Szabo was usually about the crew having fun with the skit, but one time it ended up in a seriously crazy situation. This happened the next year in Alaska while we were getting footage for Creatures of Habit 4. For a few years in a row, we'd head up to Valdez, Alaska, usually in April when the conditions were best for great snow and getting some blue sky days. We were riding and filming heli-accessed backcountry, working with Chet, our go-to helicopter pilot. Chet was solid — he'd take us wherever we wanted to go in the endless snowboarding zones of Valdez.

We did some first descents — meaning we rode our snowboards down mountain zones that hadn't been ridden down before — thanks to the relationship we'd built with our pilot, Chet, over the years. We pushed the limits of what we could get away with in the heli-ski world, but Chet trusted us, and we trusted him. Sometimes he'd just hover over a drop-off point, and we'd have to jump straight out of the helicopter to the snow below. Other times, he'd fire his gun from the helicopter into the snowpack where we planned to land, just to test for avalanche danger. Definitely not standard helicopter pilot protocol — but that was Chet. He was a badass, and we had some great times, doing things way outside the normal playbook — but man, it led to some epic stuff.

He'd thread us through tight snow canyons, banking the chopper back and forth at 45-degree angles as we swooped through them. We also got unreal views of the mountains as we flew to our next peak drop-off location. One minute, we'd be flying 20 feet above the snow, following the terrain and then suddenly, the mountain would drop off and we'd be thousands of feet in the air with nothing but open space below us heading to the next peak to ride. It was the closest thing to flying like a bird — it was absolutely unreal.

One evening at a restaurant bar, Jon Freeman ran into a local guy who had a helicopter. It looked like one of those old-school bubble copters from the early James Bond movies — the same type of chopper that Freeman had already used in a few clips for Double O Szabo #2 that we had already filmed for, that he would drop in his next video. Perfect. The universe was lining things up for us. Freeman could picture a few close-up shots with Dana and this chopper that he could splice into a scene we'd previously filmed to add more depth to the skit.

After another great, long day of filming with Chet and the boys in the Valdez peaks, Matty Goodman and I were supposed to pick up Freeman and Dana on the side of the highway after they got the footage they needed with the old-school helicopter.

Freeman and Dana — who was playing the main bad guy — decided to film a scene where Dana would shoot a rifle from the helicopter, aiming down at me for that classic action-movie gunshot effect. Except, here's the kicker — Dana was firing live ammo from his rifle. And Freeman? He was on the ground, filming real bullets flying near him to get the perfect shot from what would be my perspective, looking up at the chopper with bad guy Dana shooting down at me. That's one way to commit to a scene, that's for sure.

We saw them off in the distance shooting this stuff, but we weren't really paying close attention since it was happening about a mile from the main highway. Matty and I were just hanging out — talking, listening to music, and figuring they'd be done soon so we could head back to town, gear down, shower up, and grab food.

But time kept passing, and still no sign of the chopper. We figured they were just getting extra artsy — probably flying over another ridge to get more shots. Eventually, we just said screw it. Let them hitchhike back or catch a ride with the pilot — they'd figure it out.

We headed back to town, cleaned up, ate, and were just relaxing in the hotel room a couple of hours later when suddenly Dana and Freeman busted in — wide-eyed and out of breath.

"Where'd you guys go?! We crashed the helicopter!"

Wait...what?! No way!

Turns out, while Dana and the pilot were about 50 feet above the snow filming Dana's shots, the old-school helicopter's motor locked up. They dropped straight down onto the snow. Thankfully, they both just got the wind knocked out of them. After catching their breath, they quickly linked back up with Freeman — who had been filming from the ground not far from where they crashed.

The three of them had to work their way out of the zone they were in, about a mile from the road, through deep snow. It wasn't easy, but eventually they managed to hitchhike back into town.

Meanwhile, Matty and I were totally clueless. We figured they were still filming somewhere off in the distance, probably taking their sweet time with another shot. We had no idea they'd just survived a full-on helicopter crash.

Looking back, it's wild to think that earlier that same day, we were thousands of feet up riding insane lines from Chet's helicopter — and a few hours later, Dana and the pilot dropped out of the sky in another chopper. Luckily, they were only 50 feet up and hovering over a soft snowfield — not over rocks or high enough to make it deadly. There was even fuel leaking everywhere, but it didn't catch fire. It could've been tragic. Instead, it just became another wild behind-the-scenes moment from a Double O Szabo skit.

The Cliff Dummy Stunt

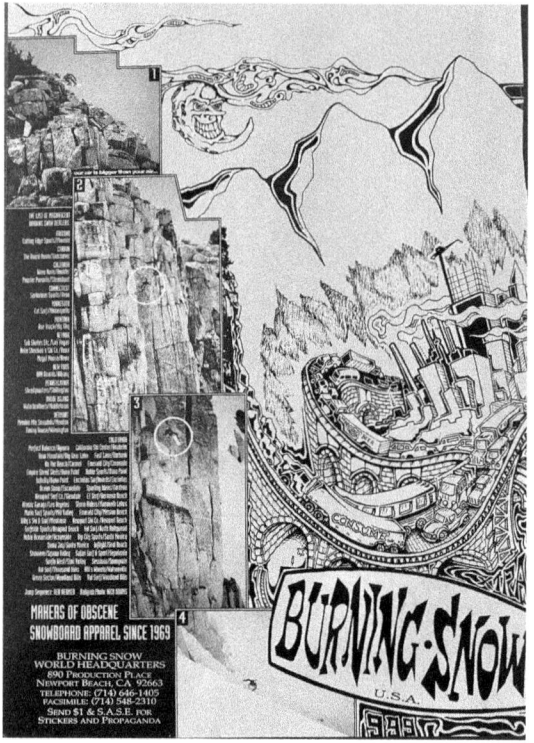

The dummy sent the 200 footer. I almost did too.

In snowboarding, when you're pushing your limits, sometimes you end up being the test dummy — whether you like it or not. The first time hitting a big jump or a cliff drop is a mix of trying to calculate the speed and trajectory needed while making sure the landing won't rearrange your skeleton. It's all part of the game.

But this time, for a Creatures of Habit video, we flipped the script. Instead of being the test dummy, we decided to make one — for a short skit that would go down in snowboard history as one of the most ridiculous, hilarious, and sketchy stunts we ever pulled off.

It was late season at Mammoth, and the plan was simple: strap a dummy onto a snowboard and launch it off a 200-foot cliff for the perfect long-shot drop. A full commitment to chaos — just to see how it would all play out.

A crew of about ten of us — Matty Goodman, Steve Graham, Dana Nicholson, Tom Burt, and some local Mammoth friends — made the grueling hike up into the backcountry to bring this absurd idea to life. Jon Freeman was behind the camera, ready to capture whatever magic or mayhem was about to go down.

This wasn't some Hollywood production with careful planning, rehearsals, or safety measures. No, this was raw, real-deal snowboard skit filmmaking, where we just winged it and figured things out as we went. That's what made it so damn fun — waiting to see how it would all come together in the end.

The idea was to film me riding toward the cliff — then cut to the money shot: a wide shot from a distance showing the dummy making the insane drop. I'd be wearing the same gear and riding the same board at the top and bottom of the cliff to sell the illusion. It was late in the season, but there was enough snow to make it happen. We made sure the snow led all the way to the edge so the dummy could launch clean off the lip.

Freeman set up his shot at the top, pointed the camera at me, and said:

"Are you going big?"

Without hesitation, I pulled down my ski mask at the edge of this monstrous drop and said:

"I'm going big — last cigarette, boys."

That was the cue.

Except…there was one small problem.

The snowboard that was donated for this skit was a beast — a massive 180cm plank that felt like a non-maneuverable missile strapped to my feet. That alone made it awkward as hell to control. But the bigger issue was the snow track itself.

The track led straight to the edge. No room to turn, slow down, or stop. The moment I hopped sideways to get the drop-in shot, the board locked in — and suddenly I was tracking directly toward the cliff. I couldn't steer that beast, and the snow conditions didn't help the situation either.

This was supposed to be a dummy stunt, but in the blink of an eye, it nearly became my final stunt.

I had zero options. The board was too big to maneuver, tracking straight toward the edge, and that drop was coming up fast. There was no turning the board — no bailing out gracefully. If I went off that cliff, I wouldn't be here to tell this story.

In a split-second self-preservation move, I made myself fall over on purpose, stopping just in time before I would've launched off the cliff to my death.

I came to a dead stop, heart pounding, staring at the edge just a few feet from where I laid it over.

Instant reality check: this skit was supposed to be funny — but that almost turned tragic.

I laid there for a second, letting my brain catch up with what just happened. Then I got up, laughed it off, and brushed the snow off like nothing happened.

Let's get back to work.

With my near-death moment out of the way, it was time for the dummy to do its job.

We strapped it into that same death-trap board and sent it down the snow track. It launched clean off the cliff in perfect riding form. Freeman nailed the long shot as the dummy soared through the air, doing a 160-foot double front flip with the board angled just like a real rider going full-send. It was a beautiful disaster in motion.

Then — another disaster struck.

Instead of clearing all the way to the bottom, the dummy got hung up on a rock ledge about 40 feet above the runout, stuck high on the cliff face.

Now we had a problem.

We needed the dummy to finish the drop, but climbing up that sheer cliff face? Not happening.

That's when Tom Burt stepped in.

Besides being a legendary big-mountain snowboarder, Tom was also an expert rock climber. Once we made it to the base of the cliff, he took one look at the situation, shrugged, and said, "I can get up there." Then he just started scaling the rock wall like it was another day at the office.

Within minutes, Tom made it to the ledge, grabbed the dummy, and coordinated with Freeman to stay out of the shot. Then he pushed it off, finishing the part of the stunt that hadn't been completed — until now.

Freeman captured the final drop as the dummy dropped the remaining distance, landed in a clean layback position, and slid effortlessly down the snow, closing out this ridiculous stunt in legendary fashion.

Now came the finishing touch.

I threw on the dummy mask, the jumpsuit, and strapped into the big board at the bottom of the cliff.

Mimicking the dummy's final pose, I laid back just like it had, sliding in perfect sync with the same form and style.

Then I pulled myself up from the layback position to stand up while riding and cruised into a circle of cheering friends. I pointed back up at the cliff and shouted:

"Did you see me stick it on that lower shelf?!"

The reaction was priceless — laughter, disbelief, total mayhem after a chaotic stunt that almost didn't happen.

Freeman had every angle dialed. With some slick editing — speeding up the dialogue, slowing down the action — when the video came out, people lost their minds.

Some thought it was real. I had people ask me how the hell I managed to land a 200-foot cliff drop.

Especially with a 160-foot double front flip and a smooth layback landing off that lower shelf, all cut to the right music to keep the energy high — slow-mo on the huge drop just cranked up the insanity.

Some were convinced I actually pulled off that monster stunt.

Sometimes, just for fun, I'd say, "I have Jedi-level skills."

Then I'd let them in on the joke that it was just a dummy stunt — but it led to some classic stories and conversations from back in those awesome snowboard days.

We were just a bunch of snowboarders with no budget, no safety measures, and no regard for common sense — but we pulled off a classic piece of snowboard skit history.

The thought of almost accidentally sending myself off that cliff? Yeah, that was sketchy.

But the memory of that dummy skit? It still makes me laugh every time I think about it. I've watched it online since then — a reminder of that ridiculous, chaotic, and legendary day in the Mammoth backcountry, when we almost lost the dummy...and we almost lost me.

-Chapter 8-
Moto KillZ Snow

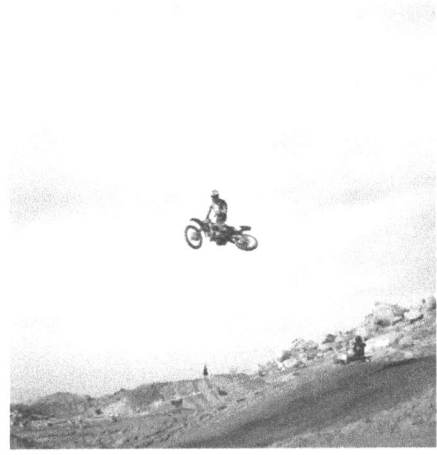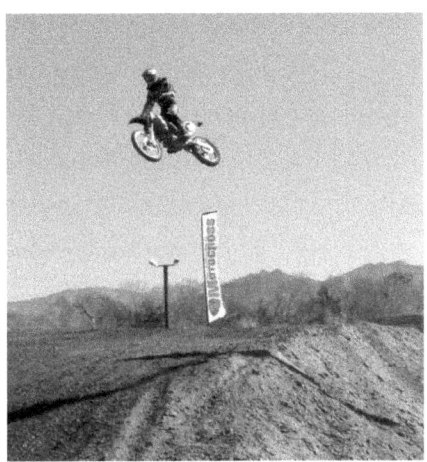

Mid-flight at Perris and Milestone MX

I had already caught the motocross bug, and a guy named Ronnie McCoy put on an event called the Boardercross–Motocross, or BXMX for short. He owned Stormriders Snowboard Shop in Mammoth — a great hardcore snowboard shop, which unfortunately closed its doors with the expansion of the Village in the town of Mammoth. That left Wave Rave as the dominating hardcore board shop in Mammoth, owned by Steve Klassen.

I have countless stories with Steve. Besides being the five-time winner of the Xtreme Verbier Big Mountain Freeriding competition and a two-time King of the Hill champion in Alaska, we've had tons of fun snowboarding together. Later in life, we started taking our kids on adventures together — like the 7-mile ride to Shadow Lake on early e-bikes from his shop, Wave Rave, with our kids in tow. We also went river rafting in Yosemite with our young children. Beautiful day on the water — parking our vehicles a few miles apart for an awesome float down the river, making some great memories, from way after our early days of riding snowboards together.

But there's one time with Steve Klassen that I'll never forget.

He took me bungee jumping out of a hot air balloon that he owned. We drove down near Bishop from Mammoth, tied a 300-foot rope to his vehicle, and went up in his hot air balloon. When I was getting ready to jump, he asked me if I was scared. I said, "No, I've done this in New Zealand off a bridge over a river — it's no problem. Let's do this."

Just as I jumped, he yelled out a very realistic, "Wait!"

As I was dropping 300 feet toward the ground over the desert, my mind started racing. I knew I was clipped into the bungee on my side, but I started wondering, Did he connect the other end to the hot air balloon? I hope so, or I'm done.

When I finally started to recoil and bounce back up toward the balloon I jumped out of, I realized it was just a twisted joke. Steve at his finest.

As I came flying back up toward the balloon, I flipped him off with both hands mid-air and yelled some joking profanity up at him. He slowly lowered the balloon, and once I was back on the ground, I unhooked — experience complete. Steve got me good.

That was a classic joke I'll never forget, from a classic guy I'll never forget.

Funny memory that just popped up. Anyway, back to Ronnie and his family — the McCoys — who had the vision to put in the blood, sweat, and tears to open the first Mammoth chairlift to the public in 1955. Mammoth expanded over the years to include 25 different lifts and became a full-fledged mountain resort, offering people a great experience for both skiing and eventually snowboarding.

Ronnie's event was the perfect mix of snowboarding and motocross, and I couldn't resist jumping in. The format was simple — no judging, no scores based on style or tricks. Just a head-to-head race format in both sports.

Day one was boardercross: a downhill snowboard race against multiple riders on a course packed with jumps, berms, and obstacles. First one through the course and across the finish line wins.

Day two? Same deal, but on dirt bikes. Each rider raced in their class on a motocross track, and just like the snowboard portion, it was all about who crossed the finish line first. Everyone raced in the class of their highest sport — pros had to go pro in both snow and moto. The overall ranking was based on your combined results from both the snowboard and motocross races.

It was a blast racing boardercross, especially considering I was more of a freestyle guy than a racer — but I held my own. The next day, we lined up on the moto course at the legendary Mammoth Motocross track.

It's one of the most iconic spots in the country — carved into the mountains of Mammoth Lakes and known for its high elevation and once-a-year access during the official Mammoth Motocross race.

I'm sure Ronnie pulled some strings to make this separate event happen at that legendary spot — which was amazing! And to make things even crazier? It was snowing!

I remember lining up next to some solid rider friends I knew well, including Mark Gabriel, who was a good snowboarder and had skills on a dirt bike, and Eric Litzenberg — aka Litzy (RIP 🏂) — who also had good snow and dirt skills.

Litzy passed away from testicular cancer. Ironically, he had joined the One Ball Jay club.

An old pro snowboarder friend, Matt Cummins, co-founded the wax and accessory brand "One Ball Jay" in 1986. He named it after his friend Jay, who lost a testicle in a skateboarding accident. The name stuck and became a legendary brand and part of snowboard culture for almost 40 years. Litzy became an unexpected member of the "One Ball Jay" club — but not in the way anyone would ever want. He had a testicle removed after doctors discovered it was cancerous. At first, we all believed he'd caught it in time and just figured he was now in the One Ball Jay club — no big deal. He was hopeful. We were all hopeful.

But cancer has a cruel way of flipping the script. It spread, metastasizing quietly at first, then aggressively, like a wildfire igniting and racing through his body. No matter how hard the doctors tried to contain it, the flames kept rising. Eventually, they couldn't be put out. We lost Litzy to that fire.

I've known a few guys who've ended up in the One Ball Jay club from sport injuries gone wrong. Life has a twisted sense of humor sometimes.

But back to the race…When the gate dropped, I went handlebar to handlebar with Litzy, battling for position.

Everything was covered in snow, except for the brown dirt part of the track where the bikes had already been practicing — and it actually made for amazing traction.

As intense as the racing was, I kept getting distracted. The snowfall was unreal — riding at full speed with the flakes streaking toward my goggles felt like jumping into hyperspace in a Star Wars scene. It made the whole race surreal, and I had to force myself to stay locked in and focus on the track instead of getting lost in the beauty of the moment.

I wasn't winning the motocross event — Some of the pro moto guys had me beat, but because boardercross on snow was my strength in this dual-sport event, my combined score across both races put me in a podium position.

Honestly, it was one of the most fun events I've ever done — the perfect blend of two sports I loved, wrapped into one incredible weekend.

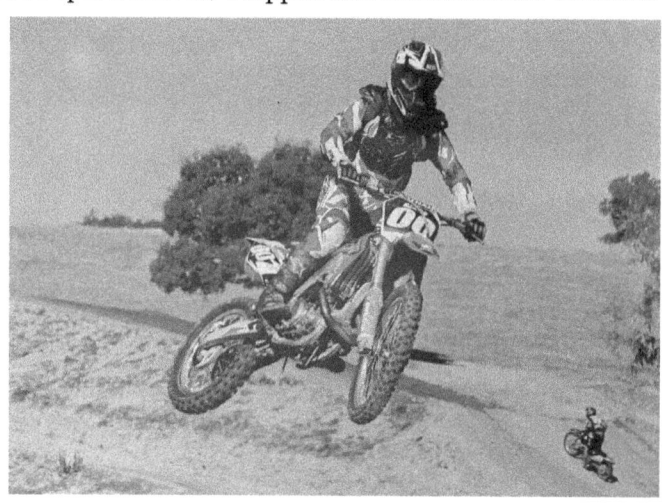

Passing the Torch

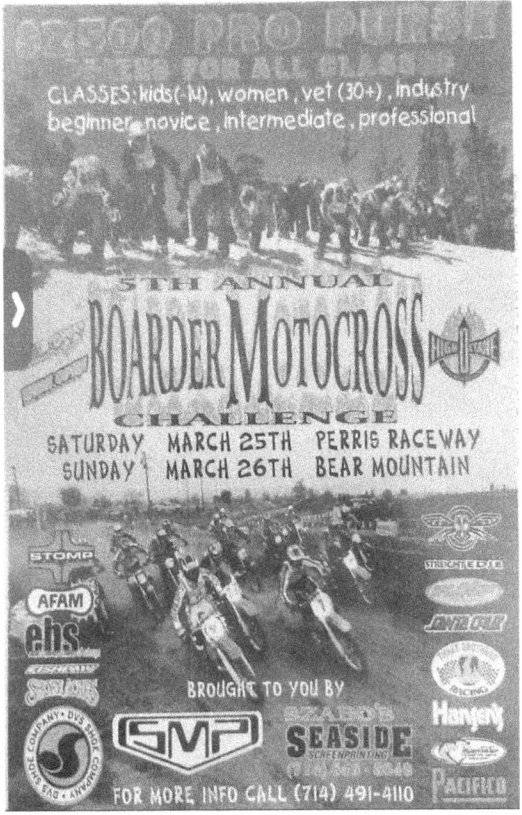

BXMX Flyer — ran it, raced it, six years strong

When the next season rolled around, I called Ronnie McCoy and asked when Boardercross Motocross was happening again.

His response? "I don't have time this year. I'm too busy running my shop Stormriders, and my kids are a handful."

I was stunned. "What?! You have to make it happen! That was the best and most fun event I've ever done, and I was looking forward to it all year."

Then Ronnie hit me with it. "Then YOU put it on."

I laughed. "I guess I'll have to. Someone's gotta do it."

And that's how I ended up running the event for the next six years in Southern California. I set up the snowboard portion at Bear Mountain once, and at Mountain High the other five years. The motocross race was always at Perris Raceway, which was a great track.

Running the BXMX was a ton of work — a good chunk of money up front to secure the venues and insurance, tons of logistics, some promotion, and plenty of nail-biting, wondering if we'd even have enough snow by the time the event rolled around. It ended up being a late snow season event to avoid conflicts with other scheduled events. I ran ads, printed flyers, hustled for sponsors, and every dollar I brought in from the entry fees went straight to the pro prize purse.

My friend Wing Lam, who owned "Wahoo's Fish Tacos," even stepped up and catered the event for free — providing tacos to all the riders. It was a win-win, since after you ate his tacos at the BXMX, you'd definitely end up at his restaurants later craving more.

Luckily, the sponsors stepped up big, throwing in a ton of prizes for all the different levels of classes, so the podium (top 3) riders could enjoy solid rewards for doing well in the competition in all of the divisions.

In total, I was able to race four out of the six years I put it on. But honestly? Organizing the whole thing was brutal. Tracking results, managing scoring, dealing with logistics — it was a grind. But at least with the race-race format, there was no judging bias — you finished where you finished, and that was that. For us, no complaints, no politics — just a great time doing two different great sports together in one unforgettable event.

In the last year that I put on the event, Dusty Walters got tangled up with another rider in the pro division during the motocross race and ended up in a coma for nearly two weeks.

The workload of running the BXMX was already overwhelming on top of all the other things I had going on, and after six years, I decided to call it quits.

Unfortunately, no one else stepped up to take over the event, so when I walked away, BXMX disappeared with me.

Still, I'll always believe it was one of the best crossover sport events. No judging bias, no subjective scoring — just pure adrenaline racing and a simple race-race format, that's it. "You get what you get, and you don't get upset." A lot of people told me how much fun they had doing the event. I know this is true because I had a blast too!

Dirt Killz Snow: The Beginning of the End

My snowboarding career was in a great place. I was doing what I loved — riding, filming, and pushing the limits of the sport. In the earlier years, in the late '80s, competitions were the only way that sponsors recognized value in a snowboarder.

By the 1990s, I had been part of the freeride pioneering era, where we were able to show sponsors that snowboard competitions weren't the only way to promote their brands. Instead of standing on a podium, riders like us proved that magazine shots, video parts, groundbreaking riding, and image-building were just as — if not more — valuable. We made names for ourselves by riding terrain in ways no one had done before. In magazines and videos, we would have memorable images, showcasing the boards and gear and showing product that snowboarders wanted to buy. It was a win-win: we got to ride great stuff, and the companies backing us got authentic, high-impact exposure for their product.

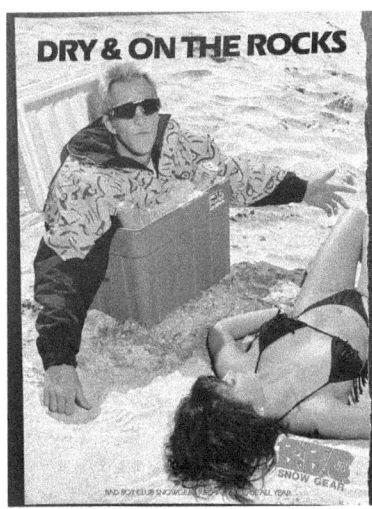
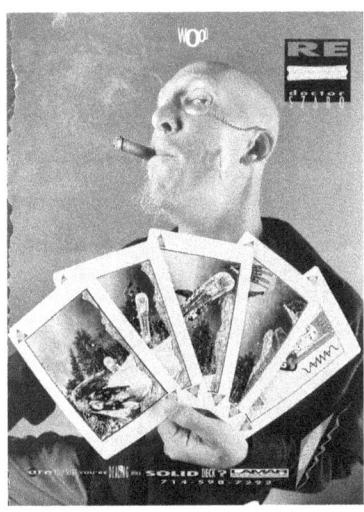

Lifestyle ads, before it was a thing

121

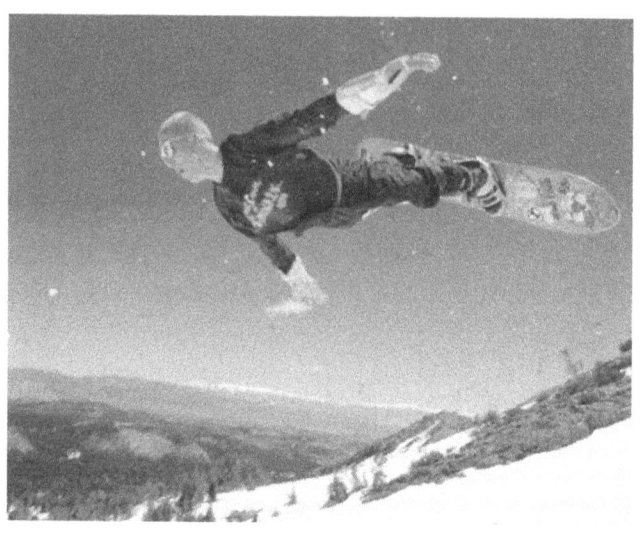

Pilot Z, coming in for a landing

By the mid-'90s, the level of riding was evolving rapidly. Tricks like the cork — which was a backflip with a full twist — were starting to blow up. It was one thing to go upside down, another to spin on your snowboard, but combining flips and spins? That was next-level. These days, watching my friend Marko's kid, Dusty Hendrickson, throw quad corks — four flips with four twists — is mind-blowing. I can't even wrap my head around it. At the time, even landing a single cork felt like stepping into a whole new realm of snowboarding.

I had no problem doing huge single backflips, and I was comfortable spinning up to 720°, but that extra layer of complexity — the flip with a twist at the same time — was something I hadn't figured out yet. Looking back, I wish I had taken my parents up on an offer they made when I was 11 years old. They told me they'd put me in gymnastics if I wanted to go. I shut it down immediately.

"I'm a skateboarder," I told them. "I don't do gymnastics."

At the time, it seemed ridiculous, but now I see what a difference it could have made. Gymnastics teaches air awareness — the ability to control your body in flight, adjust body positions, and recover from mistakes — just like a cat landing on its feet. With that level of control, who knows what tricks could have been mastered.

Regardless, I still had that *corked spin trick* on my mind. I told myself that if the right jump lined up, I was going to go for it.

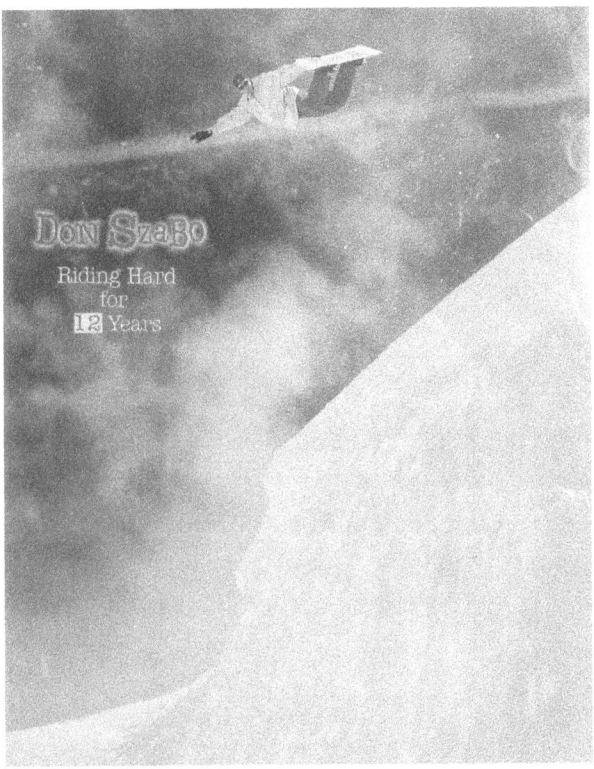

Riding Hard for 12 years until I couldn't

The Jump That Changed Everything

A fresh foot of snow had hit the local mountains in Southern California, so I made my way up to Big Bear. The plan was simple: shred with friends, find some fun lines, and maybe hit the right jump to try a corked spin for the first time.

The session started off great — flowing down the mountain, slashing fresh turns, and linking up with some of the local crew. Then we got to a jump that I knew well. I had sent big, laid-out backflips off it before. It was the kind of jump that let you land as far down the mountain as you wanted, at high speed, without getting wrecked. With fresh snow covering the landing, it felt like the perfect setup.

A couple of guys hit it first, launching into the sky and disappearing out of sight over the landing. I stood at the top, watching — then dropped in. As I picked up speed, I knew I was going to try a corked flip.

I hit the lip, initiated the backflip, and started twisting. But mid-air, I realized I didn't fully understand how to combine the flipping and spinning together in the right way.

This was before *foam pits* and *resi mats* — before the progression tools that let riders learn tricks more safely. Back then, if you wanted to land something new, you just had to go for it and hope for the best. And this? This was not the best.

I completely miscalculated the rotation and landed sideways, instantly launching into a high-speed, head-over-heels cartwheel. The impact was brutal. At one point, my right arm jammed deep into the snow, and as my body kept flipping, the force ripped my shoulder right out of its socket.

When I finally came to a stop, sitting dazed in the snow, I knew something was seriously wrong.

I looked down at my right arm — and it was clear. The head of my shoulder wasn't in the socket anymore. It had dropped deep into my armpit.

A few years earlier I'd felt this exact pain before.

I landed in sticky, slushy snow that stopped my board cold and launched my upper body forward. My left arm jammed into the snow, and as I flipped over it, I tore all the ligaments and tendons clean apart. That was my first major shoulder injury.

The year that followed sucked. My shoulder kept popping out — snowboarding, skateboarding, wakeboarding, whatever I was doing. If I pushed even a little too hard, it would dislocate again. I got used to asking friends to help pop it back into place, no matter where we were. Eventually, I had no choice. I went in for surgery to tighten things up and fix it. That repair held, and I was able to ride again.

My right shoulder had just been torn to pieces in almost the exact same way.

And I already knew the deal.

Once those ligaments and tendons are gone, your shoulder becomes unstable. It'll keep popping out, again and again, until you fix it. This wasn't a tweak or a strain — this was full-blown, season-ending damage. Surgery would be the only way back if I wanted to ride at the level I was used to.

I'd been through this before. I knew what it meant. Surgery. Rehab. A long road back.

But I'd done it once. Time to do it again.

The Shoulder Struggle & Moto Obsession

After this shoulder surgery, recovery wasn't just about getting strong again — it was about surviving the mental battle. This wasn't my first rodeo. As I mentioned, a few years earlier, I had gone through this same process, but it didn't make it any easier.

This time, I was living in Huntington Beach with Seth Enslow, one of the original freerider maniacs. Seth wasn't just another motocross rider — he was a stuntman. Seth's story is legendary. He wasn't just one of the first true freeride pioneers — he embodied the very essence of going big.

Back in those early days, we liked chasing adrenaline that most people couldn't fathom. But Seth operated on another level; he lacked a fear switch. While we assessed risks, Seth was already wide open, hitting jumps only the pros would consider. He'd either stick the landing and leave us in awe, or crash so violently it was sometimes a miracle that he walked away. That was Seth — pure heart and chaos on two wheels.

Crusty Demons of Dirt wasn't just a motocross film — it was the beginning of a revolution. The raw, explosive energy behind it started with Jon Freeman, the same creative force who brought us the Creatures of Habit snowboard films — the very films I'd snowboarded in for a handful of years.

One day, Dana Nicholson threw out a game-changing idea to Freeman.

He said, "We should make a freestyle and freeride motocross video similar to Creatures of Habit — high energy, great music, skits, and insane freestyle motocross riding." That single pitch lit the fuse.

The concept shattered the mold of traditional motocross footage and gave birth to a new era — freestyle motocross as we know it. With Crusty Demons of Dirt, they didn't just document dirt bike riding; they created a movement, blending adrenaline-pumping stunts, rebellious style, and raw storytelling into a cinematic experience that electrified riders and fans alike. It launched a worldwide phenomenon of going bigger, riding harder, and pushing the boundaries of what was possible on two wheels — and that progression is still charging forward today with the next generation of freestyle and freeride motocross riders.

Seth originally lived in Pennsylvania. He came to California with $1,400 cash, a dirt bike in the back of his truck, a snowboard, and not knowing a single person. He met up with Bubba (RIP🏍), a classic character from the Crusty Demons of Dirt skits. From there, he got introduced to Dana and the Crusty crew — and the rest is history.

Now, here I was, living with Seth a few years after the original Crusty revolution, watching him head out to ride dirt bikes all the time while I was stuck on the couch and rehabbing my shoulder — it was killing me.

I had always loved motocross, but over the past few years, I had become obsessed with it.

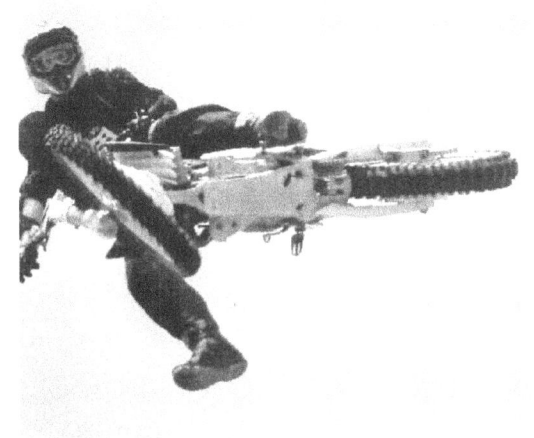

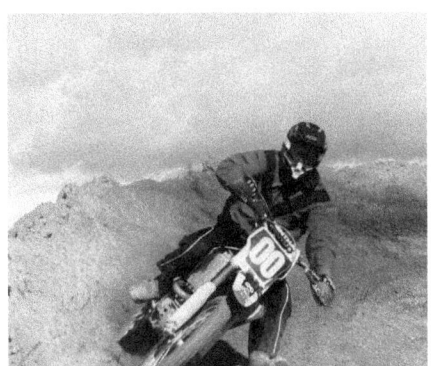

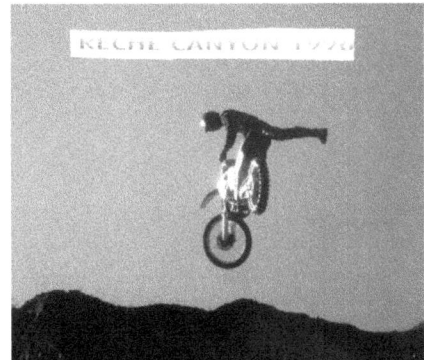

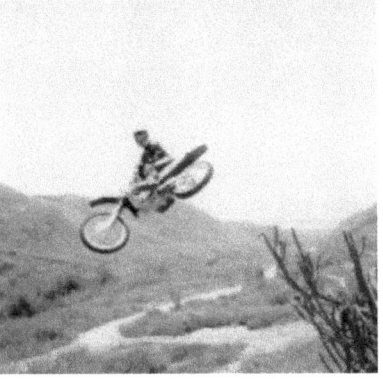

Moto's power and suspension — what a rush

The power. The suspension. The raw adrenaline. There's nothing like it. When you're on a dirt bike, with all that horsepower under you and the throttle in your hand, it's like being handed the keys to another dimension. You can go as fast, as far, and as big as your mind will let you. That feeling — when everything clicks, and you launch into the air with full confidence in your bike and your body — it's unreal.

After two months of healing up and finally starting to feel like myself again, I was sick of sitting around. I needed that feeling back. That rush. That freedom. That pure, unfiltered ride where anything felt possible. That's what I was craving again.

One day, Seth came home and said, "Z, we're going to go ride G-Spot. You wanna go?" I didn't hesitate. "Hell yeah, let's do it."

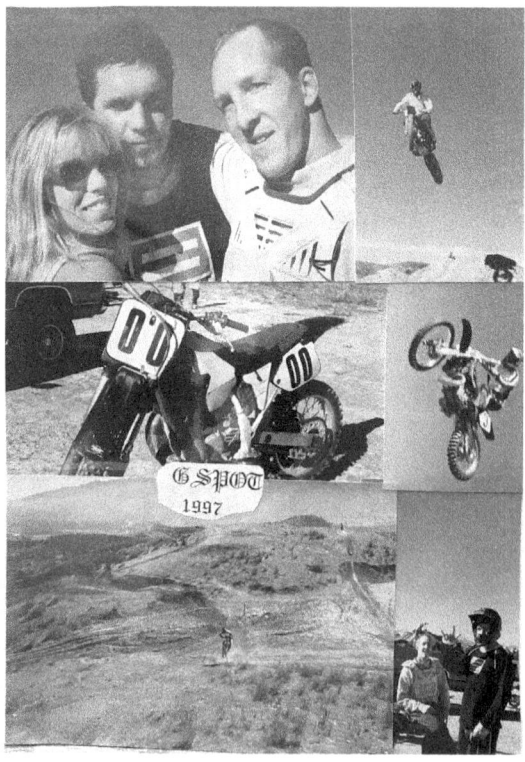

G-Spot with Seth — beginning of the end for snow

Dirt KillZ Snow

The G-Spot moto area and track was legendary. Built by Marc Matson, it was one of the best private, lock-and-key local motocross spots around. Killer terrain, epic views, and perfectly built jumps — and we had access to this great place when it all lined up.

But I was about to learn the hard way why my doctor told me to wait four full months before pushing my surgically repaired shoulder. I thought I could get away with riding again at the two-month mark — since I was feeling pretty good, and had gone through a similar surgery a few years earlier — but I was wrong.

I wasn't even riding that hard — just rolling with the guys, having fun on the track. I overjumped a decent-sized jump, landed out past the downhill transition, and came down hard in the flats. I didn't crash. But the impact? It was brutal for a shoulder that wasn't anywhere near 100%. I heard and felt it the second it happened — my shoulder tearing apart everything the surgeon had worked so hard to fix.

I rode up to the crew, heart sinking, and said, "I just destroyed my shoulder surgery from two months ago. I can't ride anymore."

The doctor confirmed it. All that pain, all that healing — gone in a second.

Now I was facing another surgery. Another setback. But this time, I wasn't taking any chances. I waited the full four months. I followed every rehab instruction to the letter. I was determined to come back stronger than ever.

By the next snow season, I thought I was finally ready. My first trip of the season was to Canada. I was easing into it, just cruising through some moguls, when suddenly I felt that all-too-familiar clunk. My shoulder dropped straight into my armpit again. I knew that terrible feeling all too well, and this time, we couldn't get it back into socket up on the mountain. It was stuck — locked deep in my armpit. This was not a good situation.

Ski patrol had to sled me down. By the time they finished the paperwork, my muscles had contracted so much that my shoulder was being pulled hard into the dislocated position. The pain was unreal. At the hospital, I had to be put under general anesthesia just to get it to relax enough for them to pop my shoulder back into place. This wasn't the first time — I'd been put under for the same painful process on my other shoulder too.

Back in Orange County, my doctor looked at me and basically said, "I don't know what else I can do." He admitted I'd pushed it too soon before, but now he wasn't sure how to make it strong and stable enough to hold up to the kind of abuse I was going to keep putting on it.

He referred me to the specialists at Kerlan-Jobe — the elite doctors who worked on NFL and MLB players, the top athletes. They ran deep scans and figured out that my last dislocation wasn't the usual forward one — it had blown out the back. A whole different kind of shoulder instability. This new surgery would involve an additional incision through the back of my shoulder on top of the front incision done multiple times before. This will tighten ligaments and tendons on both sides of my shoulder and create real stability — something that could hold up to the punishment I was sure to dish out to it.

It was my third major shoulder surgery on the same arm, and another four months of rehab to try to get back in riding shape. And another snow season just slipped away.

Meanwhile, my sponsors were upfront with me — without contest results, magazine coverage, video parts, or even their product shots, they couldn't keep paying me.

And they were right. This was the second winter in a row that I couldn't ride.

No new footage, no photos, nothing they could use — and nothing I could show for being the pro athlete I still felt like inside, but physically couldn't be..

It was crushing. I had worked for years to get to where I was, and now I was watching it fall apart. Not because I gave up — but because my body just couldn't keep up after all the damage I'd done to it.

Still, I couldn't walk away without a fight.

That summer, once my shoulder finally felt solid again, I booked a trip to New Zealand with one of John Freeman's filmers. We went heli-boarding, and the snow was great. I went big — charged lines, dropped cliffs, did everything I could to prove I still had it. I thought we got some great footage and that everything would be fine.

And then…we found out after the trip that his video film camera had a light leak. Every roll of 16mm film that we shot was ruined. There wasn't any usable footage from that trip.

That was the final blow. After everything I'd fought through — all the surgeries, the pain, the lost seasons — that moment crushed me.

I just didn't have it in me anymore to keep chasing something that kept slipping through my fingers.

Maybe it all happened for a reason…

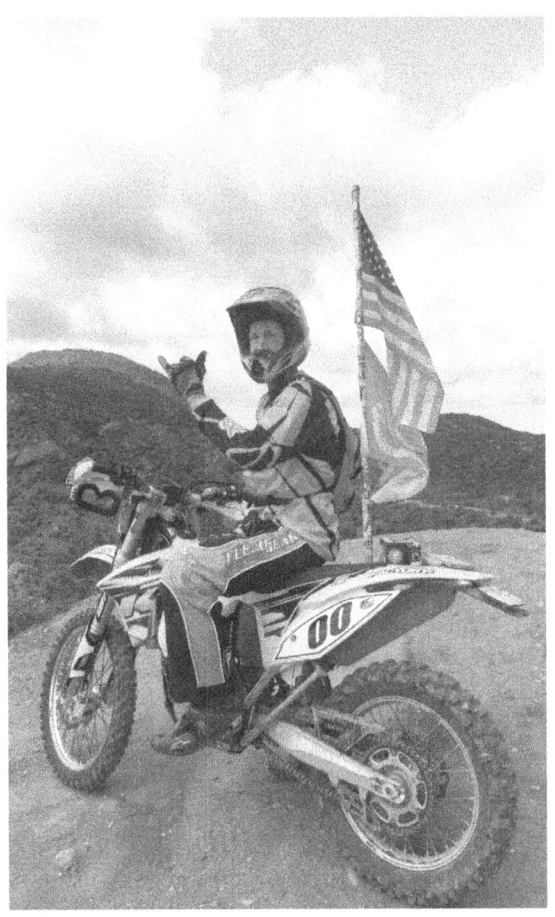

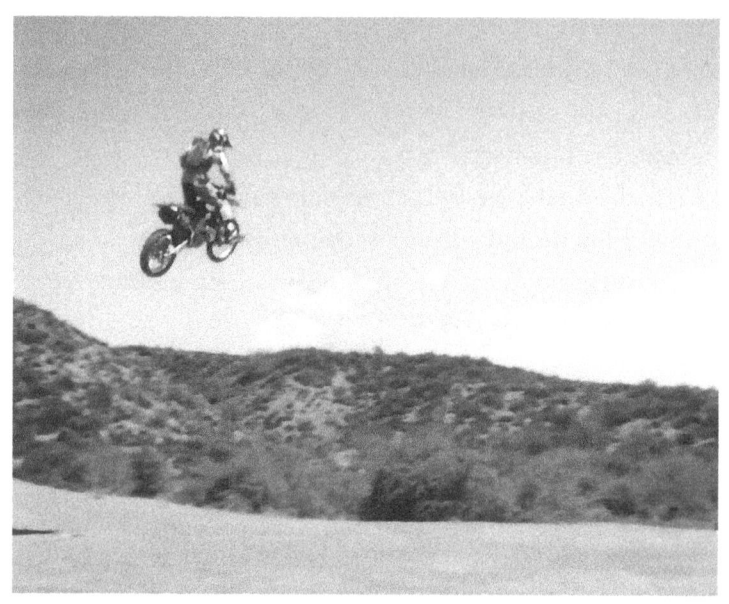

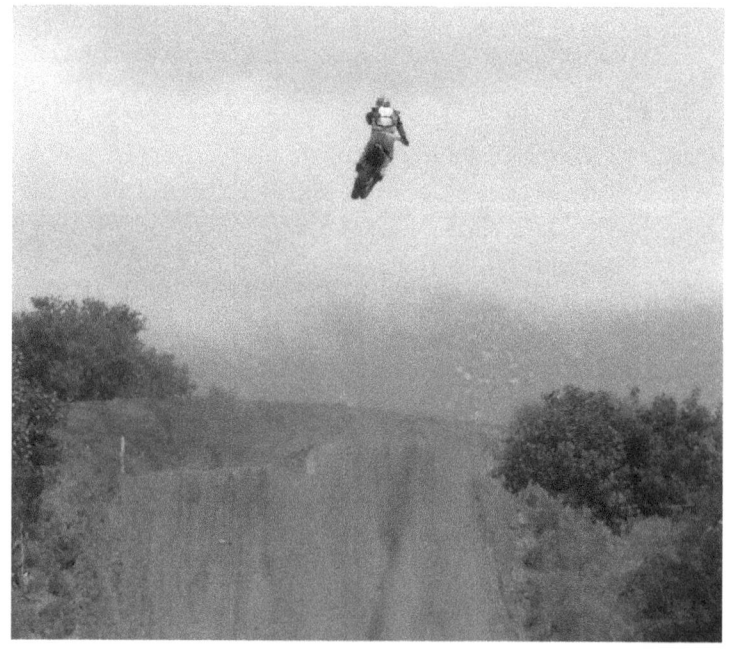

Chapter 9

Transition Time

After the disaster in New Zealand, when all my snowboarding footage was ruined because of the film camera light leak, I knew deep down it was the final nail in the coffin for my pro snowboarding career. It felt like the universe was telling me it was time to switch gears.I had spent my life pushing limits, and after over 10 years of doing what I loved to do on the snow for a living, it was clear I needed a new direction.

Motocross had become my latest adrenaline obsession, and back then, action sports were growing fast. The Gravity Games — and especially the X Games — were the biggest platforms for action sports at the time. I landed a side gig as a freestyle motocross judge, which put me right in the middle of the scene with some of the best FMX riders in the world. I wasn't throwing the tricks myself, but I had a good eye for technical difficulty and could appreciate the skill required to execute them.

The first judging opportunity came through Gravity Games, which was run by my old pro snowboard friend Rob Giustina. It was a great gig — traveling, hanging with a solid crew, and staying close to the action. Eventually, I transitioned to judging for X Games, where I judged guys like Nate Adams, Travis Pastrana, Mike Metzger, Brian Deegan, Ronnie Faisst, and Carey Hart, to name a few. These weren't just motocross riders — they were pioneers of Freestyle Motocross (a.k.a. FMX), pushing the limits of what tricks were possible on a dirt bike. These guys were on an entirely different level — perfectly in sync with their machines, throwing massive tricks at heights that seemed impossible.

X Games had become the dominant force in action sports competition, and every year, it grew bigger. For two years, I was part of that, watching FMX history unfold right in front of me. I was judging when Travis Pastrana landed the first-ever double backflip on a dirt bike in a competition — an absolutely insane moment. I also judged one of the wildest FMX events ever attempted: motocross jumps on snow at the Winter X Games. The riders had to use spiked tires for traction, but the bikes didn't handle like they did on dirt. The whole thing seemed sketchy, and sure enough, Brian Deegan ended up breaking his femur during the event. That was enough for Winter X Games to scrap the whole concept. FMX on snow was a bad idea, and Deegan paid the price to prove it.

At one of the LA X Games, another judge that day, Robbie Maddison, looked at me and asked, "Who are you, mate? I don't recognize you as an FMX rider." I told him straight up — I wasn't. I was an ex-pro snowboarder who had transitioned into motocross for the love of it and had been invited to judge because of my experience in action sports. He didn't seem to know what to make of that, which I understood. FMX was its own world, and I wasn't fully embedded in it the way these guys were.

Shortly after that, X Games made some management changes and started occasionally showing judges on TV. I wasn't invited back as a judge. It made sense — they wanted their judges to be current or former FMX pros. I respected that.

Robbie Maddison, by the way, went on to do some of the craziest, most amazing stunt moto riding in history. If you haven't seen what he's done, look him up. It's legendary.

I was now out of the X Games scene. I didn't want to try to snowboard professionally anymore, but I wasn't ready to step away from action sports.

Also during this time — since my shoulder injury — Black Flys and Fleshgear, two companies I had been sponsored by, offered me an opportunity. Since I wasn't pursuing snowboarding professionally anymore, they asked if I wanted to rep their products to motocross shops. Fleshgear sold moto gear, and Black Flys sold sunglasses. It wasn't a bad gig — traveling, meeting shop employees, buyers, and owners of motocross shops, and staying connected to the industry in a different way.

I took the job, and soon I was on the road hitting up moto shops across Orange County and the Inland Empire. And wherever I went, my two road dogs, Lucky and Bailey, came with me.

Lucky was truly a lucky dog. A buddy of mine who installed car stereos found her abandoned in a house in Compton. He had been doing a job up there when he heard whining from an abandoned house. He came across this puppy — alone, surrounded by dog poop, in an empty, run-down house. Somehow she had been left alone and would've died soon. He scooped her up and took her with him, unsure of what to do next.

He stopped by my place in Huntington Beach, where I was still living with Seth, and told us the story. He didn't know if he could keep her. At that point in my life, I figured I could use some company. "I'll take her," I said. She needed serious medical attention — worms, scabies, the works. Fortunately, I had a friend who worked at a pet hospital and helped get Lucky treated. That was the beginning of our journey together.

Not long after that, Bailey came into my life from a steel yard in the Inland Empire. The workers were kicking around this poor stray puppy that had been scrounging for food during their breaks. He was just looking for some scraps, some kindness — but instead, he was being treated like trash. Soon, my other dog, Lucky, had a partner.

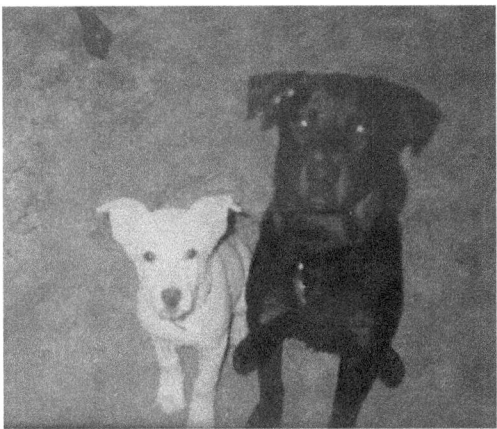

Lucky and Bailey — they were both '97s

I had always liked the idea of having two dogs — they could keep each other company. Just like that, I had my crew: Lucky and Bailey. I always referred to them by their birth year, the same way you do with cars, bikes, and boats. They were '97s. I was a '66 — the same birth year as Vans skateboard shoes.

With Lucky and Bailey, I was stepping into a whole new chapter of life. It was a big shift from my snowboarding days of jetting around the world with no real responsibilities. But even as life changed, one thing stayed the same: I still needed that adrenaline rush — and motocross became my adrenaline sport of choice.

Repping on the Road

Repping for Black Flys and Fleshgear took me to all kinds of shops, but Chaparral was the big one. It was the 800-pound gorilla of Southern California moto shops — a massive, 160,000-square-foot powerhouse that moved a ton of product. It was a great account to have financially, but dealing with their buyers was a different story. They were always swamped, always in a rush, and getting them to sit down and focus on what I was presenting was a challenge. I understood — it was business, and they had a lot on their plate — but it was never my favorite place to deal with.

On the other hand, Three Brothers Racing in Costa Mesa? That was my favorite shop — full of cool people that worked there and a great vibe inside.

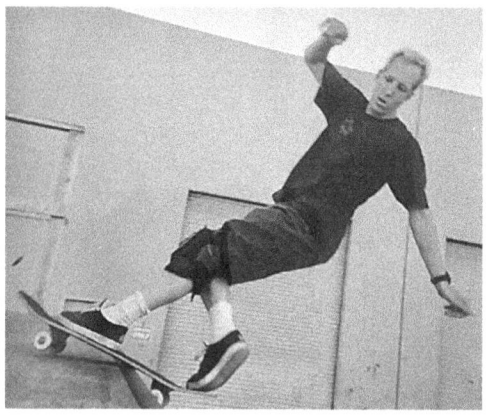

Black Flys had a fun ramp to Sk8 when I rolled by there

Three Brothers Racing — A Cool Moto Crew

Three Brothers Racing was right near the Black Flys warehouse, so it was easy to swing by and check in. The shop was originally run by three Brazilian brothers who had come to the U.S. chasing the American dream — and they made it happen. They were some of the most welcoming, down-to-earth guys you could meet, always greeting you with a smile.

Quite often when I visited the shop, I'd chat with a guy working behind the counter — a cool dude with a full leg cast, walking on crutches. He looked like the Marlboro Man — tough as nails. We'd talk about gear, riding, and whatever else was on our minds.

One day, I rolled in and noticed his cast was smaller — now just up to his knee. He was moving around better. He told me Three Brothers was having a big desert ride over Labor Day weekend and asked if I wanted to go.

"I'd love to," I said, "but I don't have a dirt bike right now."

"No worries," he said. "I've got two '97 Honda CR250s — one's my race bike, one's my practice bike. You can ride the practice bike."

I looked at him — this guy still had a broken leg, and he was planning to ride? That was insane. He can't ride like that.

At the same time, he was probably looking at me thinking, This snowboarder rep sells me glasses and moto gear but doesn't even have a dirt bike? He probably can't ride for shit.

When we hit the desert, it was about 20 trailers deep — Three Brothers Racing had a serious crew. We geared up and took off with about 15 riders. Right away, we were up front, pushing it. As we wove through technical rock sections, I noticed John lifting his leg high over rocks and obstacles, protecting his bare toes from hitting things. The guy was riding hard — with a broken leg and toes sticking out. That was next-level.

I looked over and said, "I like your style. You're a badass."

That trip cemented our friendship and was when I truly bro'd down with John Brewton. From that point on, we rode together for over 15 years, pushing each other on and off the tracks and trails. Three Brothers Racing became more than just a shop — it became like family.

Lights Out to Life-Flight Out

Motocross is all about speed, flow, and that perfect connection between rider and machine. And then there are days when things go completely sideways. This was one of those days — one I'll never forget, even though I can't remember an entire week from what happened that day.

I was out riding one of my favorite motocross tracks called Racetown, a place we hit regularly. There was a jump at the back of the track — a 50-foot step-up, followed by a 60-foot tabletop that most riders would roll across after hitting the *step up*. That was the standard way to hit it.

But not for me.

I had taken this jump to the next level. I'd seen a pro rider send it way beyond the normal step up landing zone, and after watching him do it, I decided that was the new standard. Instead of landing on the step-up and riding across the tabletop, I was launching from the takeoff all the way to the final downside, landing at the end of the table top, 110 feet away. On the throttle hard in fourth gear.

I'd done it dozens of times, flawless landings, no problem. But on this lap, fate had other plans.

As I approached, completely committed, I had no idea that another rider had crashed in my exact landing zone. There was no flagger to signal that a rider was down. Nobody knew. The crashed rider had managed to scoot himself toward the edge of the track, but his bike was still dead center in my landing zone. And from 110 feet back, I couldn't see any of this.

At around 40 mph, in fourth gear, I launched it.

By the time I saw his bike, it was too late. I slammed into it mid-landing at high speed, and the impact catapulted me over the handlebars, straight into the dirt. Lights out.

I was out cold. Instant dirt nap.

They had to load me onto a gurney, carry me off the track, and I was then airlifted to the hospital. I may vaguely remember seeing helicopter blades as they loaded me in — or maybe that's just what I like to think I remember. Either way, I was in bad shape.

A Week Lost to Concussion Fog

At the hospital, the diagnosis was three broken ribs, a punctured lung, and a concussion that wiped out an entire week of my memory.

I was told that dozens of people had came to visit me, but to this day, I don't remember anyone or anything from that week. The only evidence that I had any visitors in the hospital is a RIP tombstone I took home, made out of foam — a twisted little get-well gift from Damian Sanders, since he was always building props for his company Monster Stage back then which he still does now and produces amazing creative products.

Looking at it later, I realized how close I came to needing a real tombstone. This was a life-or-death crash. Easily could've gone the other way. But once again, I was blessed to stay on this side of the dirt.

Visiting Jon Brewton — Deja Vu with a Twist

A few years later, I found myself on the other side of the hospital bed — except this time, I was the visitor.

This was right when four-stroke 450cc dirt bikes were just starting to take over motocross, replacing the two-stroke 250s that had dominated the sport for years. The first Supercross race of the season at Anaheim Stadium was coming up, and everyone was buzzing about the change.

Our friend Chris Barrett had just gotten one of the new 450s and swung by John Brewton's house. Being a true moto guy, John couldn't resist taking it for a quick ride down the street to see how it felt compared to the two-stroke motorcycles everyone was used to riding for so many years.

That's when everything went wrong.

A car turned left in front of him, giving him no time to react. The impact destroyed him. He was left with five major injuries at once:

- Compound fracture of the right femur

- Compound fracture of the left humerus
- Shattered cartilage in his left knee
- Torn tendon in his clutch hand
- Every single bone holding up his left cheek was broken

They had to put in plates and screws to rebuild him — a plate and nine screws in his wrist, two plates in his face, a rod in his femur, and another plate and screws in his humerus.

And on top of all that? A traumatic brain injury.

I visited him every day for a week at the hospital down the street from his house in Orange County. When he finally got released a week later, I went to his house to check on him.

The first thing he said?

"Dude, I never saw you once while I was in the hospital."

I just laughed. "Yeah, well, same thing happened to me when you told me you visited me in the hospital that week I don't remember at all when I crashed too. I guess concussions cancel out visitors."

Seth Enslow — The Hardest Hit of Them All

If John Brewton had the most injuries at one time of any of my friends, then Seth Enslow had the worst single head injury of anyone I know of — and it's documented in his video The Hard Way.

I had a front-row seat to one of the most intense moments of his life — his attempt to break the world record for the longest dirt bike jump. It was December 1999, just days before Christmas, at Mike Cinqmars' (RIP 🙏) house in the high desert. The goal? To beat Doug Danger's 251-foot motorcycle jump record set in 1991. Seth was determined to make history.

The setup looked solid. I was there the day before it all went south. The jump ramp was incrementally pushed back — from 100 feet in 20-foot increments up to 200 feet. By the time the wind picked up and halted the session, Seth had done a 230-foot jump and came down deep into the dirt landing.

As I left Cinq's house that evening for Huntington Beach, I thought, "He's got this." It seemed like history was in the making.

But the next day…everything changed.

The desert wind shifted direction — it was subtle but crucial. What had been a slight headwind turned into a slight tailwind, a potentially deadly shift for someone launching off a massive ramp at 72 mph. Seth and a few friends remained in the high desert, and others showed up the next day to watch him send it again. However, they didn't recalibrate the jump for the wind shift. He approached the gap at the same speed, unaware that the gentle push from behind would alter his trajectory.

Seth launched high — around 40 feet — and overshot the downslope landing, slamming into the flats at the 245-foot mark. The impact was devastating. His face struck the handlebars with such force that it crushed his skull above the right eye, causing him to fall from the bike while still moving at considerable speed. It was the kind of crash you don't just get up from, one that's unforgettable whether witnessed firsthand or later in his video, The Hard Way.

He got airlifted to Loma Linda Hospital, and surgeons had to peel his face down from ear to ear to repair the damage. They inserted two titanium plates to replace the crushed part of his cranium and put his skull skin back together with 55 staples. It was a brutal surgery, just days before Christmas. Not the holiday he had envisioned, but we were all so grateful that he was still alive.

Seth Enslow survived what could have easily been a fatal crash. That's what set him apart — not just his willingness to go bigger than anyone else, but his resilience to take the hit and get back up. He was an extremely committed rider, going all-in every time in those early years of pushing the limits and really going big on a dirt bike. That world record might have slipped through his fingers that day, but he proved something more significant — that heart and fearlessness can carry a man farther than any measuring tape ever will.

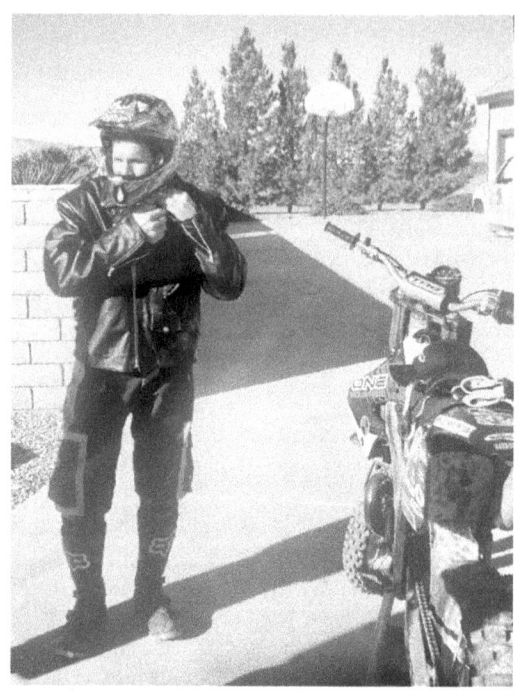

Seth, gearing up the day before disaster

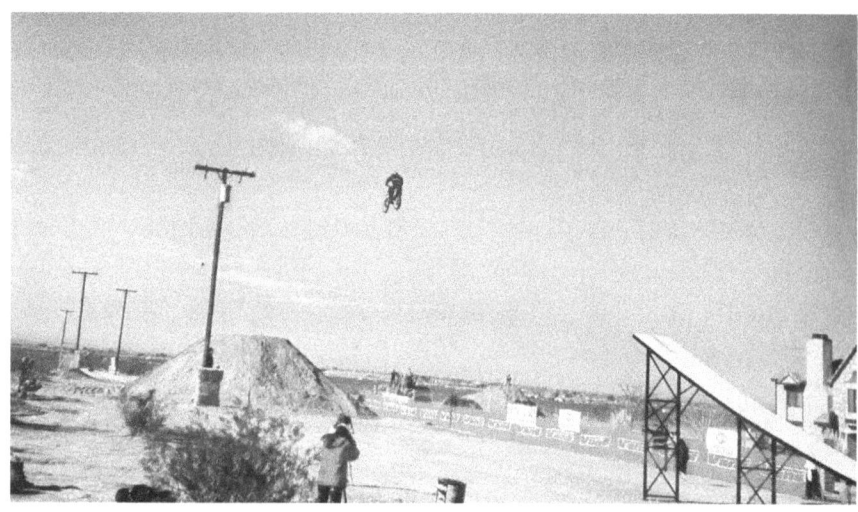

The world record was his the next day, until the wind said otherwise

A Business Proposal

Some friendships are meant to weave in and out of your life, crossing paths in the most unexpected places. For years, Jon Seck and I had been running into each other in the most random ways. The first time was back in the '80s at Arnold's backyard ramp on the west side of the Valley. Back then, I was skating any backyard ramp I could get access to, always on the hunt for the next session.

Years later, in the early '90s, I found myself on a spur-of-the-moment trip down to Ensenada in Mexico to go surf. I saw him again when we were out one evening, and I recognized his face immediately — long hair, a bit of a wild energy, and a striking resemblance to Anthony Kiedis from the Red Hot Chili Peppers. This was before cell phones, so I actually grabbed a pen and a napkin, wrote down his number, and labeled it: Jon, looks like Anthony Kiedis. I told him I'd hit him up sometime.

We became good friends and spent a lot of time together back in California — surfing locally and taking trips to Costa Rica and different spots in Mexico. We lived an adventurous life, packing in unforgettable experiences. But the wild surf trip to Hawaii — that one could've been a book on its own...

In 1999, Jon came to me with a proposal.

At this point, he had been working in the screen-printing industry for a few years, and he knew everything about the process — the machines, the inks, the drying techniques, the logistics of turning a blank surface into a finished product. He had been selling print jobs to customers, and he felt good about the business.

The owner of the shop he worked for wanted to sell. Jon didn't have the money to buy the shop, but he had the experience. He came to me, pitching the idea that if we bought the business, we could build something successful together. He made it sound like the perfect opportunity — low risk, high reward.

At that point in my life, I had been jumping off cliffs — literally and figuratively — for years. This was just another one. The only way to know if the landing was solid was to take the leap.

Taking the Leap

We met with the owner at the shop. He made it look easy. Turn on the machines that push the ink through the screens, run the material through the dryer — and just like that, hundreds or thousands of stickers or prints are ready to go. He ran through the billing, the customer list, and how the clients would come with the business. It all sounded like a machine that just needed someone to keep it running.

Jon was nodding the whole time, fully convinced we were about to start printing money, as the previous owner described it. Within days, we agreed to buy the business. We drafted up a contract between us, signed it, and just like that, we were off to the races.

Too bad it wasn't that easy.

The moment the deal was done, reality came crashing in. Running a screen-printing shop wasn't just about printing. It was quoting jobs, getting the jobs, managing work orders, handling accounting, dealing with shipping, ordering materials, keeping customers happy, and making sure everything ran smoothly day in and day out. The previous owner, who had made everything look effortless, disappeared after he had the money in his hands.

Jon, for all his knowledge about printing, wasn't a business operations guy. He knew the process and how to sell print jobs, but when it came to actually managing the day-to-day grind, it fell on me. I was now the one holding it all together, learning how to run a business from the ground up with no experience.

Would we stick the landing on this cliff jump, or were we about to freefall, hit the bottom, and splat? One way to find out.

The Reality Check

That first year was brutal. I had gone from having some freedom to being completely tied down. Before this, I was still working as a rep for Fleshgear and Black Flys, traveling, making connections, and living life on my terms. Suddenly,

I had real responsibilities — not just a sales rep business and dogs to take care of, but now a shop that needed constant daily attention to keep from sinking.

I remember Artie, my Black Flys manager, checking in week after week, asking if I had made it out to my accounts to see what they needed. I kept telling him I couldn't. I couldn't leave the shop. It needed me 100% of the time, every day. It got to the point where he asked if I could at least make it out to Chaparral in the middle of the week every week or two. I couldn't even do that.

Finally, he had to cut me loose. "We're going to have to let you go, Z," he told me. My Black Flys and Fleshgear accounts were handed over to Mike Bishop, who was already on the road repping other stuff — and just like that, my other financial lifelines were gone. All I had left was this struggling shop that was barely staying afloat.

Jon and I worked long, hard hours trying to figure it out, but there were moments when it felt like we were drowning. I remember one afternoon, after months of grinding, we finally took a break. We drove down to the beach, just a few miles away, and saw everyone out there enjoying life — good surf, warm sun, people laughing, having the kind of summer we used to have.

We just stood there for a moment, taking it all in.

Then we turned around, got back in the car, and went back to the shop to keep trying to figure out how to keep it going.

Sink or Swim

It wasn't just the workload. We were struggling to get proper pricing, losing customers tied to the previous owner, and failing to meet some deadlines and commitments as we tried to get our processes in order. Business was slipping through our fingers, and we were barely keeping our heads above water.

Jon said he'd go out and find new business, tapping into old connections and anyone who might throw us a lifeline. I didn't know if it would work, but at that point, we had no other option.

Then Jon came through. He was reaching out to potential clients — on the phone, face-to-face — seeking anyone in need of promotional items. His network of friends and acquaintances proved to be valuable, connecting us with key buyers and significantly boosting our business.

We identified our individual strengths: I managed shop operations, ensuring production ran smoothly amidst the controlled chaos, while also bringing in a respectable amount of business when time permitted. Jon's strength in sales was undeniable. By focusing on what we each did best, we transitioned from merely surviving to actively climbing out of our financial hole. Orders began rolling in, production stabilized, and we offered competitive pricing, quality products, and good turnaround times to our growing clientele.

Within a year, we had transformed the shop into an operation more successful than it had ever been under the previous owner, with business thriving and momentum on our side.

With things running smoothly, Jon got info from some friends planning a surf trip to Tahiti with a crew of guys he had been surfing with. He had been bringing it up for a while, and now, for the first time in a long time, it actually felt possible.

After a year of nonstop grind, stress, and uncertainty, we looked at where we were, how we had turned things around, and decided — let's do it. We deserved a vacation after all that.

A week in Tahiti. Clear blue skies, good waves, and nothing but an awesome trip awaiting us.

It sounded like a dream.

What could go wrong?

Well…we'd find out soon enough.

Tahiti: Big Wave Adventure

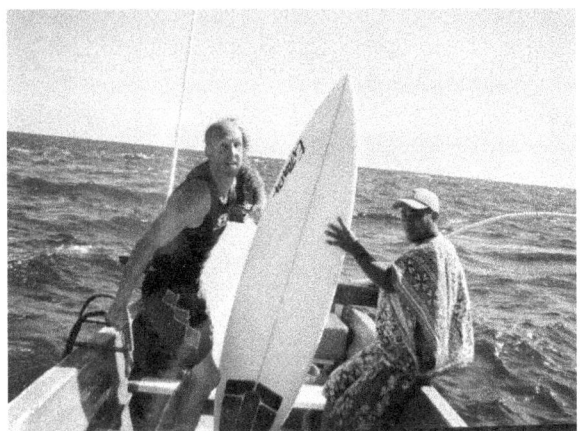

Chasing waves by boat, a mile off shore

In early 2000, I went on a surf trip to Tahiti, a journey that etched itself deep into my memory. It was the kind of adventure that every surfer dreams of but few get to experience. There were seven of us on this trip, a mix of friends and friends-of-friends. Some I knew well, others were strangers united by a shared love for chasing waves. Our meeting point was LAX, where the excitement buzzed in the air like static electricity. As I watched the guys arrive, lugging two or three boards each, I could already tell this wasn't going to be an ordinary trip. They debated board sizes, wave conditions, and strategies for surfing different waves.

"If it's *double overhead*, I'll ride my bigger gun," one said. Another chimed in, talking about boards for more playful surf.

I had brought just one board: my trusty 6'6" tri-fin. It was the board I rode everywhere, and as always, I intended to make it work. While they dissected the nuances of wave-riding gear, I knew that success out there wouldn't be about the board — it would be about the rider and, more importantly, their mindset.

Our destination wasn't just any wave. Tahiti is home to Teahupo'o, one of the world's most infamous breaks. Known for its thunderous power and machine-like perfection, it's a wave that demands respect. Teahupo'o is a wave that breaks left and seems to defy physics, with its thick, hollow barrels crashing over a shallow reef. Even the best surfers in the world tread lightly here. Photos of its beauty and brutality grace the pages of surf magazines, but nothing prepares you for seeing these kinds of waves up close.

For our trip, we headed to Moorea, a smaller island in Tahiti, where we'd surf Hapiti. This wave was a cousin to Teahupo'o — not quite as heavy, but still challenging and hollow. Hapiti was also less exposed, and locals had made sure it stayed off the mainstream map, a treasure hidden from the surf tourism masses. No contests, no promotions. It was raw and preserved, just as they wanted to keep it.

To get to Hapiti, we needed a boat. The break was a mile out at sea, far beyond the reach of the shore. We met a boat driver named Jo-Jo and piled into the boat with our boards, and set out to get some surf. The waves greeted us with an unrelenting double overhead swell, a size that never let up the entire trip. In fact, each day, the waves grew bigger and more menacing, but that just added to the challenge.

The first to test Hapiti's power was my business partner, Jon. He paddled for a wave — a steep double overhead — and went all in. But Hapiti wasn't forgiving. Jon said he was in a critical part of the wave in the tube but got into the wrong position, and the wave picked him up and threw him *over the falls*, churning him like laundry in a washing machine. When he resurfaced, his watch and surf hat were gone, and his shorts were barely hanging on. He paddled back to the lineup pale as a ghost, but I admired his grit. Despite the beating, he didn't back down.

For me, the challenge was exhilarating. By this time in my life, I was riding a lot of motocross and had grown used to catching 100 feet of air on my dirt bike. That kind of mindset — of committing fully and trusting your abilities — translated seamlessly to the water. To drop into Hapiti's steep cylinders, you had to go all in. The reef below was so visible through the crystal-clear water it looked like you were about to land on it. But I knew better. I trusted the ocean, my skills, and my ability to adapt.

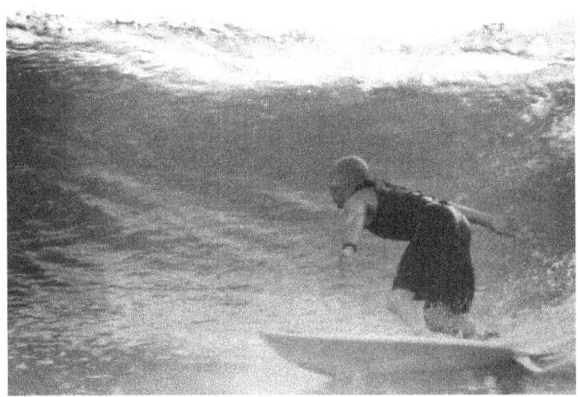
Surf happened, surf cameras didn't, random shot instead

When my turn came, I spotted a wave, paddled hard, and launched into it. The drop felt almost weightless, like freefalling into the unknown. I landed my heelside bottom turn and carved into the face of the wave, which roared with power and precision. It was mechanical perfection, a wave that was like a canvas, and I felt that majestic rush once again, drawing lines freely like an artist. I kicked out of the wave at the end, grinning ear to ear, and paddled back for more.

Not everyone shared the same mindset. After Jon's tumble, our entire crew froze — not one of them caught a wave the whole trip. They just sat out there like human buoys, bobbing in the lineup but never committing. It was like they'd come armed with the perfect boards but forgotten to pack the courage to match. Jon and I, on the other hand, caught wave after wave, laughing like kids. For us, it was a playground, and the ocean had gifted us unlimited access.

By the final day, the swell had grown into something monstrous. Hapiti was now a solid *triple overhead* — a massive, hollow beast that seemed to breathe in the distance. There were no other surfers in the water that day. Everyone else had decided it was either too dangerous or simply insane. But Jon and I weren't backing down. We rode out with the boat driver, jumped into the lineup, and prepared to face these giants.

Jon caught the first wave, a towering triple overhead. He dropped in and disappeared down the face, swallowed by the sheer scale of it. I watched in awe as he carved through the wave and out of sight. Now it was my turn.

As I waited, I saw a massive wave looming on the horizon. I paddled furiously, trying to get outside, but it was no use. The wave broke in front of me and created a wall of whitewash that was four times overhead. I held onto my board with everything I had, but the force ripped it from my grip and snapped the leash. Suddenly, I was alone, tumbling underwater — and when I surfaced, my board was gone.

Wave after wave came, and I dove under each one, conserving energy and letting them pass. When the set ended, I swam toward the channel, hoping to make it back to shore. But the ocean had other plans. No matter how hard I swam, I drifted farther away from the shore. Realizing there was no use fighting it, I did the only thing I could: I floated.

Lying on my back in the warm, silent water, I felt an odd sense of peace. With no board, no noise, and no sign of land, I simply existed — weightless and calm. Time seemed to stretch endlessly, and for about twenty minutes, I embraced the solitude.

Then Jon's voice pierced the quiet. "Szabo, get in! Quick!" His urgency snapped me back to reality. I looked up to see him reaching down from the boat. I grabbed his hand, hauled myself aboard, and listened as he explained what had happened. From their vantage point with binoculars, they'd seen me vanish and feared the worst. The channel we had to navigate the boat through was closing fast with the growing swell, and timing our return would be critical.

On our way back, we spotted my board floating in a calm area inside the impact zone. With Jo-Jo's boat driving skills, we scooped it up and navigated safely through the channel. By the time we reached shore, my heart was pounding, but I couldn't wipe the grin off my face.

Surfing heavy waves four times my height might have been a bit ambitious, but I wouldn't trade the experience for anything. Tahiti had tested me, humbled me, and reminded me of why I loved the ocean, the adventure, and the thrill of pushing myself beyond the limits.

Beyond the Waves:
Tahitian Connections and Adventures

Tahiti wasn't just about the waves. As incredible as the surf trip was, the experiences we had on the island itself were equally unforgettable. The locals we met through our boat driver quickly became friends, and they opened up their world to us in a way that made the trip even more special. Their kindness and generosity turned our time on Moorea into more than just a surf trip — it became a connection to a culture that embraced the ocean, the land, and the people around it.

One of our new friends was a talented woodcarver who crafted intricate pieces of art from the island's native wood. His carvings were stunning, the kind of pieces that felt alive with the spirit of Tahiti. He sold them to tourists, but with us, it was more than just a transaction. We bonded with him, and by the end of our trip, I had several pieces of his artwork — a reminder of the beauty he created and the friendship we shared.

Another local was a snorkeling guide who took us on an unforgettable underwater tour. The reefs surrounding Moorea were like an underwater paradise, alive with vibrant coral and tropical fish darting in and out of the crystal clear water. It was breathtaking — an awe-inspiring blend of nature above and below the surface.

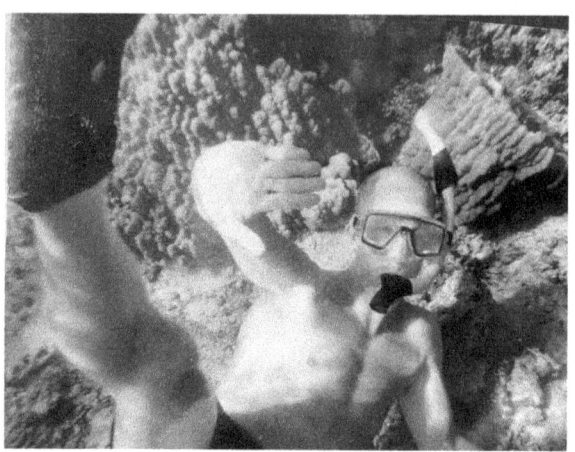
Snorkel dork, under the sea

During the snorkeling trip, the guide noticed something about me. I could dive deep and hold my breath longer than most, and that caught his attention. He offered me a challenge — something he usually did himself but thought I could handle. He handed me a large cow leg bone, still bearing a bit of meat, and explained what I needed to do.

"Take this down to the anchor," he said, pointing to a spot 20 feet below the boat. "Hold it steady, extend it out, and wait. The sharks will come."

The prospect of sharks didn't faze me. It was thrilling. I dove down, gripping the anchor to steady myself underwater, and extended the three-foot bone toward the surface. Sure enough, a six-foot shark appeared, gliding effortlessly through the water. It latched onto the bone and gave a few hard tugs, pulling at my arm — but nothing I couldn't handle. From below, I could see the people above, peering down from the boat or snorkeling at the surface, watching the scene unfold. It was surreal, sharing this moment with a predator of the sea, yet feeling completely in control.

Later that week, Jo-Jo and our Tahitian friends invited us to a local party. It was an invitation that came with a bit of risk, as we would soon learn. The party wasn't meant for outsiders — it was strictly locals-only — but our new friends wanted us to experience the true heartbeat of Moorea. They vouched for us, bringing all seven of us to the gathering.

When we arrived, tensions were heating up. Some of the locals weren't happy to see a group of white outsiders among them. There were a few heated words exchanged between our friends and the others, and for a moment, it seemed like things might escalate. But ultimately, cooler heads prevailed. No fists were thrown, and the situation settled down. It was a glimpse into the pride and protectiveness the locals had for their community — a reminder that while we were welcomed by some, we were still guests on their island.

Despite the occasional hiccup, the trip was filled with nothing but good times and good vibes. From riding incredible waves to making connections with the people of Moorea, Tahiti had given me more than I ever expected. These weren't just memories of adrenaline-fueled surf sessions or heart-pounding shark encounters. They were moments of connection — of bonding with strangers who welcomed us into their world, even if only for a short while.

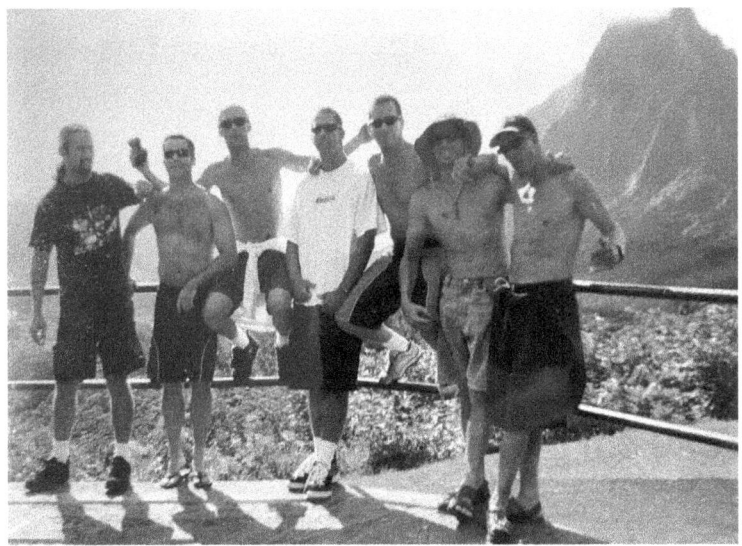

Tahiti crew, enjoying the view

It was another chapter in the life of Z, proof that the best adventures aren't just about where you go or what you do. They're about the people you meet, the risks you take, and the memories you create along the way. And Tahiti?

Tahiti was awesome.

After an unforgettable week in paradise, all seven of us packed up our memories and boarded the flight home. The island vibes, the waves, the laughs — it was everything we needed. Jon and I returned to California feeling recharged and alive, but reality was waiting. It was time to shift gears and dive back into the hustle of our screen printing business in Orange County. The trip may have ended, but momentum was building, and the next chapter of my life was about to unfold

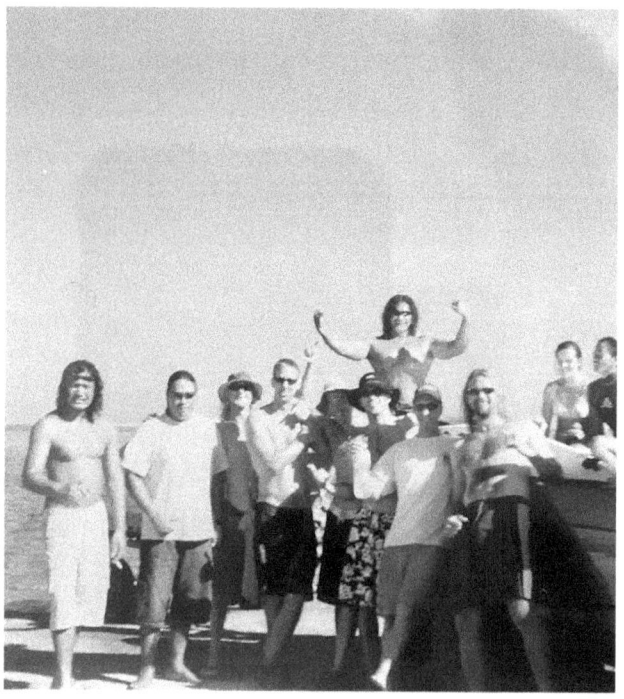

Good Vibes with Tahiti friends

-Chapter 10-.
Love of My Life

So as I was running my dogs, Lucky and Bailey, up and down Dog Beach in Huntington Beach after another long day at the semi-new print shop — which I'd finally gotten the hang of running — I jogged toward the cliffs like I often did to unwind. As I was heading to my usual end of the beach, I passed a beautiful woman. We both smiled as we went in opposite directions, but I couldn't shake the thought of her. Before reaching the cliffs where I would usually run my dogs, I turned around, hoping to see her again, and a few minutes later, I caught up to her, now heading in the same direction. Slowing down, pretending to be a bit tired from running with Lucky and Bailey, I said, "Hi, cute dog!" Really, she was the cute one to me, but it was a good way to start. That's how I met Heather, the love of my life, in the summer of 2000.

As we walked and talked, I learned she was a schoolteacher, out walking her parents' dog to get some exercise for both herself and their dog. She was also giving her parents a break, since they were older and didn't have anyone else to help with their dog. My dad had already passed away the year before, and being from a small family myself, I could relate. I told her about the print shop I was running, which was always a handful to keep going. I mentioned how I'd come out to get some exercise after another hectic day at work.

I ended up walking her to her car and getting her phone number, saying I'd give her a call. That night, as I fed the dogs, showered, and settled in, I thought about her and how natural the conversation had felt on the beach. It felt good knowing I'd see her again.

The next day was busy, and so was the one after that. Running the print shop was nonstop controlled chaos, but we always delivered. Still, I couldn't stop thinking about Heather. Two days after Dog Beach, I gave her a call.

"Took you long enough," she said, half-joking.

"I figured two days was the sweet spot — any sooner and I'd look desperate," I shot back.

She laughed, and after a good little conversation, we set up our first date.

I picked her up at her clean, cozy duplex in Belmont Shores, and we walked to a local restaurant she recommended. She looked cute in a black shirt with a little bird icon on it, and the whole night felt easy — just walking, eating, and talking with a cool girl. We walked back to her place, kissed a little, but she wasn't one to go too far on the first date, and that was fine by me. After a great evening, I headed home and got ready for another busy day at the shop.

We kept going out — not doing anything fancy — but it didn't matter. I just enjoyed being with her. We'd walk or ride bikes along Belmont Shores, or she'd come up to Huntington Beach and I'd show her some of my favorite places to eat, walk, hike, and bike or go to the beach. Each time we hung out, I felt more connected to her.

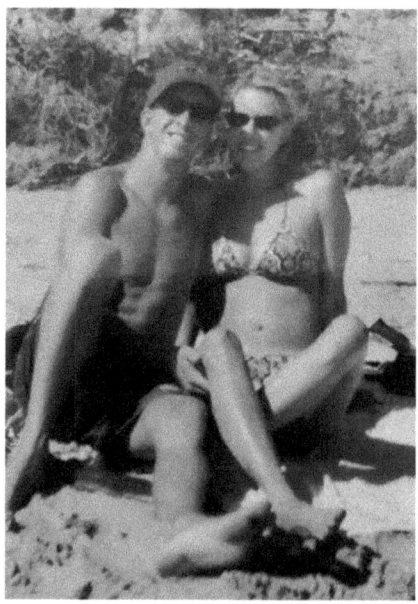

Good beach vibes with Heather

Not long after we met, I found out we shared the same birthday, though she was four years younger. It felt like another sign that we were meant to be together.

One night, I invited her over for dinner at my place, which was close to the middle school where she taught. She usually commuted 20 minutes from Belmont Shores to the Huntington Beach–Westminster border, so it worked out great. I set the table, cooked a nice meal, and after dinner, we walked my dogs, Lucky and Bailey, around the neighborhood. It was another simple but perfect night.

Heather ended up staying over so she could get enough sleep to make it to school the next morning, and after that, we started spending more and more time together. It just kept getting better the more we hung out.

In addition to the walking and biking, we loved hiking down in Laguna Hills. Laguna Beach was beautiful for walking along the ocean and window shopping in the artsy town on PCH. We'd catch movies, comedy shows, live music — always enjoying whatever adventure we chose, often throwing some good food in the mix. Through all those months, it felt easy and seamless just being together.

There's one classic story about us and garlic. We both loved it; we didn't mind the "stinky together" part at all. I'd heard about The Stinking Rose in Beverly Hills, a garlic-themed restaurant, and we looked it up — this was back before you could just pull up everything on your phone. It sounded like the perfect spot for garlic lovers like us, so we made the trip an hour north up to Beverly Hills. The restaurant had an old-school vibe but was packed with people enjoying this quirky little piece of garlic heaven. We ordered garlic appetizers, a garlicky salad, our main course was garlicky with some garlic bread on the side. Dessert wasn't garlic, but I had ordered a piece of cheesecake and I washed it down with some milk, which was my go-to drink with dessert. After we left, overstuffed and satisfied, Heather drove us home. Halfway back, though, my stomach wasn't happy. I rolled down the window at freeway speed and let my dinner take a joy ride outside. When we got home, I noticed her Jeep had a frothy white pinstripe down the passenger side. I had her come around to the other side of her car and we both burst out laughing hysterically! My stomach had given her Jeep Cherokee a new splattered pinstripe paint job it seemed. After our laughing calmed down, I was able to hose down the side of her car and we turned in for the night. Just another good time together and a classic story that I won't forget.

During the winter, we'd hit the mountains to go ski and snowboarding together. Heather tried to pick up boarding, but she took some hard falls on her butt. I was able to guide her from behind, holding her arms and showing her how and when to lean and turn. Since she was also "regular foot," meaning that she stood left foot forward, so taking her through the turns was easier, and it was nice holding her and helping her learn this new sport. It wasn't my usual fast-paced ride down the hill, but I enjoyed spending this time with her. Eventually, she switched back to skiing. On her skis, she could go at a fast pace down most runs. We would be able to enjoy all that the mountain had to offer. We would ride all over either the local mountains, Mammoth, and even up to Tahoe on occasion. We'd spend the whole day dancing across the slopes together, her on skis and me on my board, loving every minute of these days together on the slopes.

Heather was a trooper out in the desert too. We would go camping and riding motorcycles with friends away from the city under the stars, out in our own world.

Besides my daily driver truck that I used for day trips to different tracks and trails to ride moto, I had a Ford E350 van for the trips where I'd camp out with my dogs, my dirt bike, and friends.

Sometimes we'd go meet the crew from Three Brothers Racing in different desert locations or with Damian and friends to Dumont Dunes. Dumont was all sand dunes, wide open without rocks or trails, just massive dunes to carve moto lines however you wanted.

The girlfriends and friends would hang out in camp while the guys went riding, scouting lines and jumps in the dunes. In the evenings, things got wild — gasoline poured and lit on the sand to fire up the night sky, sometimes startling a friend or two, or someone launching over the campfire just for laughs. It was all part of the fun. Making memories in the desert was a blast. Heather fit right in with everyone, and people loved her. No matter what came our way, she and I always found a way to handle it together.

We were a great team.

One time at Ocotillo Wells, Heather borrowed a 90cc fat-wheel bike to ride alongside me and behind me on single-track trails. We were riding on a pretty basic trail, parallel to Pole Line Road. I rolled up another hill with her following me and I saw a steep drop in front of us. I signaled with my hand for her to stop, but she went right past me, not wanting to tip over if she stopped. I watched her go by me and hit the drop, landing about 12 feet down, front wheel first. For a split second, it looked like she'd pull it off, but then she tumbled over the bars.

My heart stopped, but when I got down to where she crashed, she was mostly okay with just a sore ankle. She was able to get back on her bike and just ride down Pole Line Road that regular vehicles would drive down, and we made it back to camp. That night at camp, I still remember her with her foot propped up on our cooler and some ice in a bag over her slightly swollen ankle that wasn't really hurt very badly, thank God!

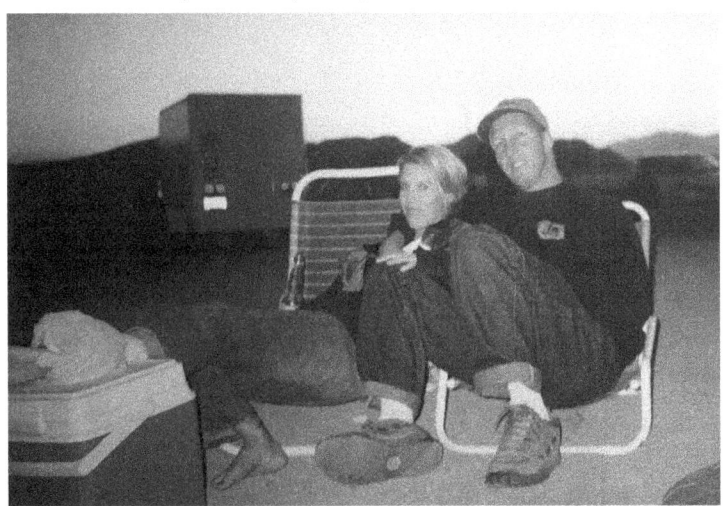

Heather's ankle on ice after her crash

I remember seeing her nose-dive off that cliff trail on the dirt bike and being so worried for her! I knew I loved her, and I didn't want her to get hurt. We relaxed that evening on a nice desert night. I still have the picture of her with her foot up being iced after that crazy adventure riding with her that day. I'm so glad she was OK!

Glamis Crash

Glamis — where the sand seems to stretch to infinity and the sound of engines fills the air from all around. It was the early 2000s, and while the place wasn't really my scene, it still had its pull. The dunes attracted every kind of dune buggy, each more outrageous than the last, flexing horsepower and custom builds to a roaring audience in different pockets of the sand dunes. But I wasn't there for the show-and-tell that some people thrived on.

Motocross tracks were always a blast — especially when it came to big jumps — but my heart was also in the technical side of riding. I loved navigating obstacles, *threading through* rock gardens, and chasing the rush of pinning it down trails. I was constantly hunting for features to click, blip, and flow with, or steep climbs to charge straight up. Wide-open sand was fun every once in a while, but with no features to work with, it felt kind of bland and repetitive — what I really craved were *sharp, intricate lines* through challenging, ever-changing terrain.

Still, I wasn't one to sit out an adventure, so I agreed to go with a buddy there. That day, I found myself leading a crew of six moto friends, carving flowing lines through the rolling dunes. The sheer vastness made the ride feel almost endless, but then I spotted a jump that called out to me. Years of snowboarding had honed my eye for lines, and after riding moto on and off for years, I could already picture the arc of this jump in my mind.

A 70-foot gap loomed between takeoff and landing, and I knew exactly how I wanted to hit it. Rolling over the jump once to size it up, then I came around again, this time pinned in third gear, and sent it. Clean landing — smooth as butter.

We flowed deeper into the dunes, the crew trusting me to show them the way. That's when I saw the next one — a bigger version of the last jump. This jump screamed fourth gear, wide open, and a 100-foot gap to clear to the crest of the landing. I couldn't resist. I rolled up slowly and over the takeoff to scope the line. I could see the landing 100 feet in front of me — yep, I got this.

When I hit it for real, I came flying into the takeoff in fourth gear. But the suspension compressed more than I expected from the speed and transition. Oh no — my *skid plate* scraped the sand on the way up, stealing just enough speed. The arc of my flight changed instantly. Instead of landing clean down the backside, I came up short and slammed into the steep upside of the dune before the landing.

The impact ripped through me, but all I could feel was my left ankle screaming in pain. My friends raced over as I sat there, trying to process what just happened. Through clenched teeth, I said, "Take my boot off before my ankle swells, or you'll never get it off." It was a brutal kind of urgency, but they managed to wiggle it free. That's when my leg dropped, unnaturally bent at 90 degrees. My tibia bone was poking through the skin of my shin, right in the middle of my lower leg. I had snapped both my tibia and fibula clean in half.

Two of my friends sped off to get help, while the others stayed with me. When they came back, they had a makeshift first-aid kit for the situation: two one-foot-long 2x4s and a roll of duct tape. We splinted my leg right there in the dunes, wrapping it tight, then hauled me back to camp before driving to Brawley Hospital out in the desert.

At the hospital, the news wasn't great, but it wasn't unexpected: I'd need a titanium rod inserted straight through my tibia from knee to ankle to hold everything together. It would be the first of two rods that leg would eventually endure. "Good times," I thought, half-laughing through gritted teeth.

When I finally got a phone call out, I called Heather. I kept it simple, though I knew she'd hear the weight in my voice. "I messed up," I told her. "I miscalculated a jump and crashed pretty bad. They're putting a rod in my leg."

And Heather? She didn't hesitate. She drove hours into the desert to find me recovering in a hospital bed, far from home and in rough shape. When she walked into my hospital room, it wasn't just relief I felt — it was love, pure and strong. She came to get me, to take me home to Orange County where I could start recovering and piecing myself back together.

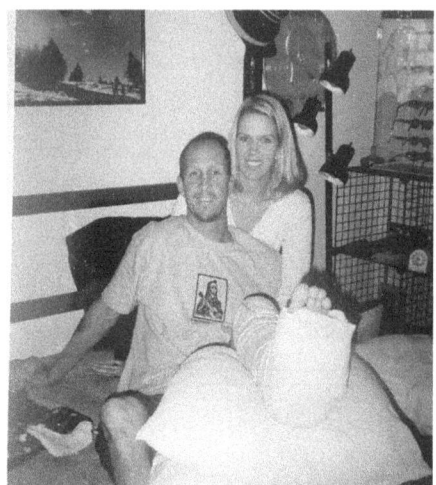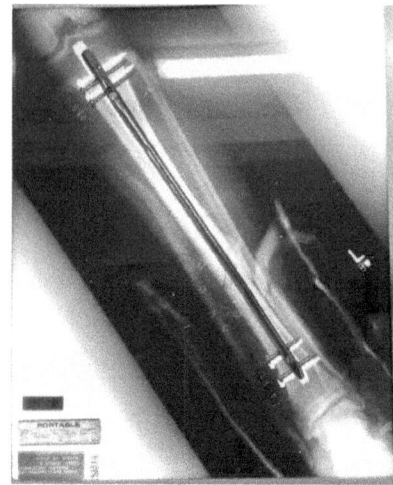

Rod in my leg, Heather by my side

Heather was my partner, my anchor. No matter what happened, we had each other's backs. That day, she didn't just bring me home — she reminded me why she was my rock through the ups and downs of life. I could tell we were meant to be together. It just felt right.

After nearly two years with Heather, filled with incredible times and unforgettable memories, I knew I wanted to spend my life with her. I had the idea to take her to Costa Rica — a place I'd been a few times on surf trips with friends. Costa Rica had everything: beautiful landscapes, warm ocean water, great weather, and even some surf. But this trip wasn't about riding waves; it was about us and the future I saw together.

Before I even mentioned the trip to Heather, I had a few things to figure out. I'd talked to my mom several times about Heather, telling her how I knew she was the one. Mom had met Heather many times, and they got along right from the start. Heather could hold her own in any conversation, carrying herself with a natural warmth and ease. She was a schoolteacher, and people took to her instantly — students, colleagues, pretty much anyone she met. Her students always told her how much they loved having her, whether it was for English literature or her art class. Everyone saw what I saw in her, and that meant a lot to me.

One day, my mom surprised me.

My dad had passed away in 1999 from stomach cancer. He'd been a huge influence on me — he was a feisty guy who refused to go to the doctor when his stomach hurt. I remember him not being able to join our small family for Thanksgiving dinner, and he was gone before Christmas. I thought he was going to live to 100, and maybe he would have if it wasn't for the devil disease, cancer.

He was one of the original health nuts before it was a trend. Growing up in Reseda, I remember him making "date shakes" every morning — blending bananas, dates, wheat germ, fish oil, raw eggs, and milk. He'd pour it into cups for me and my sister Karen, insisting we have some before heading to school. These days I've kept the habit with my own protein shakes a few times a week, loaded with healthy ingredients.

One day, when visiting my mom, she pulled out her wedding ring and offered the diamond for me to use for Heather's engagement ring, giving me her blessing. I didn't hesitate. "Thanks, Mom! This is awesome! I love you!" I said.

With the diamond in hand, I borrowed one of Heather's rings to get the sizing right. After all, I was Double O Szabo — always ready for a mission — and this was a great one.

I also went to speak with Heather's parents. Her dad, Ed, was a character — a classic old school salesman type, but not the slick or slimy kind. He was down-to-earth and he sold products to big companies with charm and honesty.

Her family was a lot like mine. Both of our parents were older, even though my dad was eighteen years older than my mom. I told Ed that I wanted to marry his daughter and make her very happy. He had gotten to know me over the past couple of years and liked me. After hearing my plan, he gave me his approval, and I shook his hand firmly, saying, "Thank you. She makes me so happy, and I plan on doing the same for her."

With everything set, I asked Heather if she'd like to go to Costa Rica that summer. She'd soon be off for her school break, so the timing was perfect.

We flew into San Jose, picked up a rental car, and kicked off the adventure. First, we explored the mountains and volcano areas. We didn't have much of a plan, so when we got lost, we'd stop and ask the locals. We spent a few days exploring ancient sites and did some horseback riding in that area, then packed up and headed to the jungle.

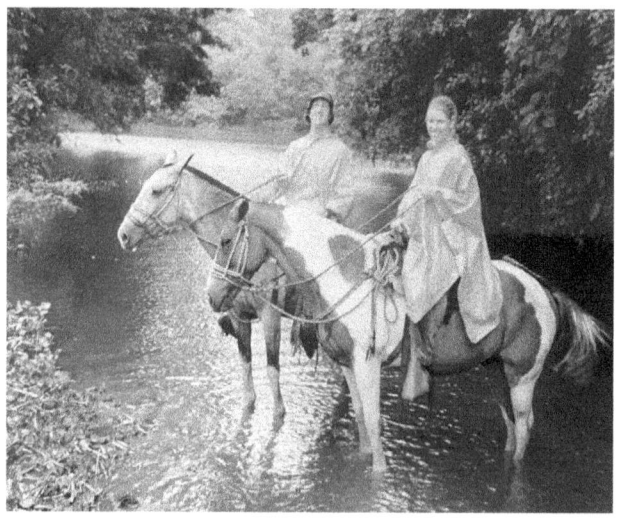

Hoofing it with style in Costa Rica

In the jungle, we were surrounded by massive trees and lush greenery. We crossed old rope-and-wood bridges that swayed and bounced with every step, giving you that adrenaline rush each time. We saw monkeys, exotic birds, and heard all kinds of wildlife in the dense jungle. At one point, I half-expected Tarzan to swing by — but he never did.

We did some zip-line tours — Costa Rica is known for them. Some ziplines were incredibly high, soaring above the jungle, while others wove tightly between the trees. We'd relay from one zip-line to another, sometimes climbing down rock faces or trees to reach the next part of the adventure. After a couple of hours, we'd come down pumped and ready to enjoy some good food and jungle vibes at a restaurant built right into the landscape. Eventually, we'd relax back at our place, soaking it all in.

After a few days, it was time to head to the beach town of Tamarindo. I constantly checked to make sure I still had the engagement ring safely hidden, especially as our bags got tossed in and out of hotels and the rental car. Luckily, everything stayed on track as we made our way to the next destination.

When we got to Tamarindo, the warm ocean breeze and laid-back vibe of the town welcomed us. Our place had bright, colorful tiles with a touch of Aztec flavor that matched the Costa Rican style perfectly.

After settling in, we went out for dinner at a spot right on the beach. As the sun set, we took a nice walk along the shore, holding hands and just enjoying the moment.

As the timing felt right, I gently pulled her hand, turned her to face me, and dropped to one knee. I pulled out the ring I'd been carrying for seven of our ten days in Costa Rica and asked her to marry me.

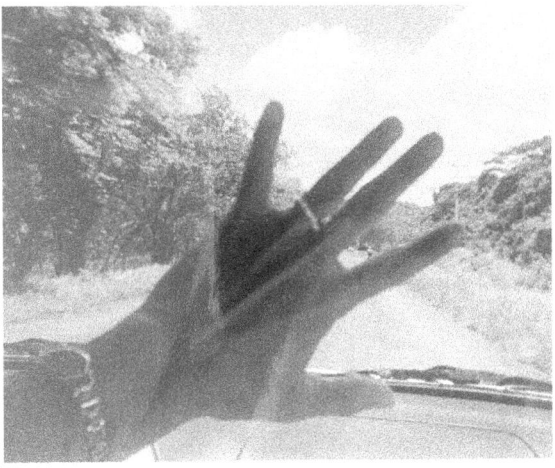

Mission accomplished, OO seals the ring deal

She said yes.

We hugged, we kissed, we laughed — and that moment marked the start of a whole new adventure together.

The rest of our trip was a blur of happiness, making plans, and soaking up the beauty of Costa Rica. We came back engaged, ready for everything life had ahead of us.

After getting engaged, we started planning to move in together. Since my house was just down the street from the middle school where she taught, it made perfect sense for Heather to move in. But first, she had to clear out her duplex in Belmont Shores, and a garage sale seemed like the best way to lighten the load.

It was early Saturday morning in the summer of 2002, around 6 a.m. We spread her furniture and other stuff across the front lawn. People were already starting to show up, scanning everything.

As we were getting everything set up, Heather offered to grab us some coffee and donuts from a spot just down the street.

She asked me to stay out front and handle the garage sale while she was gone, figuring I could hold down the fort.

Not long after she left, a guy pulled up and immediately looked like he'd struck gold. His eyes went wide as he scanned the tables, chairs, lamps, and all the garage-sale furniture.

"This is perfect!" he said, almost like he couldn't believe his luck.

He explained he was moving into a new place and needed furniture to fill it up. "How much for everything?" he asked.

Without giving it too much thought, I threw out a number that seemed fair.

He must have thought so too because he immediately said, "I'll take it!"

He pulled up his big flatbed truck and started loading everything up.

By the time Heather came back with our coffee and donuts, most of her stuff was gone.

She looked around, wide-eyed, and asked, "Where's all my stuff?"

I handed her the wad of cash, thinking she'd be happy, but she raised an eyebrow. "You sold it all for this?"

She laughed, shaking her head, realizing she'd left me with a little too much responsibility.

In the end, though, we both appreciated that we didn't have to sit around all day.

We enjoyed our donuts, packed up what little was left, and headed home — to start our new life together.

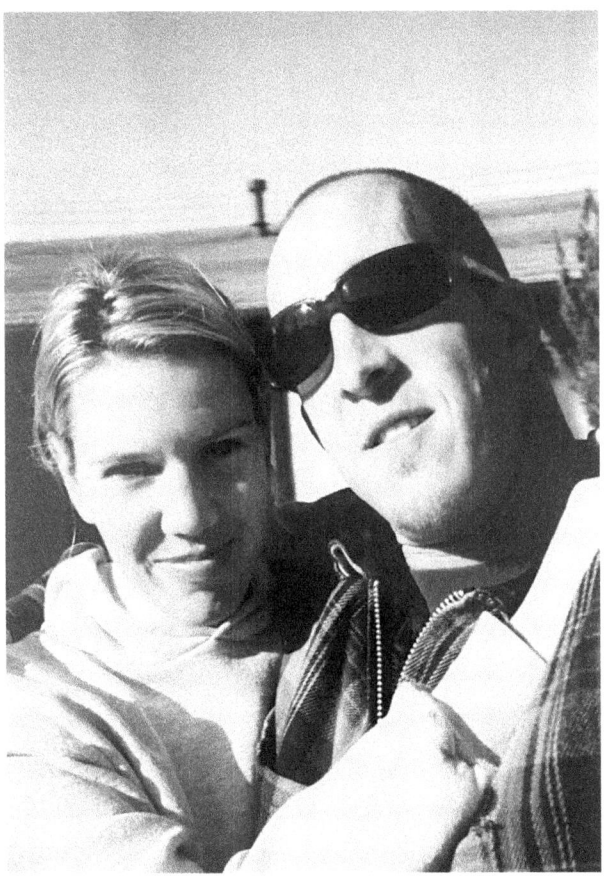

Start of our new life — my house, now our home.

-Chapter 11-
Married with Children

Living with Heather felt so natural. My home became our shared space, and her teaching job was only a mile away, making her commute easy. A quick zigzag down the side streets would bring her to her parents' house, just across the main road. Everything seemed to align perfectly.

It felt like the universe had lined things up for us, almost as if by magic. I'm not one to believe in magic, but I do believe things happen for a reason.

The following year was full of shared adventures and quiet moments that strengthened our bond. Heather poured her heart into teaching while I stayed focused on running the print shop. Outside of work, we enjoyed our time together but also kept our individual interests. I was still riding motocross for that rush of adrenaline, and she spent time with her close friends. She often visited her parents just down the street, and everything felt easy.

We'd spend holidays together, visiting her parents or having my mom and sister Karen join us. Sometimes we'd host; other times we'd meet at their places or dine out. Our families were small, but those gatherings were filled with quality time, weaving into the rhythm of our lives.

We started planning our wedding for the following summer. After checking out a few places, we agreed on the Pageant of the Masters venue in Laguna Canyon. It was beautiful, nestled in a special area that already held meaning for us. Laguna was like a world apart from Huntington Beach even though it was only 30 minutes south. While Huntington was beautiful with its grid of streets and rows of palm trees, Laguna had a natural, untouched quality. The rolling hills, lush trees, and winding roads created an earthy charm, with Laguna Canyon as the centerpiece. Heather and I spent time hiking in those hills, going to the beach, window shopping, and eating out in that beautiful area. It became the perfect spot to start our life together.

The big day arrived, and everything was set. My best men and Heather's bridesmaids stood by our sides as we prepared to say our vows. Earlier that day, we had taken some incredible photos down by Laguna Beach. Our photographer found the perfect spot, capturing the ocean's beauty alongside Heather's radiance in her wedding dress. She looked stunning, her dress and makeup highlighting everything I loved about her. Once the photos wrapped up, we hurried back to the venue, ensuring we had the rings ready and were set to begin the ceremony.

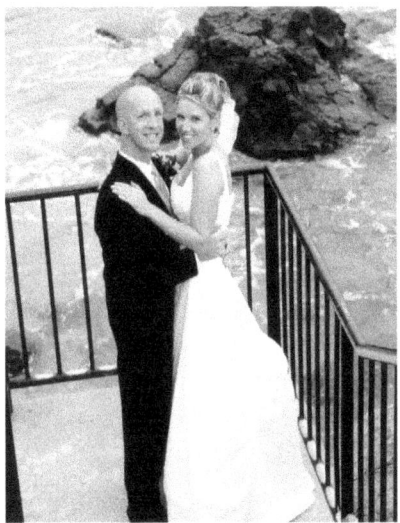

Wedding day vibes in Laguna

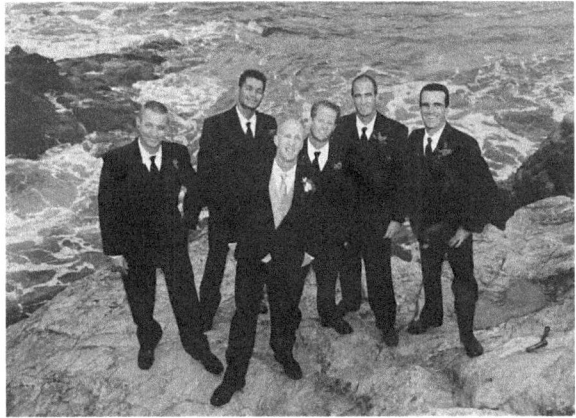

Locked in with the best man crew on the rocks

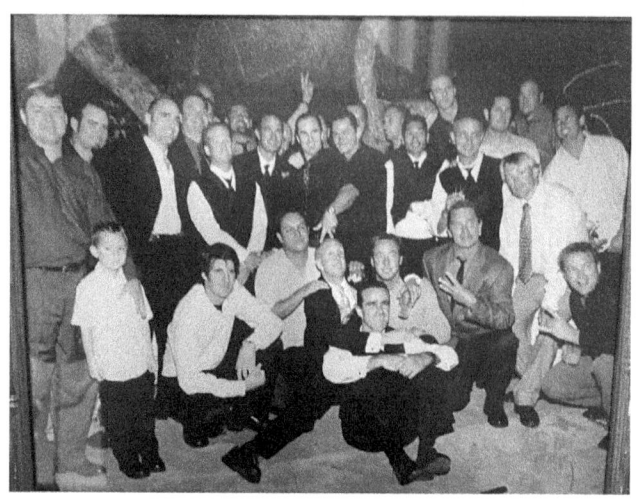

All the boyz on wedding night

The ceremony was beautiful, with the Pageant of the Masters venue comfortably hosting our 100 guests. Family and friends filled the space with familiar faces from different chapters of our lives. We stood together, surrounded by love and support, committing to one another, "till death do us part."

After the wedding, we headed to Kauai for our honeymoon, staying in a cozy condo owned by my friend Wing Lam, founder of Wahoo's Fish Tacos. I remembered when Wing had just one location in Costa Mesa back in the late '80s — a hard-working guy with big dreams. Wahoo's became iconic by serving health-conscious meals with bold flavors, clean ingredients, and an action sports vibe. It now has over 60 locations and counting.

Wing gives back to the community in so many ways — from donating thousands of meals to those in need, to supporting the Surfrider Foundation, and inspiring the next generation by speaking at multiple colleges. He shares his story with students and entrepreneurs, showing how passion, adaptability, and community involvement can drive both business growth and lasting impact. Proud of him and all that he does.

Wing's condo was perfectly located on Kauai's coast, giving us access to explore both the drier northern areas and the dense, tropical south.

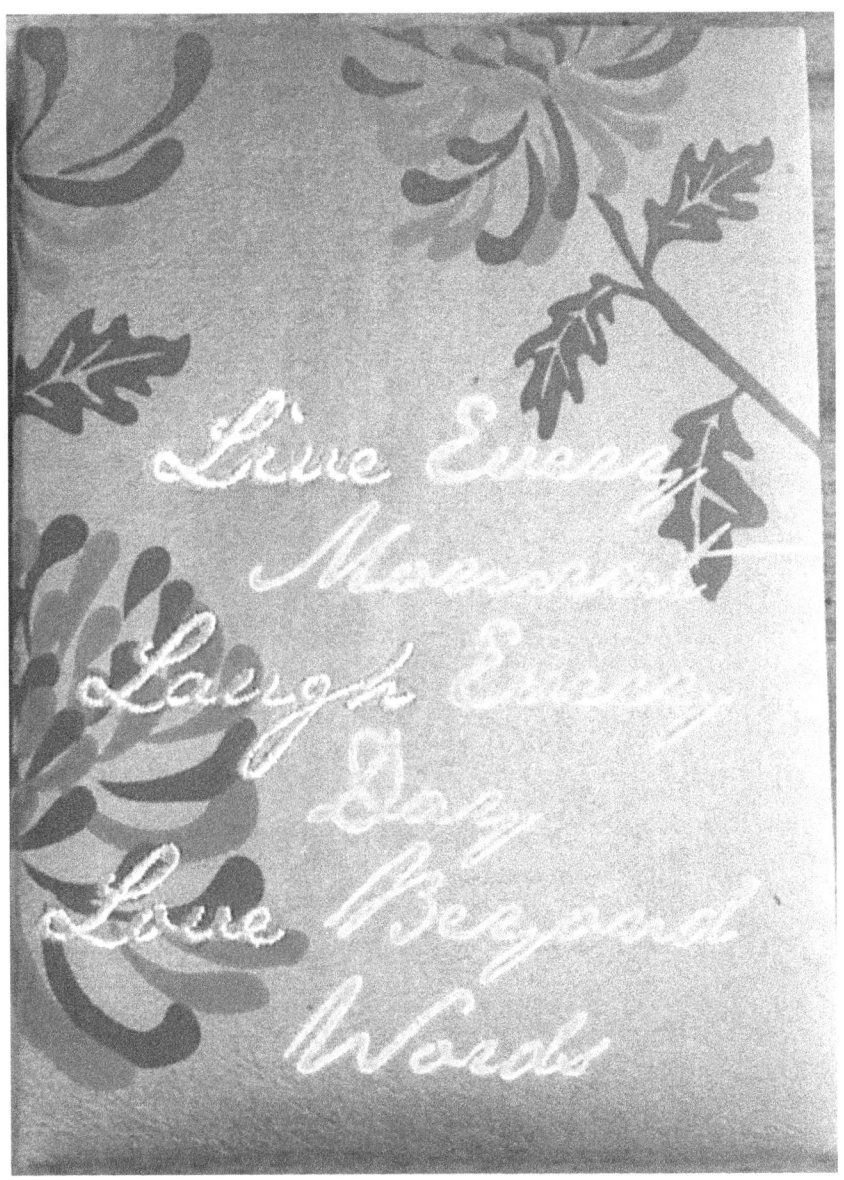

This love and life book was for Heather. The love that we shared lives on in these pages.

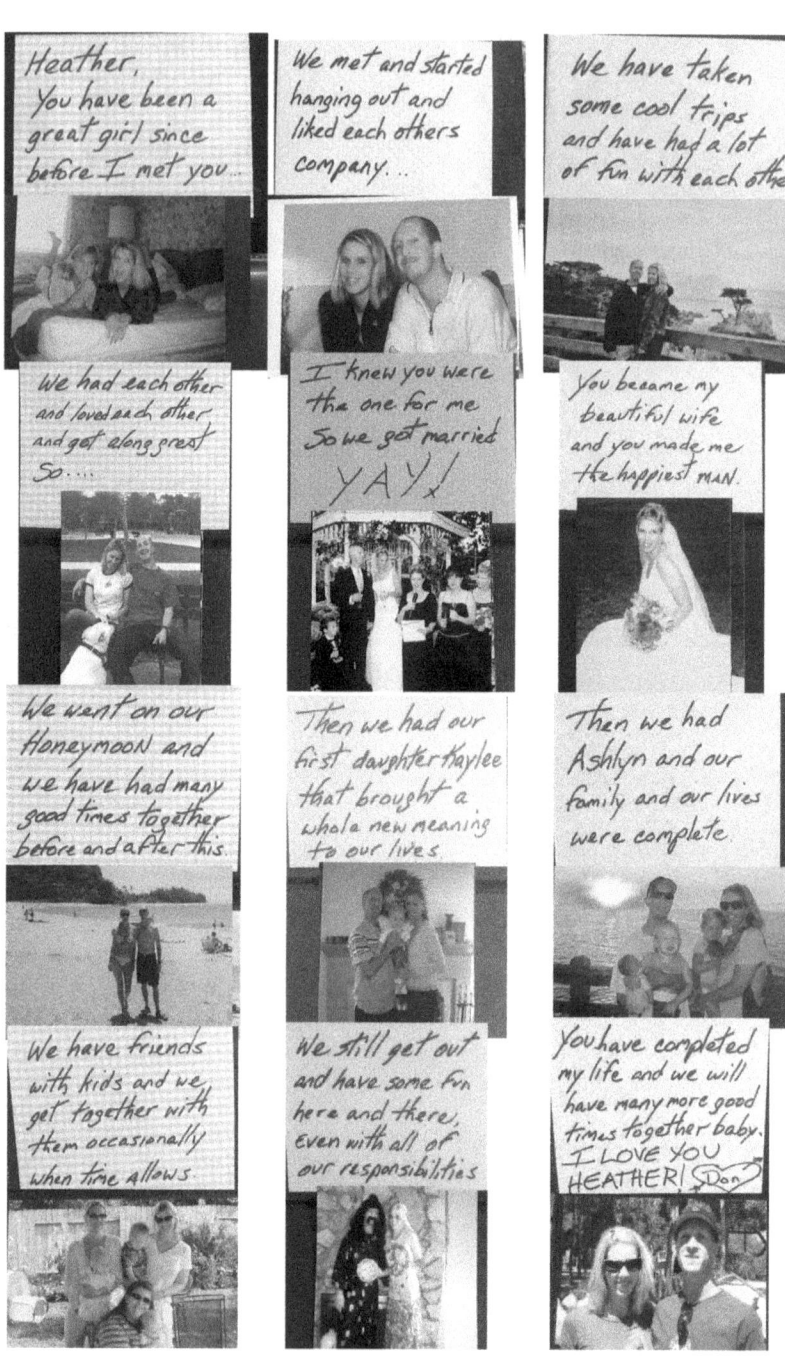

12 Photos and words in the book — one love story

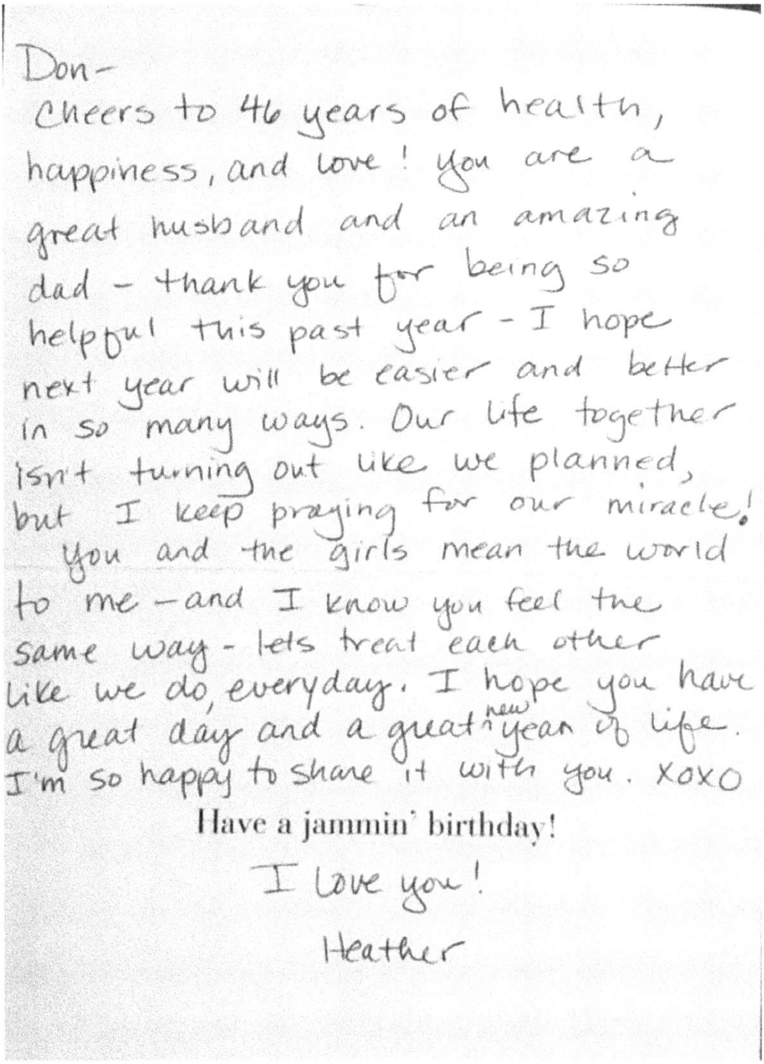

Don—

Cheers to 46 years of health, happiness, and love! You are a great husband and an amazing dad — thank you for being so helpful this past year — I hope next year will be easier and better in so many ways. Our life together isn't turning out like we planned, but I keep praying for our miracle! You and the girls mean the world to me — and I know you feel the same way — lets treat each other like we do, everyday. I hope you have a great day and a great new year of life. I'm so happy to share it with you. XOXO

Have a jammin' birthday!

I love you!

Heather

This letter still brings back emotions. Her words were filled with love, hope, and honesty — even as life was writing a different ending than we hoped for.

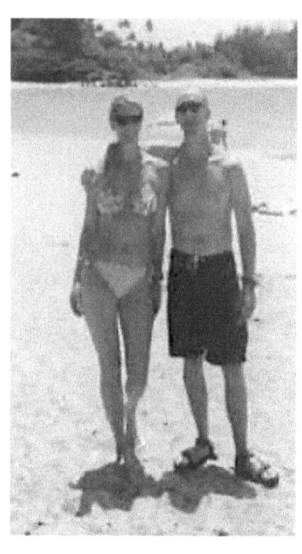

Kauai was sweet

From snorkeling in the warm, colorful waters filled with fish and coral, to hiking, chasing waterfalls, horseback riding, enjoying great meals, and soaking in the beautiful surroundings — it was the kind of trip that let us slow down, be present, and simply enjoy each other. Just the two of us, no distractions — starting our new chapter in a place that felt like paradise.

After our Kauai honeymoon, we returned to Orange County with the last bit of summer still in front of us. Heather didn't have to get back to work immediately, thanks to her teaching schedule, which allowed her summers off. Though I had to run the shop during the week, we still managed to steal time for each other. We'd catch the sunset after a quick walk, bike ride, or hike. Going down to the beach where we'd met became a special part of our routine. Sometimes, Heather would bring her parents' dog along, and we'd head to Dog Beach with my dogs, Lucky and Bailey, letting them run leash-free. Watching them frolic and do what dogs do was such a simple pleasure. Closing out the summer this way felt comfortable and natural — like the two of us were exactly where we were supposed to be, taking care of each other with love and respect.

What once seemed like the worst thing to happen — my devastating shoulder injuries and surgeries that eventually ended my snowboarding career — now felt like a twisted blessing. Those injuries had led me down a different path, one where I'd found Heather. If I hadn't been injured, I wouldn't have been jogging along the beach with my dogs that day or running the print shop Jon and I owned. Life has a way of working itself out in ways you don't expect. Sometimes you think you know your path, but there's another plan you can't see, waiting for you just around the bend.

Heather and I had planned on having kids. We discussed our future and thought we'd aim to have our first baby in early summer so she could enjoy her maternity leave over the summer break when she wasn't teaching. True to plan, in June 2004, we welcomed our first baby girl, Kaylee. We'd initially settled on the name Kylie, but after running into my old friend Seth Enslow and then remembering that he had a daughter named Kylie, I decided I couldn't go through with it. I've always been a little quirky like that — even down to what I order at restaurants — I don't like having the same thing as anyone else. So Heather and I came up with Kaylee, and it fit perfectly. Kaylee was a beautiful baby, but loud right from the start. We quickly learned that life with a newborn meant disrupted sleep, but every bit of it felt worth it for the joy she brought that summer. Heather was a natural mom, handling those early months like she was made for it.

When Thanksgiving came around, we packed up and headed to the desert with our Three Brothers Racing family, a tradition for us. Heather enjoyed hanging out with the other wives and moms, and we all gathered in a big camp circle, making the most of those long weekends together. Now that we had a baby, staying in just the van wasn't enough, so we brought our new *toy hauler* for a bit of desert luxury.

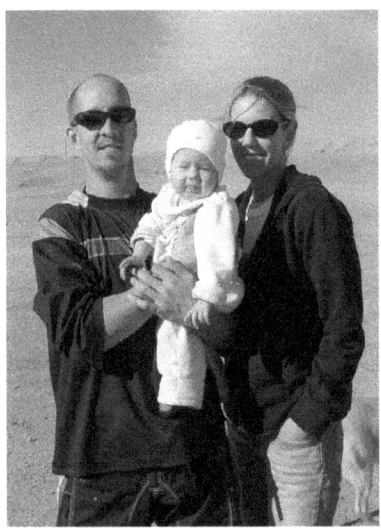

Desert dayz with baby Kaylee

Kaylee's first birthday arrived, and we hosted a party at our place. Friends came over, and it turned into a laid-back gathering, with some beers and a lot of laughter. I proudly showed everyone the thatched structure over our above-ground jacuzzi — a mini oasis that my friend John Brewton helped me build. I remembered a moment when Kaylee, just six months old, was in a floaty beside me in the jacuzzi. At one point, I turned away to grab something, and when I turned back, she had flipped upside down. My heart nearly stopped, but I quickly righted her, realizing those few seconds had felt like an eternity. That moment stuck with me — a reminder of the delicate balance between life's joy and worry. At her party, Kaylee seemed more interested in the wrapping paper than the presents. She even got frosting all over her face, looking as cute as ever.

By then, our shop was running smoothly enough that Heather could take the entire year off instead of just three summer months for her maternity leave. It was a blessing to have that time, and the business allowed us the flexibility to spend time together and take trips throughout the year. We took Kaylee to Yosemite, a place of unmatched beauty that we'd visited many times. The granite rock, towering trees, and landscapes painted by nature herself — it was a place we loved sharing with her. We also took her on more camping trips to the desert, and soon enough, Kaylee was walking, talking, and joining us with Lucky and Bailey on outings to the local parks. Life felt complete and joyful.

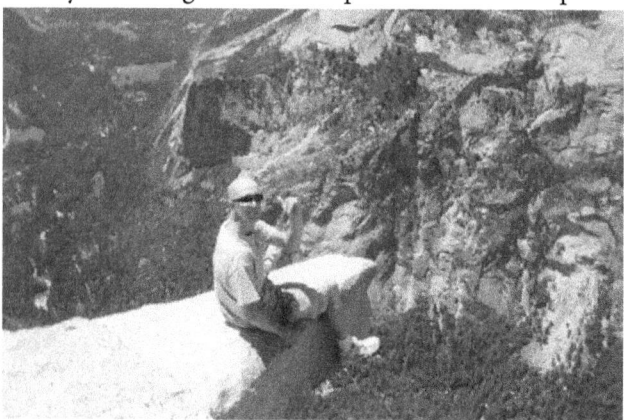

Yosemite's Half Dome — over 2,000 feet straight down beneath me

We knew we wanted another child to complete our family — a sibling for

Kaylee to share her life with, just like our dogs had each other, and Heather and I had each other too.

In the summer of 2005, I found our dream home in a great neighborhood in Huntington Beach, just a mile from the ocean. It was a beautiful two-story house with a three-car garage, a bonus room above it, a pool, a built-in jacuzzi, and a barbecue. We could envision raising our family there, and it was in an excellent school district for our kids. Heather had concerns about the pool, so we agreed to install a locking fence for safety — something her dad generously offered to cover.

Settling into that house felt like another step toward the future we had dreamed of. In July 2006, our second daughter, Ashlyn, was born. Kaylee, now two years old, proudly embraced her role as the big sister, wanting to help tuck Ashlyn into her crib and do "big girl" things. Watching her become a loving, protective sister felt like our family had come full circle, each piece falling into place just as it was meant to be.

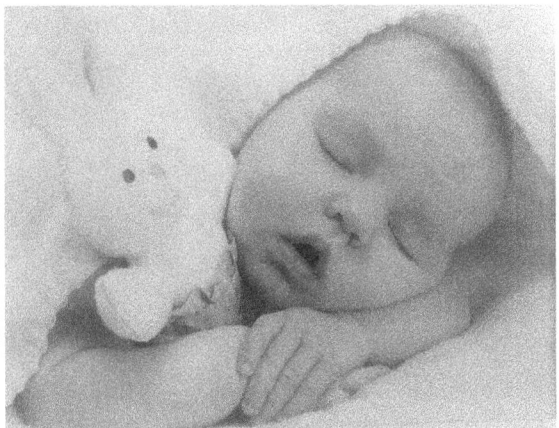

Baby Ashlyn, too cute

Kids and Sports

Life was moving in a whole new rhythm. We had found the house we'd always dreamed of, and with two beautiful daughters and Heather by my side, life had become something I could never have pictured back in my sports-only days. The love for my family — the love for my kids — was an experience like nothing I'd ever known. Watching our daughters grow, each new stage felt like a new adventure. We'd take walks, share family dinners, and spend countless hours at parks where they'd swing, climb, and laugh — just being kids. Those playgrounds became places where we'd all let loose; even I couldn't resist joining in on the fun sometimes, channeling the old kid inside me.

In our Huntington Beach neighborhood, just a few houses down, was a family with two daughters the same ages as ours. It was like we'd hit the neighborhood lottery. We had a beautiful house, and a great local school right around the corner where we could walk our daughters to kindergarten and grade school — what a score! Every morning during the week, Heather was off to teach her students, and I would walk the kids to school. The neighbor family's mom, Michelle, would sometimes have her kids ready for me and the girls to scoop up and walk to the school if she couldn't walk too. Seeing the four of them — our daughters and theirs — walking together, laughing, and sharing stories made those mornings special. Their eyes sparkled with the kind of wonder that only young kids have, and it was clear this was the beginning of some special friendships.

Heather had to teach her own students, but my flexible schedule let me be there to walk the kids and still manage the business. Sure, some days were busier than others, but we made it work. It was all part of the blend — the give and take that made family life flow.

In those years, I felt that natural urge to share my love of sports with our daughters. Snowboarding was still my passion on the slopes, and while I was excited to introduce Heather to it, we both soon realized skiing was more her style. But that didn't stop us from hitting the slopes together, each in our own way, carving down the mountain, finding our rhythm side by side.

Those memories — of young love and awesome days in the mountains — still warm my heart from those early years with Heather, when everything just seemed to click. Now reflecting on the early days with our daughters, I still remember them scootering around on the sidewalks out front. They'd put their right foot forward at first, until I stepped in and taught them the "regular foot" stance — left foot forward, right foot pushing — just like their dad. It was my way of getting them ready for skateboarding and snowboarding.

To me, skateboarding was like dancing — only better. Dancing was never my thing, but on a board, I felt right at home. Soon enough, the girls were riding around the neighborhood with me — one at a time at first as they started to skate on their own, and then both of them on their own skateboards. Circling the block together, my heart couldn't have been happier.

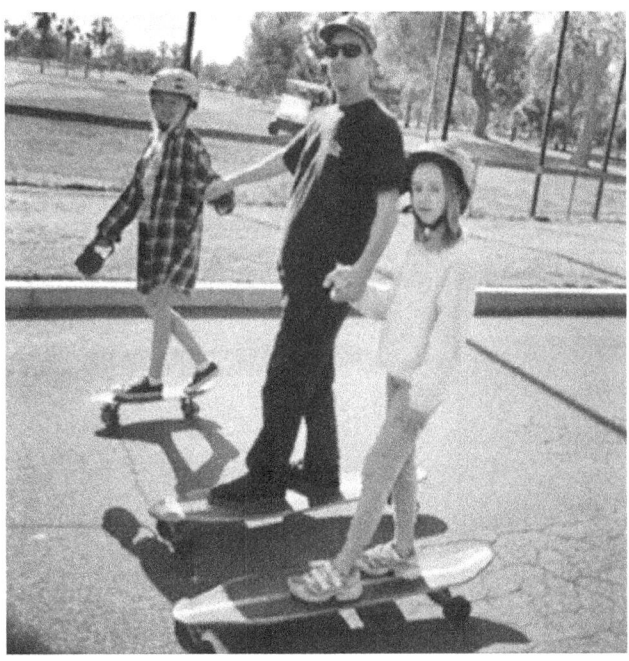

Taught girls to ride regular foot — easier to teach 'em

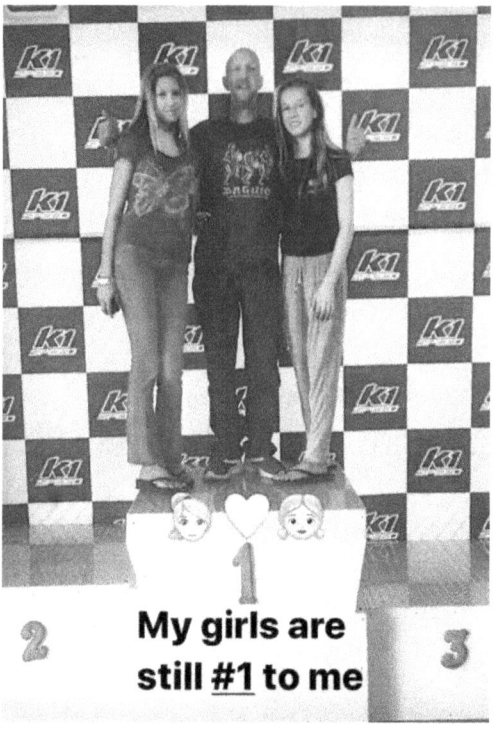

My girls are still #1 to me

Life had its rhythm — keeping the shop running smoothly with a dash of controlled chaos, Heather teaching, and our family adventures all blended together in a life that felt full and complete. The years clicked by, with holidays and visits to the desert with friends and family. Thanksgiving with the "Three Brothers" desert crew became a tradition, a blend of familiar faces and the wild unknown of the desert — bonfires, motorcycles, and stories swapped under a sky so clear it made you forget the city ever existed. The desert had a way of drawing out adventure, whether it was someone's bike breaking down or someone running out of gas on the trails. No matter what came up, we always had each other's backs and made it back to camp in a circle of trailers that felt like a little world all our own.

Taking Kaylee and Ashlyn out on their little *quads* was another joy. Sometimes we'd ride loops near camp, or I'd take them on mini destination missions out in the desert. Watching them navigate, throttle, and brake — seeing them on their own little adventures — was heartwarming. Sharing those experiences with my daughters filled me with pride and happiness.

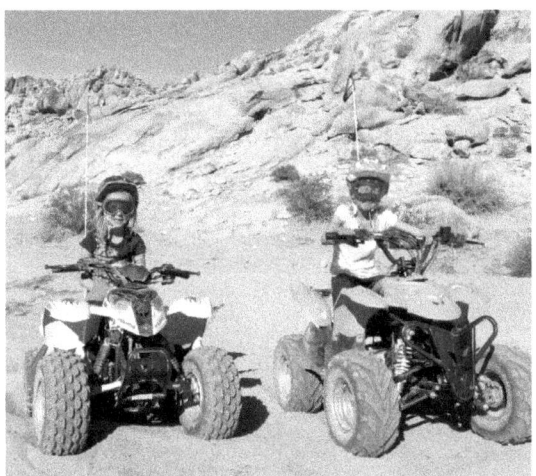

Kids on Quads

Those 3 Bros campouts were special and they had become a big part of our lives. They'd host campouts where customers and friends gathered — up to thirty trailers deep — sharing food, rides, and stories. My daughters loved the "yummy meat," as Ashlyn called it. The brothers would grill up Brazilian-style barbecue, and everyone would hang around grabbing bites hot off the grill as we talked about what had happened and what was coming up.

Ricardo, the owner and my good friend, became like family to us. We'd known each other for almost 20 years, bonded not by business — though we did make stickers for 3 Bros — but by shared passions. When Ricardo passed away in 2024 from a heart attack while on the track at Glen Helen Raceway, it left a hole in the community. He went doing what he loved, riding his dirt bike. His celebration of life was packed with hundreds who, like me, had camped, ridden, shopped at 3 Bros, and shared memories with him. We mourned a man who had given so much to all of us, and though it was a goodbye, it was also a tribute to the life he'd led — his heart and life throttle wide open. Love and miss you, my friend. Ride In Peace 🙏.

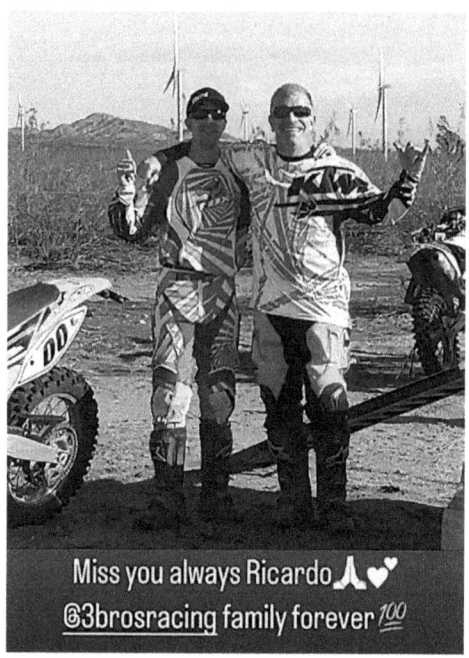

Miss you always Ricardo 🙏 💙
@3brosracing family forever 💯

25 years of friendship. Ride In Peace, Ricardo

The outdoors became our family's playground. In winter, we'd head to the local mountains — sledding in the early days, then we would go snowboarding in Wrightwood or Big Bear. When the girls were a bit older, they learned to snowboard and ski. Heather would sometimes join on skis, though she'd let me take the girls up by myself many of the times. We had friends like Todd Proffit, an old local pro from my snowboarding days who worked at Mountain High, which meant lift tickets on the house — something we appreciated, since life had shifted from sponsorships to family expenses. Ashlyn took to snowboarding. Kaylee did at first, but she ended up feeling more at ease on skis, like her mom. We made a pretty good crew on the slopes — two snowboarders, two skiers, and one tight-knit family.

We'd also make trips to Yosemite National Park to camp and hike almost every year for a few years. Standing before those granite cliffs, shaped over millions of years by Mother Nature, left me awestruck every time. I remember one year taking Ashlyn to a waterhole up there. I gave her a demonstration of how to dive between two rocks into the clear, cool water. I came to shore, and I knew she could do it — her gymnastics skills had blown me away time and again. With my phone camera ready, I said, "Hit it!"

I watched her make a graceful dive, nailing the right spot perfectly. The photo I posted on Facebook drew some comments from friends worried I'd put her in danger. They didn't get it. They couldn't see the skill it took or the calculated risk involved. To me, life wasn't about playing it safe all the time — it was about seeing things differently, looking at challenges from unique angles, and embracing the flow that action sports had instilled in me.

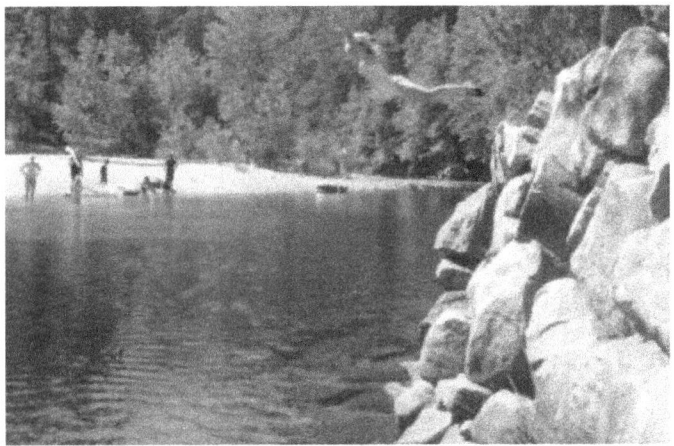

Calculated risk, perfect dive — Ashlyn nailed it at 7 years old

Not everyone gets it — the mindset, the calculated risk, the thrill of pushing boundaries. Most people live inside the lines, but that's never been me. Watching Ashlyn make that dive felt like passing down a part of who I am, a love for taking on the extraordinary. It's a memory I hold close — a reminder that my daughters inherited not only my passion for sports at the time, but also the resilience and drive to see life from a different perspective.

Chapter 12

Heather, The Final Goodbye.

The day Heather's sister Barb called her with a suggestion would forever change the trajectory of our lives. Barb had read about the BRCA2 gene and urged Heather that they should get tested, given their family history. Both of their parents had battled breast cancer and won, so it felt like a necessary precaution. Heather agreed, and soon after, they both underwent genetic testing.

The results were a mixed bag. Barb was in the clear — no sign of the BRCA2 gene, no looming threat of cancer. Heather, however, wasn't so fortunate. The test revealed that she carried the BRCA2 gene, a genetic marker that significantly increased her risk of developing breast and ovarian cancer. Worse yet, the doctors found a small lump in one of her breasts. Although it was caught at the earliest possible stage — Stage Zero — it was enough to set off alarm bells.

The medical team recommended an aggressive approach: a double mastectomy and an oophorectomy to prevent ovarian cancer. Since we already had the two kids we wanted, this felt like the safest way forward. At the time, it seemed like the best plan to put this threat behind us and give Heather a clean slate. We clung to the idea that catching it so early meant nothing could go wrong — and nothing was brought to our attention to suggest otherwise.

Heather and I even tried to keep things lighthearted when discussing her double mastectomy with close friends, joking that she got a "free boob job" out of the deal. It felt reassuring to believe we were beating cancer before it could even start.

But life has a cruel way of showing how little control we really have. What we thought was the end of the battle was only the beginning of a far darker fight. We were wrong in thinking we'd outrun cancer.

This was the prelude to a nightmare we couldn't yet imagine — a nightmare that would surface two years later with pain in Heather's neck and back. The devil we thought we'd defeated came roaring back to claim her, to take her from this world and from all of us who loved her.

Looking back, those early moments of diagnosis feel so naïve, so full of misplaced optimism — and with no info shared with us that anything could go south later. At stage zero, it seemed impossible that anything would go wrong. But cancer doesn't play by the rules, and its return was as relentless as it was devastating. This chapter of Heather's story begins with hope — but it doesn't end that way.

Two years after Heather's surgeries, life had lulled us into a fragile sense of normalcy. But one morning, Heather woke up with pain in her neck and back — a deep, relentless ache that grew worse by the day. At first, we didn't think much of it. The doctors dismissed it as a likely pinched nerve, suggesting she take it easy and wait for it to subside. But the pain didn't go away. It followed her like a shadow, dragging her down little by little. It wasn't just a pinched nerve, but we wanted to believe it was nothing. We wanted to believe we were still free of cancer's grip.

A few weeks later, we joined friends on a camping trip to Ocotillo Wells. Heather loved the outdoors — the freedom of the open desert, the hum of quads and dirt bikes, the connection we shared with friends out there. But that trip was different. Her pain had become so unbearable that she couldn't climb the ladder to the high pull-down bed in our toy hauler. Watching her struggle broke my heart. We had to make a makeshift bed on the floor, in the space where the quads and bikes were usually parked during transport. I remember holding her hand that night and whispering, "Babe, you need to go back to the doctor. Something isn't right." She nodded, but I could see the fear in her eyes.

When we returned home after the trip, she was finally able to schedule a PET scan. I'll never forget sitting in that sterile hospital room, staring at the scan results. Her neck and spine lit up like a Christmas tree — a glowing map of devastation. Cancer. Stage Four. After everything — the surgeries, the optimism, the belief that we'd caught it early enough to win — this happened.

The doctors explained that even with Stage Zero breast cancer, all it takes is one rogue cell, one microscopic invader slipping through the cracks, to plant itself elsewhere. And now it had spread, insidiously, into her bones. Hearing those words felt like a dagger to the heart. The Cancer Devil, as we began to call it, wasn't done with her. It had returned to finish what it started.

Heather's decline was brutal.

It was like watching the most vibrant person I'd ever known being devoured from the inside out. We went from skiing, snowboarding, hiking, and biking together — thriving in the wild, living our best lives — to facing the crushing reality that even walking around the neighborhood was too much for her.

At first, we cherished those simple walks, hand in hand, around the block. But as the months rolled by, one day, halfway through our usual route, she stopped and said, "I don't have the energy to make it back to the house." My heart sank. I told her, "Stay here. I'll go get the truck and pick you up." I drove her back home, praying for strength, knowing this was only the beginning of her battle's end.

As her energy faded, so did her ability to move freely. Soon, stairs became too difficult. Our bedroom was upstairs and I made her as comfortable as possible, but even going up and down for meals became too much for her. I became her caregiver — feeding her, helping her with even the smallest tasks, holding her hand through it all. For six months, I was basically at her bedside, watching her fight a battle she couldn't win.

Those months were so difficult, and yet they were also some of the most loving moments we ever shared. I saw her vulnerability, her bravery, her sheer will to hold on despite the odds. But the Cancer Devil had its claws in her now, and it wasn't letting go. Every day, I watched the woman I loved all these years — the woman who had been my partner in every adventure, my anchor in every storm — fade a little more. It was the most helpless feeling in the world.

Heather's pain became my pain, her struggle my struggle, her battle our battle. But no matter how much I willed her to stay, to fight, to beat the odds again, cancer is cruel and unrelenting. It doesn't negotiate. It doesn't care about love or memories or dreams. It just takes. And in the end, it took her from me.

This chapter of our lives was defined by love and loss, resilience and heartbreak — but most of all, it was a testament to who Heather was. Strong, brave, and full of grace, even as cancer tried to break her.

We thought of our daughters, knowing they didn't fully understand the gravity of the situation. They had known Michelle's daughters since they were toddlers. They'd spent countless hours playing, riding bikes, swimming, and watching movies together. When things got tough at home, I was thankful the neighbors were there to help take care of them — to give them some normalcy while I cared for Heather.

But nothing could replace the strain of watching Heather slip away, knowing my role was to be by her side while everything else slowly fell apart.

Stage 4 cancer is no joke. It was metastasizing — meaning it would continue to spread until some part of her body failed, shutting everything down.

Then came the day before Easter 2015.

Heather had a massive seizure in bed. I was right there, as I had been for months. I called 911. The paramedics arrived quickly, stabilized her, and took her away.

At the hospital, I looked into Heather's eyes. Her body was there — but she wasn't. There was a blank stare, an emptiness. The doctor confirmed it: only 10% liver function and 10% kidney function. She was being kept alive by machines.

We agreed she would be removed from life support at midnight, the night after Easter — after everyone had their chance to say goodbye There was no reason to prolong it. She was already gone — just still physically here, connected by tubes and machines.

I stayed with her, held her hand, talked to her — though she couldn't hear me. I called her parents, my mom, my sister, her sister, a few close friends. Everyone had a chance to say goodbye.

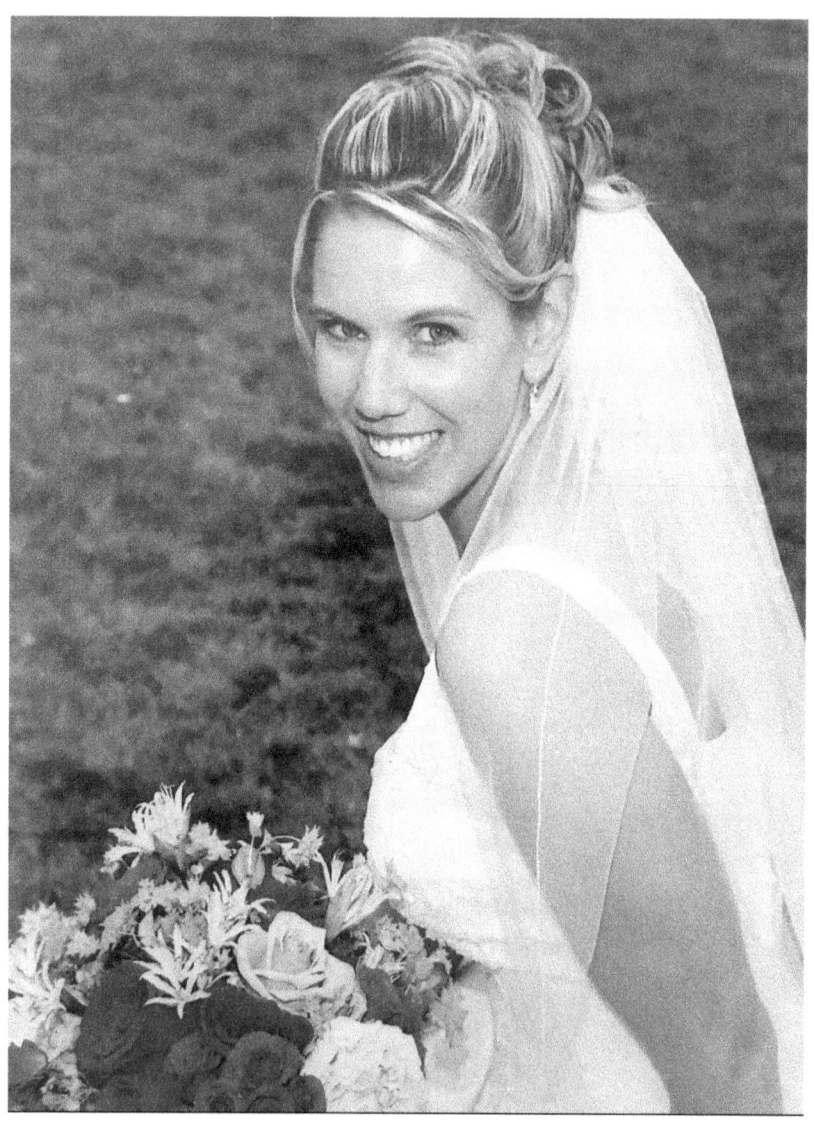

Remembering Heather

The next day, Easter Sunday, I brought our girls to see her. They spoke to their mom, but there was no response. At nine and eleven years old, they couldn't fully grasp what was happening. I could see the confusion in their eyes. They handled it the best they could, but they were struggling inside. I didn't know how to explain it to them. I didn't know how to say that their mom wasn't coming home.

Family and friends came throughout the day. We cried. We told stories. We laughed through the tears. But Heather was already gone. Her eyes were open, but she was just a shell — an empty vessel. It felt like her spirit had already left, and we were simply sharing one last goodbye with the body she left behind.

Late that night, after everyone had gone, the hospital staff came in and removed the equipment. They turned everything off.

Heather passed quietly, peacefully — and I was left with only memories.

At that moment, I truly understood how precious life is and how quickly it can be taken away. The woman I had loved for fifteen years was gone. It wasn't fair. It was impossible to understand why someone so kind and loving had to suffer like that.

But she was free. Free from pain. Free from the Cancer Devil. She had been called to a better place.

The next few days were a blur. I tried to hold it together for our girls, for our family. But inside, I was shattered. I had lost my partner, my best friend — and I didn't know how to go on without her.

But I knew I had to. For our daughters, for her. And to honor the life we had built together.

Heather's passing marked the end of one chapter of my life — and the beginning of another.

A chapter that would be defined by resilience and strength…at least for a while.

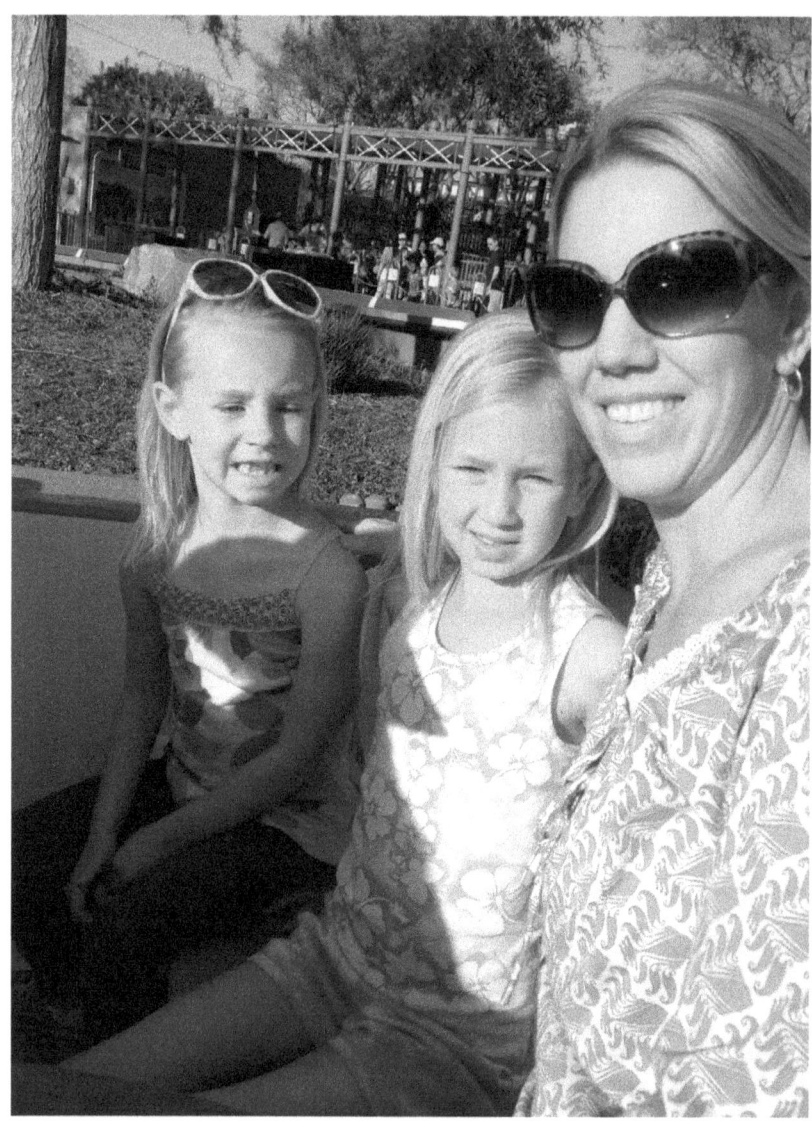

God saw you getting tired when a cure was not to be. He wrapped His arms around you and whispered, "come to me." You didn't deserve what you went through so He gave you some rest. God's garden must be beautiful — He only takes the best. And when I saw you sleeping, so peaceful and free from pain, I could not wish you back to suffer that again.

-Chapter 13-
Life After Death

Heather's passing was the kind of loss that rearranges your soul. The days immediately afterward blurred together, each one a strange mixture of heartbreak, numbness, and necessity. There was no manual for how to navigate this. My first step was honoring her memory. Together with her parents, we made arrangements for Heather to be buried next to her brother Jeff, who had tragically taken his own life a couple years earlier.

Jeff's story was one of quiet devastation. He had once been a truck driver — a solid career — until alcoholism and a DUI took it from him. Banned from driving an 18-wheeler, he moved back in with Heather's parents, but the emptiness followed him. Isolated and without purpose, his life unraveled until one day, he ended his pain. Now, he and Heather rest side by side — a haunting reminder of how fragile life can be.

A separate funeral celebration was held for Heather just north of Dog Beach, where we had first met. That place, once a symbol of our beginning, now marked the end of her life on this earth. But it was also a celebration. Friends and family came together to remember her and to honor her legacy. The stories they shared of her kindness, her humor, and her strength were a testament to the incredible woman she had been.

Afterward, we returned to what had been our family home. A small group of close friends, neighbors, and our children gathered with us, and together, we released balloons into the sky.

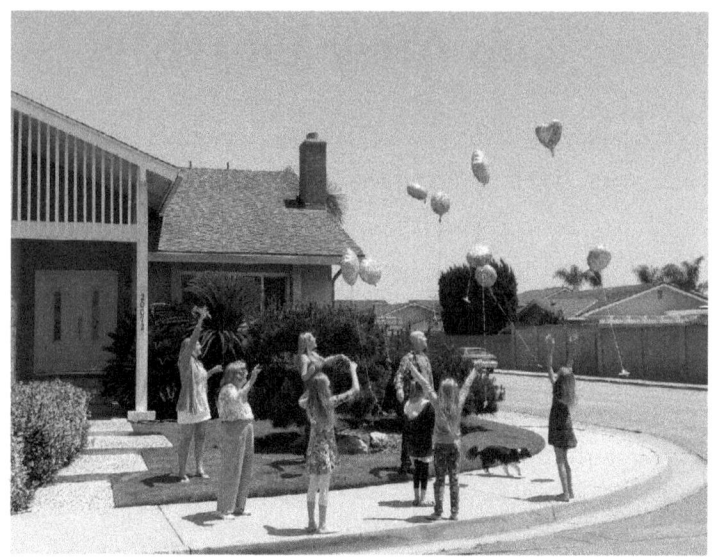
Releasing balloons, Heather's spirit is free.

Watching them drift higher and higher, I thought about Heather's spirit soaring beyond the pain that had consumed her final years. I was relieved she was finally out of the suffering I had watched grow worse and worse until it consumed her completely.

But it also ruined me — heart and soul. The love of my life, my partner in crime — I died inside along with her. I had watched the vibrant, beautiful woman I fell in love with slowly wither away as the Cancer Devil clawed at her life. After the Stage 4 diagnosis that confirmed it had spread to her neck and spine, chemotherapy took all her beautiful blonde hair. That didn't bother me — she was still the same beautiful soul I had loved for 15 years.

A few months later, the doctors found a cancerous tumor in her brain. They zapped it, but the treatment created hundreds of smaller cancer cells that spread across her brain. Not the best outcome, in my opinion, but we were just going with what the doctors said to do.

We did the best we could to live a non-fatal, loving family life together. Along with our regular local adventures, we made it back up to Yosemite.

We looked up at the massive granite walls of Half Dome and El Capitan — carved by glaciers millions of years ago — as they stood tall and timeless. We enjoyed Yosemite Falls, Vernal Falls, and so much raw, natural beauty. It's just incredible.

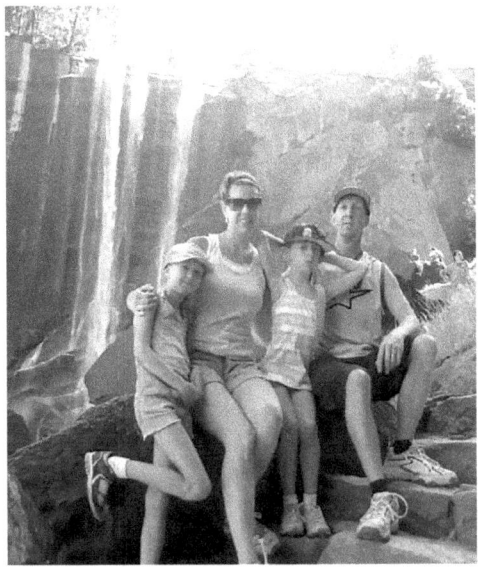

Our last beautiful trip to Yosemite together.

We also made a trip to San Francisco. Ghirardelli's chocolate shop was a highlight for our young daughters, and there were plenty of cool sights and stops along the way that made for great memories. Nothing like seeing the Golden Gate Bridge up close to remind you how awe-inspiring the world can be.

As Heather became bedridden, those trips became sacred memories. I did my best to be there for her — mentally and physically — until the end came and the Cancer Devil finally took her life. And though I felt relief that she was no longer in pain, watching her suffer mentally and physically was pure torture for both of us. You wouldn't wish it on anyone — not even an enemy. She was so brave and carried herself with strength until the very end. She was truly amazing.

But the world doesn't stop for grief. Life began to demand movement, even as I felt frozen. My daughters missed their mom deeply, but they adapted in ways that both comforted and pained me. Across the street, the neighbor family became an unexpected refuge. Their warmth and kindness enveloped my daughters, offering them a kind of surrogate home. The mother, Michelle, became like a maternal figure. It was hard to watch them attach to someone else, but I couldn't deny the stability and love it gave them.

For me, that stability came in moments of connection with the things I loved. I turned to nature, sports, and trying to create new memories with my girls.

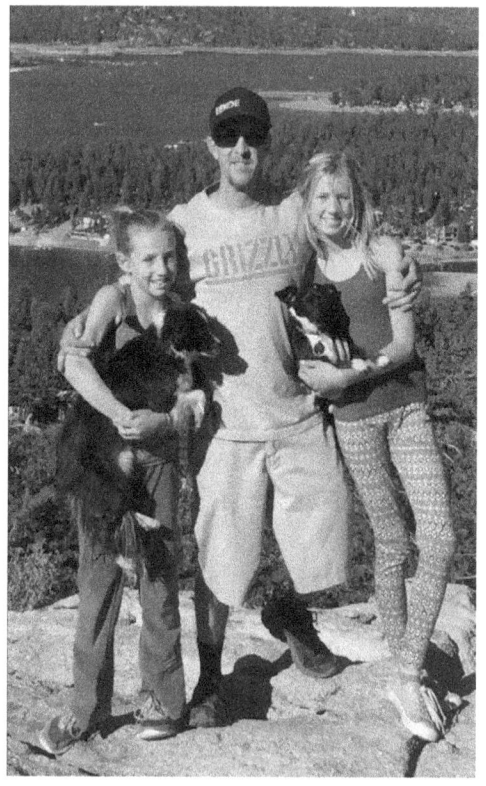

Top of Castle Rock in Big Bear with my crew

When summer came, I'd ask them, "What do you guys want to do?" Their answers were usually vague and indecisive — "I don't know" — so I took the lead. We loaded into the truck for day trips, or packed the motorhome and headed out to places like Castle Park in Santa Barbara and beyond. Places where we could just escape and be together. Mountain biking became my newest passion, and I wanted to share it with them.

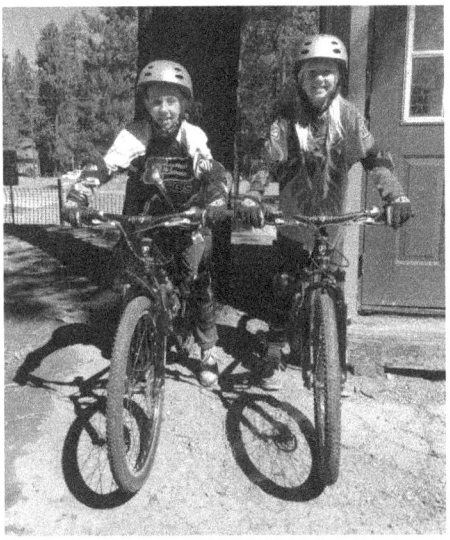

Back at it with the girls, Snow Summit style

Riding the trails with my daughters wasn't just about mountain biking. It was about sharing a piece of myself — the part that had always kept me going. After losing Heather, everything changed, and we were all trying to find our footing in this new world. At home, the girls were often distracted by routines, devices, or each other. But out on the trails, they were present. They were listening. And in those moments, we were connected in a way that didn't happen as often anymore.

Teaching them to pick lines, handle terrain, balance their weight, use the front and back brakes properly — it was more than just instruction. It was something we shared. I saw them learning, improving, trusting me. When they made it through a section and we'd stop, their smiles said everything. Those were the moments that reminded me we were still a team, still moving forward together. Riding became more than just an activity — it became a way to bond, to heal, and to create new memories when so much of our past had been rewritten.

We camped in Big Bear, surrounded by pine trees and crisp mountain air. We ventured to Mammoth, where the trails were as beautiful as the views.

Sometimes they'd roll their eyes at me when I would point out beautiful scenery. "We know, Dad, we see it," they'd say — half annoyed, half amused. It reminded me of my younger self, traveling the world as a snowboarder, so focused on the destination that I often missed the beauty around me. At least they were taking it in, even if it was just background noise.

The girls were invited to go to Disney World in Florida with Michelle's family. A theme park every day for 10 days. I agreed and paid for the trip. I liked theme parks with my daughters — seeing the wonder and laughter in their eyes. Bless Michelle's family for taking them. That's no small task — especially for 10 days in a row.

While they were on their trip, I planned one of my own. After Heather's passing, many friends reached out. One of them was Kris Jamieson, a fellow pro snowboarder from the '90s. He invited me to Oregon. He worked for GoPro, had a camera for me and a fleet of mountain bikes. I flew up, and what a blast! It was like stepping into a time machine — back to before kids, before loss, back to a version of myself I hadn't seen in a long time.

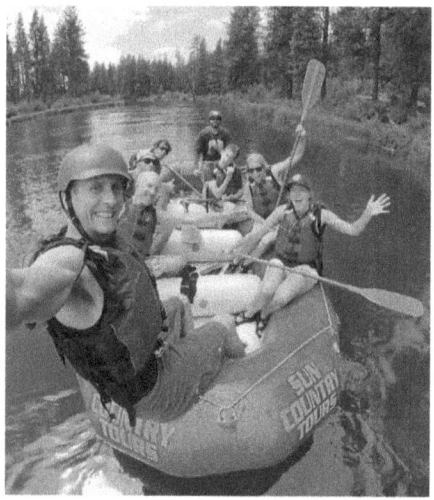

River before the rapids with Jaymo in Oregon

We rode incredible trails, tackled river rapids on a guided whitewater rafting tour, and even did some technical rock climbing. It reminded me of who I used to be — alive, adventurous, thriving.

I also reconnected with April Lawyer and her husband Chris Sheppard. April was another pro snowboarder from back in the day. Her guy was way cool, and their life in the Pacific Northwest was inspiring. She has a retail brand and shop in Bend, Oregon, called Vanilla. We all mountain biked and stand-up paddle boarded, soaking up Oregon's natural beauty from every angle. It was a trip I won't forget.

Those moments were short-lived, but they gave me a glimpse of the person I used to be.

But no amount of adventure or reconnection could fill the void Heather left. By summer's end, the high had faded, and I was left with the cold reality of her absence. My daughters grew closer to Michelle's family. Their world began to orbit around that warm, bustling household — and not me. My two little best friends were off in their own world now. I was no longer a part of it. Just another negative strike in my twisted mind that was spiraling downhill fast.

Halloween came. I went trick-or-treating with them. They were radiant — running from house to house, laughing. But when they ran to the neighbor parents to show off their candy, I felt like a ghost trailing behind — unseen and unnecessary.

Loneliness became my constant companion. Heather and I had shared something rare — a love that was genuine and unshakable. "Till death do us part" wasn't just a vow. It was our truth. Fifteen years of partnership, love, laughter, and never going to bed angry — gone in an instant.

Nights were the worst. Sleep was elusive. My mind was a battleground of memories and regrets. Prozac numbed the sorrow, but not the thoughts. Prescription sedatives forced sleep, but they couldn't touch the hollowness. My daughters deserved more than this shell of a man, but I had nothing left to give. I felt completely unnecessary in their lives.

Michelle told me more than once, "If anything ever happens to you, I'll care for the girls like they're my own." She meant to comfort me. That cut deep. She was right — they didn't need me anymore. They had a new family. A better one. I was just a lonely single dad with nothing left to offer.

My house, once filled with life and love, now felt like a mausoleum — an empty monument to everything I'd lost.

Before Thanksgiving, I was a zombie — going through the motions without feeling. At a pre-Thanksgiving party at Michelle's, I was surrounded by people, by warmth, but I felt completely alone.

When she asked if my daughters could join them for Thanksgiving dinner, I said yes, knowing it would make them happy. That night, I walked back to my empty house, and my daughters stayed with them again. I realized how unnecessary I had become in this world.

One of my go-to thoughts spun in my head: I'm home all alone, like a dog without a bone.

That silly phrase turned darker and deeper every night.

The nights grew heavier. The thoughts got worse.

One night, after 2 a.m., I got up to take more heavy prescription sleeping pills — something I always had to do just to get through the night. I stared at myself in the mirror. The man looking back was a hollowed-out version of who I used to be. The man who had once thrived, who lived a life full of adventure and love — was gone.

I hadn't smiled or felt anything in months. It felt like forever, with no end in sight.

I grabbed the bottle of sleeping pills — the ones I hated taking but couldn't live without.

"The girls will be better off," I thought. "The world will be better off. There's no reason to keep going."

"Fuck it. I'm better off gone. Things will be better for everyone if I'm not here anymore."

Without hesitation, I tilted the full bottle and let the pills tumble into my mouth like a final avalanche. I washed them down with water, each swallow a farewell to the life I no longer recognized — or wanted.

In that moment, I believed I was doing the world a favor — removing a burden that it didn't need to carry.

Where am I?

The first thing I remember is cracking my eyes open to a blurry, disoriented world. Voices surrounded me, saying my name, accompanied by the rhythmic beeping of machines. I had no idea where I was or what was happening. As I lay there, blinking and trying to make sense of it all, fleeting thoughts filled my head. I think I know what happened…is this the afterlife? It didn't look like it — I was laying under a blanket. That didn't make sense.

Then, through the haze, I saw Karen.

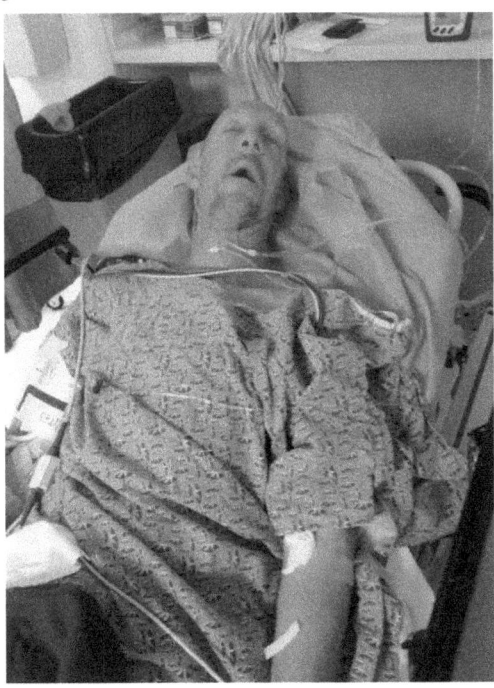

2 ½-day coma, where the darkness nearly won

My sister stood over me, calling my name. "Donnie…Donnie." She's the only one who could call me that without setting off my inner kindergartner, scarred from the year of kids laughing and comparing me to Donnie Osmond.

Slowly, my bearings started to return. Karen was talking to me, telling me what had happened. The pieces came together painfully as I realized my plan hadn't worked. My impulsive action that night — fueled by Prozac, twisted thoughts, desperation, and sleep-deprived recklessness — had landed me here. It wasn't well thought out. Just a raw, emotional fuck it moment.

I had been in a coma for two and a half days. My kids, unable to wake me up the next morning to go to school, called our neighbors — who then dialed 911.

An ambulance picked me up and brought me to the hospital. They pumped my stomach and did whatever they do for someone in a heavy sedative-induced coma. And now…I was back on this side of the dirt. Alive. Though I hadn't planned on it.

My family had visited me in the hospital during the coma, though I had no memory of it. Heather's cancer therapist who had become my therapist after Heather's passing, also came by. She later told me she had a long talk with my mom while I was unconscious. My mom told her proud stories about me — but also stories of my crashes and how they scared the heck out of her. I guess my mom even lifted the sheet and showed her my feet. My right foot is pretty mangled from a couple of different moto crashes in my past. It's not exactly pretty to look at.

My only recollection of the coma was closing my eyes at home and then opening them in the hospital — dazed and confused — trying to piece together the two-and-a-half-day gap. What a wild ride that was. I'll skip that ride next time. I've got better things to do with my life than try to end it. Not the best plan, now that I think of it — but I wasn't thinking straight at all back then…

As my mind made its way back to something resembling normal, I started to process the reality around me.

Once I was stable enough, they transferred me to a 5150 detention facility. This was standard procedure after a suicide attempt. Hospitals need to keep beds available for patients requiring immediate care, so those in my situation are sent to a facility where they can be monitored while transitioning back to everyday life.

The aftermath of the coma, combined with a Prozac-induced haze, my twisted brain, and relentless sleep deprivation, had left me in a fragile mental state. At the 5150 facility, paranoia took hold. I felt like everyone was staring at me, whispering. Some of the men there looked tough and intimidating, which only made things worse.

I was supposed to stay for a few days, but thankfully, I was able to call my sister Karen. She came and picked me up — a saving grace in that moment. I just needed familiar faces, familiar places, to start putting myself back together.

I don't know how long my daughters stayed with the neighbors while I recovered. I just know they were happy and safe there, and I was grateful for that. My mom and Karen comforted me and helped me re-enter the living world after what felt like a lifetime in limbo.

It hit me hard — how I had pushed them away during my downward spiral and didn't even think of them. All I had focused on was the misery in my mind. I had convinced myself that my kids would be better off without me — with neighbors who had promised to care for them as their own. In my twisted mind at the time, that made sense. That's how far gone I was.

In time, I started driving again, taking the first small steps toward rebuilding my life. My doctor took me off Prozac and the heavy-duty sleeping meds and switched me to lighter alternatives. These new meds weren't supposed to spin me out like Prozac did, and I wouldn't have to fight through a thick fog every day just to function. Supposedly, these would keep me going — better than nothing at all. I agreed to this lower dose of medical poison and figured I'd see how it went.

Later, I learned something that sent a chill through me — Prozac had a known risk of causing suicidal thoughts. That wasn't just fine print or some legal disclaimer — it was real. And I had lived it.

Before Prozac, my mind never wandered into those kinds of dark places. Sure, I had struggles. But I never felt completely untethered from myself. Once that drug got into my system, something changed. It didn't just numb me — it twisted my thoughts in ways I couldn't control. It was like a shadow creeping into my brain, making everything feel warped and hopeless. It amplified every doubt, every moment of pain, every buried emotion I thought I had a grip on. It didn't just cover the depression — it dug its claws in and dragged me down deeper.

I didn't realize it at the time, but I wasn't thinking like myself anymore. I was thinking like someone trapped in a chemical fog, with Prozac steering me into places I never would've gone on my own. The scariest part? It felt so subtle. I thought it was just me getting worse, not realizing it was the drug distorting my mind.

Life felt like it was idling. I went through the motions in the recovery groups that my therapist referred me to, but they didn't ignite anything in me. My engine was running, but the RPMs stayed low.

Still, I showed up. I was there for my daughters, even though they spent most of the holidays with the neighbors. I reconnected with my mom and sister Karen, spending more time with them than I had in years. They helped me piece my life back together after my mental decline into hell.

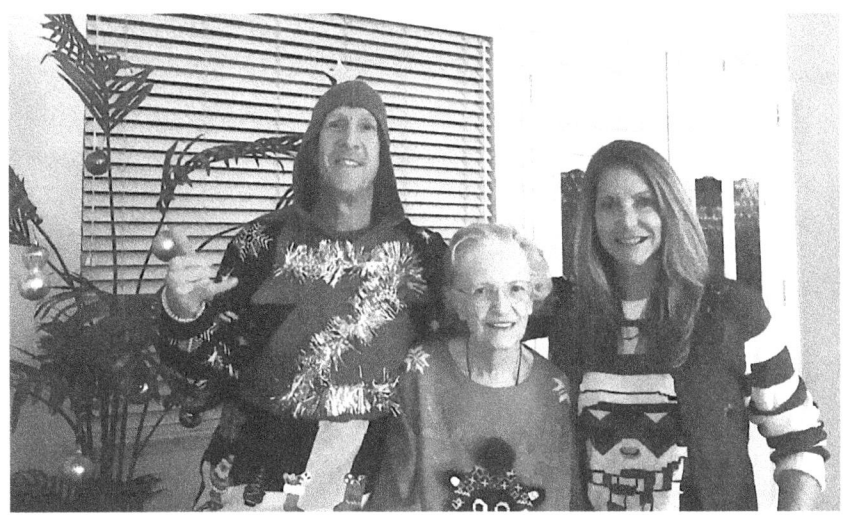
Ugly Sweater Christmas, it could've been uglier

The guilt lingered, though. I couldn't apologize enough to my daughters, my mom, and Karen for what had happened. That spontaneous, broken-brained decision could have left a permanent hole in their hearts — an unanswerable "why" that might have haunted them forever. I was so sorry for the pain I caused, but also so incredibly grateful they still stood by me, offering love and forgiveness during one of the darkest times of my life.

I should be dead, but somehow I wasn't. I had another shot at life — and this time, I was determined to make it count.

Mindset had helped me in the past, but if you forget about it and slide back into old thought patterns, the good can slip away into the darkness. And that darkness can pull you down fast. I needed to focus on recovery and commit to daily gratitude and positivity — no matter what else was going on in life.

"I'll be back," I said to myself, in my terrible Arnold Schwarzenegger voice — and laughed.

-Chapter 14-
Single-Dad-Trippin'

Life as a single dad in Huntington Beach brought its challenges, but it also brought moments of discovery and connection that I'll always treasure. My daughters were growing into their teenage years, one in junior high and the other in high school. They had lives of their own, riding their bikes to school, laughing with best friends across the street, and soaking in the carefree joy of being young. I knew their world was expanding, and as much as I wanted to still be at the center of it, I respected their need for independence.

When they weren't busy with school, friends, sports, or their own plans, we carved out time for "dad and daughters" adventures. Sometimes it was something quick and easy, like neighborhood or extended loops on skateboards or bikes, or exploring local parks and hiking trails. Other times, we'd go mountain biking whenever we could make it happen if they didn't already have other plans. I'd take them to different restaurants, walk Main Street and the pier in Huntington Beach and Newport, or hit up parks and other spots that sounded fun to them. We were a family of three now, figuring it out together.

But the motorhome? That was our magic key to new adventures. It took us beyond our usual haunts and into some of the most beautiful places across the western states. Together, we traveled back to Castle Park in Santa Barbara and indulged at Ghirardelli's Chocolates in San Francisco, just like we had done with their mom, Heather, when she was still alive.

We spent countless weekends in Big Bear, usually as a quick two-day getaway. It was close enough to pack up the motorhome on a Friday, head up the mountain, and be back home by Sunday evening. If the girls didn't have other plans, we'd load up the bikes and go. Big Bear was one of those places that felt like an escape without the commitment of a big trip. It was just far enough away to feel like we were on an adventure but close enough that we could make it happen on short notice.

Mammoth and Tahoe, that was different. Those weren't just road trips; they were special. We didn't go nearly as often, but when we did, it was for more than just the mountains and more than a couple days. It was also about reconnecting with old friends, people I had known for over 30 years. These weren't just my riding buddies from back in the day; they were like extended family. Their kids were growing up in the same world of action sports that had shaped my life, and I wanted Ashlyn and Kaylee to see them and to experience these places beyond just the trails.

As much as these places meant to me, they also became the perfect setting for sharing a passion I hoped would mean something to my daughters too — mountain biking. My latest action sports obsession.

But long before mountain biking took over, these same mountains had been a winter playground for us. Heather and I had taken Ashlyn and Kaylee up to the snow when they were younger, introducing them to skiing and snowboarding. Ashlyn followed in my footsteps, choosing snowboarding, while Kaylee, much like her mom, loved skiing. Even after Heather passed, we still had some trips to the snow, keeping the tradition alive. I even managed to score free lift tickets a few times at Mountain High, the local resort closest to home, and one time I even got passes for Michelle's family across the street who helped take care of my daughters, and we were all able to share a day on the snow together. Just a small way to give back to the family that had been there for my daughters so many times.

Snowboarding had been such a huge part of my life, but things had changed. I wasn't a sponsored pro anymore. I wasn't getting paid to ride. And now, lift tickets were usually coming out of my own pocket, and when you add two growing kids to that, the costs add up fast. On top of that, my right knee — my back leg from so many years of riding regular footed — had developed bone-on-bone arthritis from the constant leaned-over knee angle of boardsports, making snowboarding and skateboarding painful in a way they had never been before. That was a hard pill to swallow, but I've learned that when one passion fades, another one steps in to take its place.

That's how mountain biking took over. It filled every part of that action sports void I needed in my life. The adrenaline, the speed, the freedom — it was all still there, just on dirt instead of snow. It also opened the door to more opportunities for adventure with my daughters, especially in the summer when they had no school schedule. Instead of trying to plan around winter weekends, weather, and conditions, we could load up the motorhome anytime, hit the road, and explore these same mountain towns in a whole new way.

Bringing my daughters into this sport felt like the perfect way to connect. It wasn't just about the riding itself, though that was a blast. It was about being out in nature together. Feeling the wind on our faces, hearing and feeling the dirt under our tires, and taking in the beauty of the mountains. But the best part? It was just us. No distractions, no routines pulling us in different directions — just a three-person family, three bikes, and the open road of adventure ahead.

Some days we'd hit the trails, taking chairlifts up the same mountains I had snowboarded down in the winter for nearly 30 years. It was surreal, riding those same lifts with my daughters, remembering how many times I had ridden these lifts when I was having fun and chasing my own dreams. Now, I was here with them, watching them learn, teaching them the techniques of mountain biking, and feeling that deep satisfaction when they started to pick it up. Seeing them improve, gain confidence, and push themselves, even just a little, filled me with a pride that's hard to explain.

But the trip was never just about the trails. It was about everything in between — the meals we made together in the motorhome, the small-town restaurants we stumbled upon, and those quiet moments when we'd sit outside under the stars, watching the sky stretch endlessly above us. It was the nighttime movies we watched inside the motorhome, wrapped in blankets after a long day of riding, laughing about something dumb, silly, or fun that had happened earlier in the day.

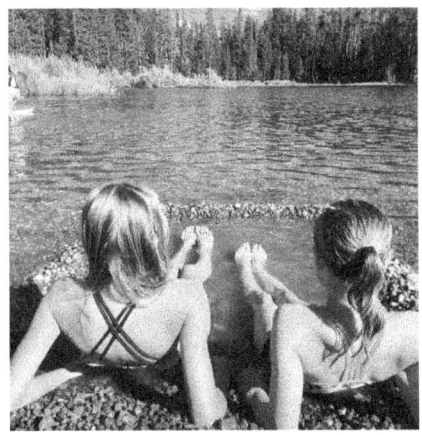

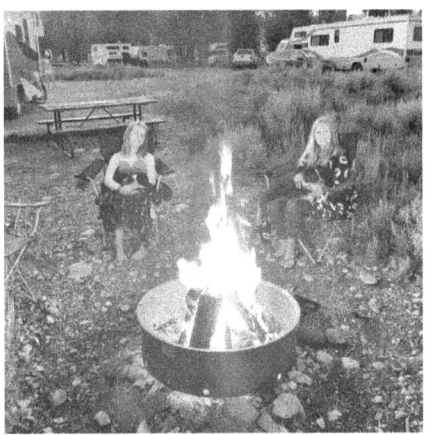

Lake chillin' and campfires rocked

I knew these moments wouldn't last, and I felt it every time. Time was moving fast. One day, they'd be grown, wrapped up in their own lives and responsibilities, chasing their own paths. But right then, in those moments, we had this.

There was something about life on the road that made everything feel lighter. No stress, no schedules — just time together, making memories. Some of the best times we had as a family of three — Ashlyn, Kaylee, and me.

Most of the time that we took off in the motorhome, the bikes came with us, and every trip turned into an adventure waiting to be had.

The Henricksens: An Action Sports Family

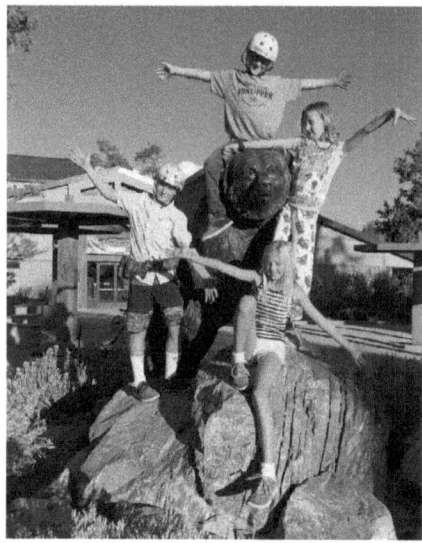

The girls rockin' with Dusty and Dillon

When we were in Mammoth, we'd visit Marko and Jenny Henricksen and their family, whose life revolved around snowboarding, nature, and action sports. I'd known Marko since the early days of Mountain High in 1985, back when snowboarding was still finding its footing. It was a small community then — if you rode snowboards, you knew everyone on the mountain that did too. That's just how it was in its infancy as a sport.

Marko's family carried that same love of the sport, but their sons, Dusty and Dillon, took it to a whole new level in their teens.

Dusty was born to ride. Even at 13 years old, it was clear to me that he had the talent and drive that set him apart from the rest.

Watching him reminded me of the first time I saw Shaun White as a kid at Snow Summit more than fifteen years earlier, shortly after my own snowboarding career had ended. I was taking some runs at Summit and remember seeing Shaun White when he was 12 years old — a wild little red-haired kid in a snowboard helmet. At the time, most people didn't wear helmets, but I saw him ripping the pipe and park and thought, "That kid is really good!" I knew snowboarding was progressing, but at the time, I didn't really care. I was in a new chapter of life, and I kept doing my own thing, just enjoying my snowboarding for the day for the fun of it, and didn't give it much thought.

Shaun White later became the most winning X Games gold medalist as a snowboarder, and he even won X Games gold in skateboarding — a truly amazing feat to accomplish in two action sports disciplines that require so much skill. To win gold in both sports is an incredible achievement for one person, and he's still ripping hard to this day and is wildly successful — a true testament to making your dreams happen by working hard at what you love to do.

There was something undeniable about Dusty's energy and skill. Something that I got a glimpse of with Shaun White, but I was way more in tune with what was going on with Dusty since he was part of a family I was good friends with. By his early teens, Dusty dominated amateur competitions with scores that outshined the pros, and he would win the local amateur skateboard contest at Mammoth Skatepark as well.

For the snowboard contests, the judges were the same for both divisions. An example of how good Dusty was — if a pro won with a score of 96, Dusty might win the amateur division with a 97. The only thing keeping him out of the pro ranks was his age.

When Dusty turned 16, he didn't just step into the pro division — he owned it. That year he became Snowboarder of the Year. Then, in 2020, he followed it up with a gold medal in the Youth Olympics. In 2021, he won X Games gold in Slopestyle and X Games KnuckleHuck competitions. It was the first time anyone from the USA had won gold in Slopestyle since Shaun White in 2009. Then Dusty represented the USA in the 2022 Snowboard Olympics. He has continued to dominate, competing in Halfpipe, Slopestyle, and Knuckle Huck competitions in recent years, and is definitely a force to be reckoned with.

Dusty is known for his innovative tricks and has mastered moves like the quad cork. He was the first to land a backside quadruple cork in a Slopestyle competition during the 2020 Burton U.S. Open. Four flips with four twists — and even now, I can't wrap my head around how he does it. He has a very creative, powerful style, and since Dusty dominates skateboarding vert ramps and bowls as well as ripping rails and street-style skating, it has enriched his style and talent to another all-around level of greatness in snowboarding.

Dusty's skills have taken him around the world and provided him with a great life, including a home he bought in San Diego at just 20 years old in 2024.. He continues to travel the world and dominate in the sport of snowboarding, along with being a ruler in other action sports. He has a very bright future and a great life.

Dillon, Dusty's younger brother, charted his own path in snowboarding. He embraced the creative side, producing viral videos like BUSTER, with 194,000 views and counting, that showcase his skate and snow skills in a way that's nothing short of amazing. Together with his friends, he produces entertaining videos and is enjoying life doing what he loves. Dillon has found his niche—blending his passion for making entertainment people enjoy with snowboarding and skateboarding in ways that are fun to watch. He has turned filming, editing, and doing what he loves into a dream lifestyle.

Watching Marko and Jenny sacrifice so much to support their sons' dreams fills me with pride. They moved from Big Bear to Mammoth in 2016 to give their boys better opportunities, and their dedication has paid off in ways that are nothing short of inspiring.

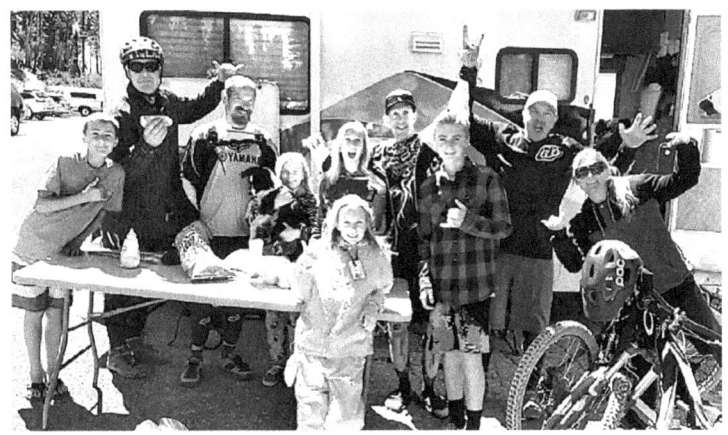

Motorhome party after MTB with Mammoth family and friends

Meeting Tahoe Longboard Chuck in New Zealand

Further north, Tahoe brought its own set of adventures and friendships. We visited Chuck Buckley, a friend I met over 30 years ago in New Zealand. Back then, Chuck and I were two young snowboarders chasing dreams of riding great mountains, riding in helicopters to access untouched powder, and doing what we loved to do. At the time, Chuck had been in New Zealand for a few months, fully immersed in the experience, while I joined for a few unforgettable weeks.

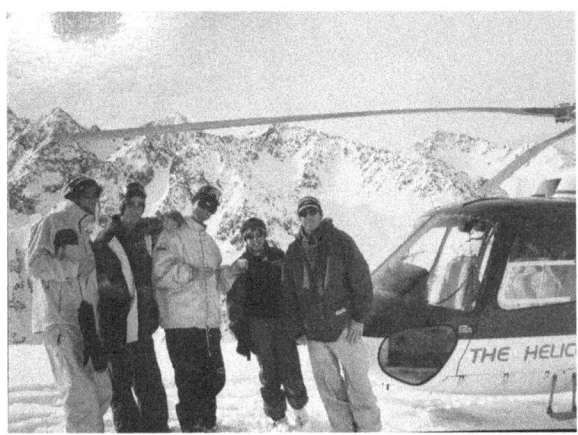

New Zealand — good snow lines, real good times

Those were the days when snowboarding was still raw, and our bodies bounced instead of broke. Chuck and I bonded, and we shared helicopter rides and fresh powder turns, jumps, and wild times on the other side of the world. He has become one of those friends who, no matter how much time passes, always feels like family. Now, Chuck runs Tahoe Longboards, a company he's built over the past two decades. When my daughters and I visited Tahoe, he welcomed us with the same warmth and enthusiasm I'd known from our New Zealand days — and the many times I have seen him since then. He even gave us a couple of TLB skateboards, showed us around his side of town, and we had dinner together. I've been crossing paths with Chuck occasionally ever since way back then, and we still meet up whenever we can make it happen. He's a great guy and a great friend.

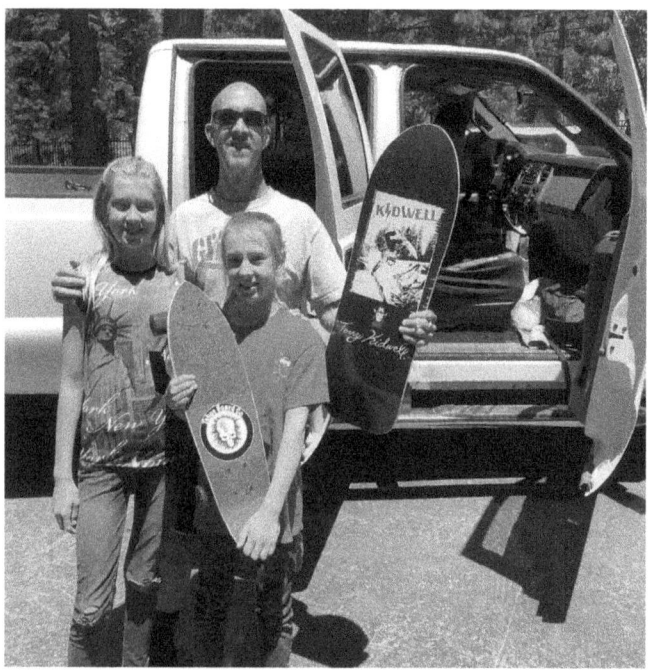

Taho Longboards, courtesy of Chuck

Recently, Chuck even pulled out some old photos when he came down to San Clemente from Tahoe to visit family. There was a picture of us and a few friends standing outside of a helicopter from 1997. Looking at moments that felt like a lifetime ago — and in other ways, like it was yesterday. He also showed me a flyer from an event we had done together with other snowboarders called Planes, Trains, and Suburbans, where we ventured in Suburbans to different snow towns across a few states to ride our snowboards, document our adventures, and have a great time. It was a reminder of the wild creativity that defined that era — and the way we were living back in the '90s. Seeing those memories come to life brought me back to a time when every day felt like a new adventure and we were ready to take on anything we wanted to make happen. Those were great times indeed.

Today, Chuck's young son Leland is already carving his own path. He started snowboarding at just 17 months old. At only 9 years old in 2025, he's not only riding with style but is already sponsored and gaining attention for his impressive snowboarding skills. I see him progressing all the time on Instagram — getting faster, learning tricks, and building confidence.

Chuck's doing an awesome job giving him every opportunity to grow — from filming him on the hill to helping line up sponsors and staying committed to getting him out on the mountain.

Leland recently won the overall USASA boardercross championship in his category and has already earned 24 gold medals. He's even started getting some TV coverage for his talent at such a young age — appearing on Good Morning America, Reno News, and Fox 40 News, to name a few.

With his natural passion, talent, and drive — and Chuck backing him every step of the way — he's on a clear path to become something special in this sport. If he keeps progressing like this, you'll definitely be hearing more about him in the years to come. Watch out — Leland The Falcon is just getting started.

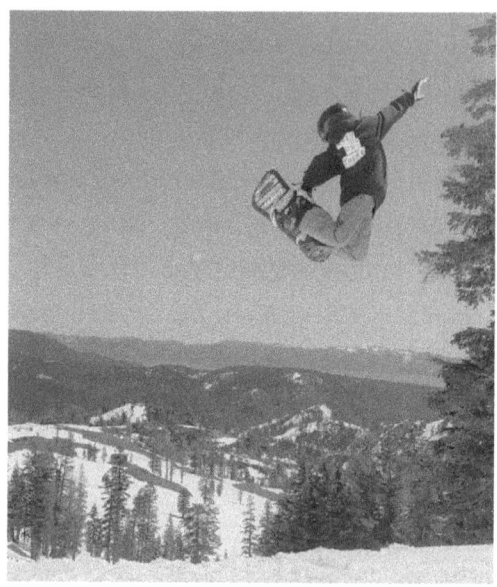
9-year-old Leland ripping!

Chuck and I still share a passion for mountain biking, and when I go to Tahoe, we try to meet up and ride down the beautiful and fun trails together. This has been a celebration of the friendship we've built over the past three decades — and we'll be watching Leland carry the snowboarding and action sports torch into the future for the next generation.

The Idaho Connection

Of all our trips together, Idaho stands out as a blend of family, friendship, and personal milestones. The natural beauty of the state was breathtaking — rolling hills, towering trees, and endless trails to explore. It was also a chance for me to see a property I'd owned for years but had never visited in person. The fourplex was part of my real estate investments. Walking through the property, meeting the management team, and seeing the place in person turned something abstract into a tangible part of life.

But Idaho wasn't just about real estate. It was about time with my daughters and reconnecting with my friend Dave Van Etten, creator of OldGuysRipToo.

com. Dave reached out after Heather passed away, wanting to interview me about my snowboarding career and how I was doing in many areas of life. That interview became a deep dive into my past, featuring links to my Double O Szabo movies, skateboard footage, and even some motocross riding. Meeting Dave and his family in person brought the connection full circle, and we all had a great time hanging out together.

A bit later, my daughters stayed with Dave's wife and kids while Dave and I hit the mountain biking trails. Idaho's natural beauty provided the perfect backdrop for our ride — a mix of adrenaline and reflection. Later, we sat down to talk about the Old Guys Rip Too interview. That site had become a collection of my action sports history — featuring everything from skateboarding to snowboarding to moto clips, to heartfelt reflections on Heather's passing and the mindset needed to stay grounded through all of life's ups and downs. At the bottom is a set of action, travel, and family photos to scroll through. Even ten years later, it remains one of my favorite ways to share this part of my story and life online.

Instagram and Facebook are a different type of sharing, I still love being part of it in this modern world. It's amazing to stay connected with people I've met all over the globe — and to make new friends in ways that didn't exist before. Previous generations didn't have this opportunity, so I feel grateful we do. We're lucky to live in a time where we can share pieces of our lives instantly, and that gift keeps evolving.

That trip to Idaho was more than just a vacation. It was a reminder of the connections that shape us, the passions that drive us, and the memories that stay with us long after the moment passes.

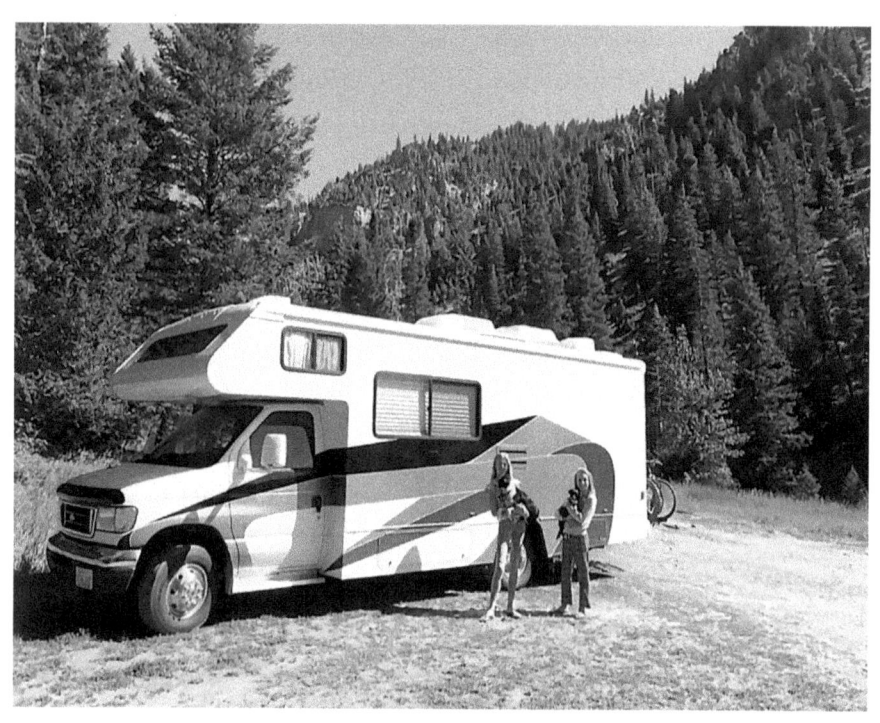

Motorhome memories, Idaho style with the girls

-Chapter 15-
Cancer KillZ

Three years after Heather passed, just as I was starting to find my rhythm as a single dad, I got a call that changed everything.

My sister Karen told me our mom had suffered a stroke and was in the hospital. She could no longer walk or take care of herself. Visiting her in that sterile, white-walled room became part of our regular routine. She eventually stabilized, but her independence was gone. And as if that wasn't enough, we got the gut-wrenching news — she also had pancreatic cancer, one of the deadliest and most aggressive cancers out there.

I had already seen what cancer could do. I watched it take my dad's life in 1999. I stood by helplessly as Heather fought her battle, only to lose it in 2015. And now, it was coming for our mom. The doctors told us she wasn't strong enough for chemotherapy — not that it was a cure anyway. It's just a brutal attack — a hope that the poison kills the cancer before it kills everything else in the person's body. And sometimes, it kills the person too.

Even people with endless resources — like Steve Jobs and Patrick Swayze — couldn't outrun it. And now, it was coming after our mom.

Cancer is like the devil itself. I hate it with everything in me.

It's taken away people I love, and most people know someone who has lost their life to this terrible disease.

But I still hold on to the hope that one day, it'll be a thing of the past. Hopefully in my lifetime — and I believe my daughters will see a world where cancer isn't a death sentence. With AI, medical breakthroughs, and genetic sequencing all evolving at lightning speed, I have to believe this disease will one day be wiped out. Just like polio. Just like the plague. Even HIV/AIDS, once a death sentence, is now manageable. The breakthroughs are coming. The world is changing — and I hope that change comes fast enough to spare others from the pain we've seen too many people go through for far too long.

But hope didn't change the reality right in front of us.

Karen and I had a hard decision to make. Mom needed full-time care, and neither of us could manage it alone. Karen had a demanding job as an engineer, and while she did everything she could, she couldn't be there around the clock — and neither could I in the current situation.

The options were brutal — put Mom in a nursing home, where she'd have professional care but lose the comfort of home, or hire a caregiver and trust a stranger to take care of her.

I hated the idea of leaving her with someone we didn't know. I'd heard too many horror stories — abuse, neglect, people wasting away with no warmth or real human connection. That wasn't going to happen to our mom. She deserved better.

By that point, I had been raising my daughters as a single dad for three years. After Heather passed, they had grown closer to Michelle's family across the street — people they had known their whole lives. Her daughters were the same age as mine, and the four of them became like sisters. They swam together, hung out, went on trips with them, and spent time at their second home in Arrowhead. They did so many things as a group, it felt like a real, complete family experience — something they all loved, and something I couldn't fully provide alone. I'd shared this earlier but it carried even more weight now. Michelle had told me more than once that if anything ever happened to me, she'd raise my girls like they were her own. And I saw how happy and at home my daughters were over there.

So, I made one of the hardest decisions of my life.

I arranged to provide monthly child support, along with anything my daughters needed — clothing, school supplies, and other expenses — so they'd be fully supported while living with Michelle's family.

I let go of our home. I sold the house, the motorhome, the Harley, the dirt bikes — nearly everything. What once filled a 3,000-square-foot house was condensed into a 6'x9' storage unit. My daughters would have stability and a full family environment across the street. And I would move into my mom's house to take care of her.

Living with her again after all those years brought things full circle. It wasn't easy, but it was a gift. We had time — real time together. We talked, we shared stories, we watched her favorite old movies around the holidays — It's a Wonderful Life and A Christmas Story. Some of those moments lit up her face and made me forget, just for a little while, that she was sick.

I took her for drives through some of my favorite scenic spots. Laguna Beach's Top of the World became a regular stop. From there, we could see Catalina Island in the distance, Palos Verdes to the north, the mountains behind us, and the ocean stretching endlessly out in front of us. Being surrounded by all that beauty reminded me that life was still happening, even in the hardest moments.

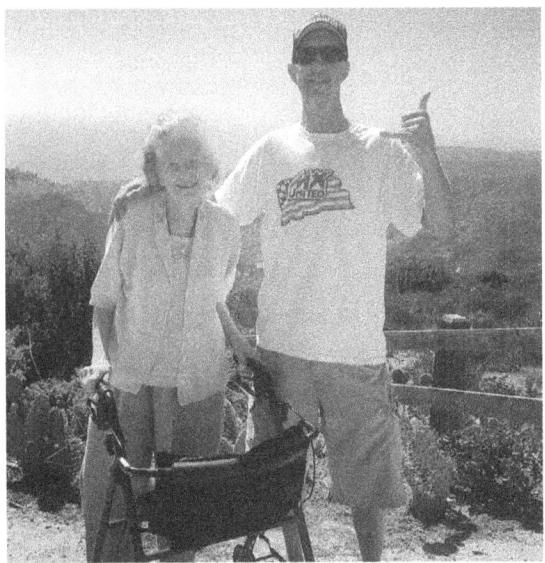

Top of World with Mom, our favorite local view

We visited San Diego, Corona Del Mar, and Huntington Beach — the city I had called home for over 35 years. We took her out to dinner when we could, holding onto the normal things for as long as possible.

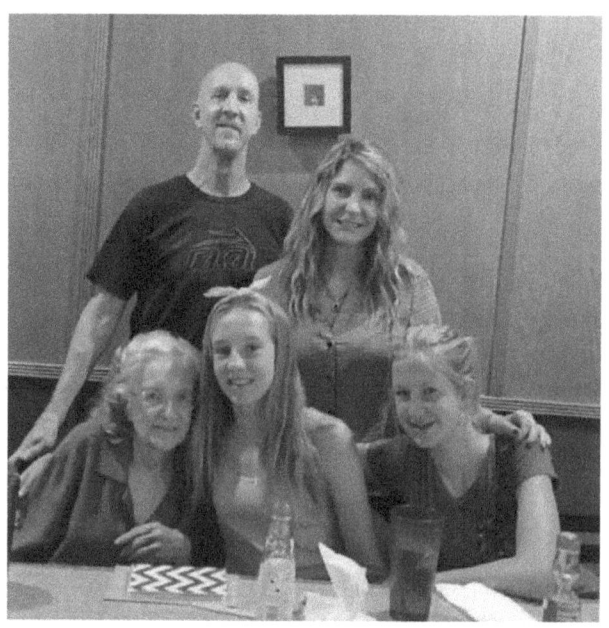

Karen and the kids with mom, before the end

And then one night, I heard it — the death rattle. A sound I'll never forget. A deep, rattling moan that chills you to the bone. I called Karen and told her to come over. We sat by our mom's side through the long night, listening to those haunting breaths that marked her final moments. By morning, she was gone.

Death has a way of changing how you see the world. It strips life down to what matters. You realize you don't get forever. You don't even get a guarantee for tomorrow. So, you have to live — really live — because at some point, your time runs out.

Our mom lived a full life. I took care of her for over two years. It was bittersweet — having that time to reconnect, only to watch her slowly be taken by this terrible disease.

To honor her final wish, my sister, my daughters, and I scattered her ashes near a small lake below Big Bear, surrounded by the mountains she loved. I keep part of her ashes in a special display in the home I live in now.

Life doesn't always turn out how you thought it would. There's that old saying — if you want to make God laugh, tell him your plans. I thought I'd grow old in Huntington Beach with my beautiful wife and daughters, in our nice home and great neighborhood. But that wasn't what was in the cards for us — not all of us together, anyway.

Losing our mom was another reminder of life's fragility. I've had plenty of close calls myself — surviving things that others didn't, and walking away when others didn't make it. I don't take that lightly. I wake up every day with a lot of gratitude.

So make your life count — every single day. Nothing is guaranteed.

Chase your passions. Keep growing. Keep learning. Be present. Take the risk. Speak the truth. Love your people. Make peace with your past. And live in a way that leaves you with nothing to regret when your number gets called.

Because in the end, it's not about the stuff you owned — it's about the life you lived, the people you loved, and the impact you leave behind.

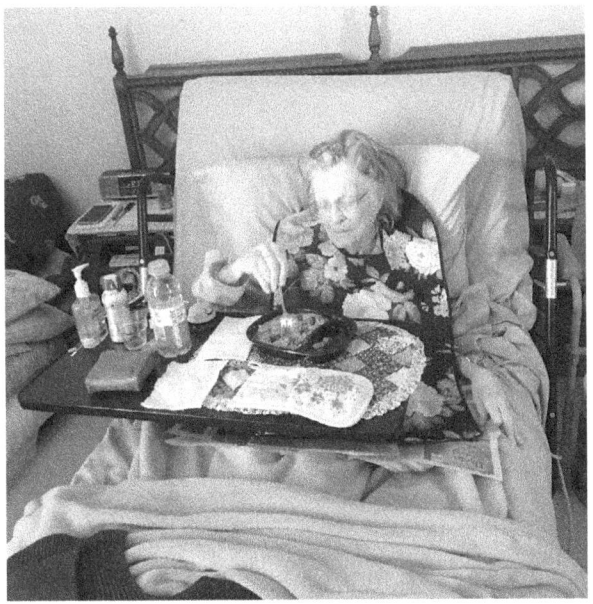

Taking care of Mom, she took care of me.

-Chapter 16-
MTB Is For Me

Spring of 2014 found me recovering yet again from another motocross injury. This time, I'd had the second rod removed from my lower left tibia — a painful souvenir of a false-neutral dirt bike failure a year before this. After the rod removal surgery, I was stuck indoors, restless and aching to break free. A couple days later, itching for fresh air and a change of scenery, I threw a leg over my Harley and rode up to Top of the World in Laguna Beach, a place where the natural beauty all around could clear any mind.

From that high vantage point, the view stretched endlessly — Catalina Island on the horizon, Palos Verdes peeking out into the ocean, and all around me, Laguna's hills dotted with multimillion-dollar mansions looking over the water. It was a stunning contrast of untamed beauty and luxury. As I took it all in, a mountain biker rolled toward me, and something about him looked familiar.

He looked at me and said, "Don Szabo, it's Steve Carrillo from Junior High! What's up?"

I blinked in disbelief. "No way!"

Steve and I had been friends back then, crossing paths often. He'd lived near SkaterCross, my old local skate park. He lived down the street from Dawn, a girl I used to hang out with. I couldn't help but chuckle, recalling how I had to stand on a curb to kiss her goodbye — eye to eye — because she was taller than I was since girls grow faster than boys in junior high.

Steve and I started catching up, and he was telling me about mountain biking. At the time, I couldn't understand why anyone would choose pedaling uphill — it didn't sound like much fun compared to the raw power and adrenaline of motocross that I loved.

"Why would you want to work your ass off going uphill?" I asked. "With a throttle, I can jump uphill further than you can jump a mountain bike. I've hit 180-foot jumps, we ride 30-to-50-mile loops on adrenaline-pumping trails, grabbing as much throttle as we want at any time. We also ride motocross tracks, catching massive air, railing berms, banging bars, and racing with friends. It's a rush that can't be beat!"

He laughed and countered with the appeal of mountain biking — being immersed in nature, building fitness, and finding a different kind of thrill. He even offered me a spare bike he had, insisting I should give it a try. Reluctantly, I agreed, more out of respect for our reconnection than genuine interest.

A few days later, we met up, and I quickly discovered how grueling the uphill climbs were. Steve absolutely crushed me on the climbs. But downhill? That was a different story. It clicked for me pretty quickly. While it lacked the raw speed and massive airtime of motocross, mountain biking had its own unique rhythm — a slower, more technical challenge of moving the bike around, picking lines downhill, and embracing the terrain. It was a new way to experience the thrill of another action sport while soaking in the beauty all around me. It was also cool that we could talk while we were riding — or at least while I was suffering on the climbs.

A few days later, Steve took me to some bike trails near Oakley's headquarters. This place had a few BMX-style jumps that we came across. His friends eyed them nervously, saying, "No way am I hitting those jumps." I laughed. The *gaps* were only 12–15 feet — child's play compared to the much bigger motocross jumps I was used to. I cleared the bike jumps with ease, earning a few raised eyebrows from the group.

I quickly realized that my motocross experience made mountain biking a natural and easy transition, just like skateboarding and surfing had paved the way for snowboarding earlier in my action sports life.

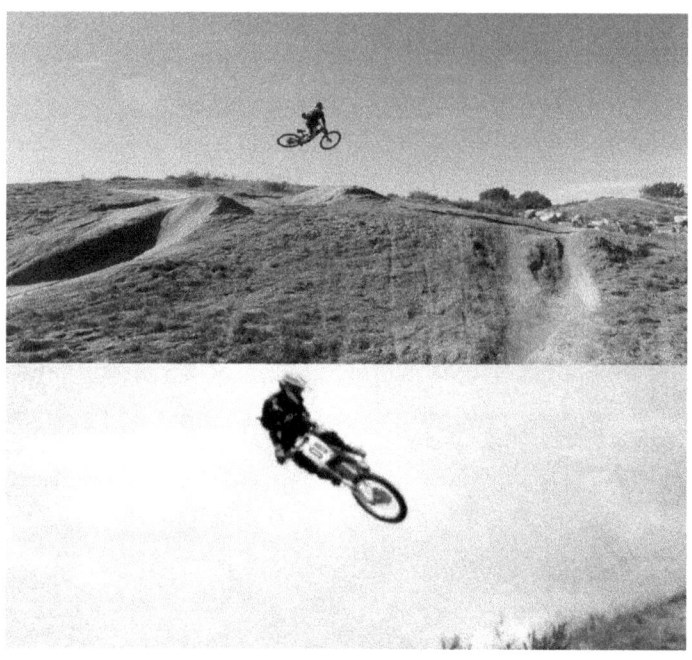

Moto to Mountain Biking just flowed easy

Summer came, and I heard that Snow Summit — where I had snow-boarded countless times — used their chairlifts for mountain biking during the summer months. The idea of skipping the uphill grind and focusing entirely on downhill riding hooked me immediately.

When I hit Snow Summit, it was a blast. They'd built jump lines specifically for mountain bikers, and it didn't take me long to figure them out. If I could see the landing, I knew how to gauge my speed and send most jumps pretty easily.

Within a few runs, I had the jump lines dialed in, and the adrenaline rush felt like coming home to another sport I loved.

I had bought Steve's extra bike from him — a used 2010 Giant Reign for $500. It wasn't the fanciest setup, and it only had 120mm of suspension, but I've always been the kind of guy who makes what I have work — and so I did.

Back in my early snowboard days, when boots, boards, and bindings were subpar, I'd tweak things just enough to make it work and then ride as hard as I could. I wasn't the type to obsess over gear; I just adapted and kept pushing forward, having fun with whatever I had.

That following summer is when I flew to Oregon and reconnected with Kris Jamieson after Heather passed away. He introduced me to newer mountain bike technology: better geometry, more suspension, and overall improved designs. By then, I was hooked on this new sport to me, so I invested in a better bike and dove deeper into my mountain biking journey.

Looking back, that chance encounter with Steve Carrillo at the Top of the World in Laguna was a turning point. Mountain biking became another chapter in my action sports journey. A different thrill that balanced parts of the two-wheel feeling of motocross and the freedom of snowboarding. It was proof that even at 47 — eleven years ago — there were still new adventures to be had, and new ways to chase the adrenaline that's basically fueled me my entire life.

Before I knew it, I'd been mountain biking for over five years. Even though it took some serious effort to grind up those hills, the thrill of bombing down, picking your lines, catching air, and pushing limits made it all worth it. There's a unique kind of flow and adrenaline in mountain biking that had gotten its hooks in me fast.

Along the way, I connected with multiple crews and built friendships inside the *MTB scene*. That community vibe was strong — people genuinely stoked for each other, always down to help fix a flat or go ride a new trail. It was a refreshing contrast to some of the other sports like surfing that I'd been a part of over the years.

I still love surfing, especially when it's about traveling to exotic locations, chasing great waves, and living those unforgettable experiences. I've had hundreds of fun surf sessions in the ocean with friends, sharing moments that stick with you. But if I'm being real, surfing comes with a very different vibe.

Paddling out into a lineup of surfers isn't always peaceful. There's a lot of posturing, stink-eye, and localism. Everyone's competing for the same wave — it's this weird mix of zen and battle. People drop in on each other, jockey for position — it can get cutthroat out there. And when you finally get your wave? Depending on the type, maybe it's a 5–10 second ride, maybe thirty seconds at a point break. But after driving to the surf spot, suiting up, paddling out, and waiting, it all adds up to just a few minutes of actual ride time when it's all said and done for the day.

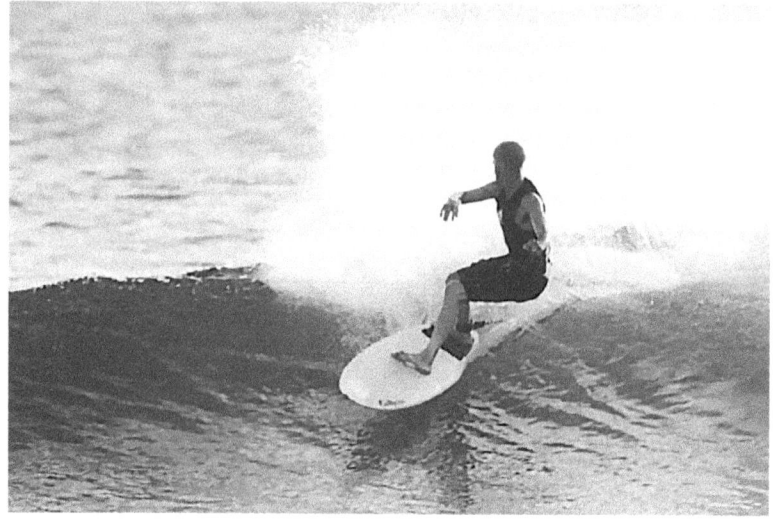

Good surf is great but you always have to wait

Again, I love it, but when I broke it down in my head, it just didn't hold up to mountain biking in terms of how much action you get for the time you have to put into it.

With mountain biking, you drive to the spot, gear up, and once you're on the bike — it's on. No waiting. No fighting for waves. Just flow. You're moving the entire time, pushing yourself physically and mentally, and getting those adrenaline hits all along the way.

Now, regular pedal bikes — what some people call analog or "acoustic" bikes — are fun, but let's be honest: climbing hills is a grind. Some people live for that kind of suffering, and yeah, it's great for fitness. But for me, it was always about the downhill. The speed, the berms, sending jumps, picking lines through rock gardens — that's the stuff I live for.

Then e-bikes caught my eye in 2019. I started seeing these full-suspension electric mountain bikes, and my curiosity was lit. These weren't clunky commuter rigs — they were legit downhill-capable machines. Suddenly, my BB gun legs would have real firepower going uphill. It was a game-changer. I could hit twice as many trails, double the number of descents, and ease the suffering on the climbs. I could ride twice as far in the same amount of time with less effort. Now we're talking.

Enter Brett Tippie

I'd known Tippie through Instagram — just casual online banter at first. We'd comment on each other's posts occasionally, throw a few likes, and slowly got to know one another. Tippie is a legend. A full-on pioneer in both snowboarding and mountain biking.

Brett Tippie has carved out a legacy that's wild, fearless, and influential. He started snowboarding back in 1983, and that passion launched him into a pro career representing Canada in over 25 World Cup events in Bordercross and Giant Slalom throughout the '90s. He capped it off by becoming the Canadian Grand National Boardercross Champion before stepping away from competition in 2000.

Brett Tippie dominated the racing scene, but since I was a freestyle snowboarder, we never really crossed paths — even though we rode snowboards during a very similar timeframe.

In 1983, he also got into mountain biking and became just as passionate about that sport. By the mid-'90s, he, Richie Schley, and Wade Simmons formed the Rocky Mountain Fro Riders — the first professional freeride MTB team. That crew helped create what we now know as freeride mountain biking: technical descents, sketchy cliff drops, lines no one thought were possible. They were doing it all on early bikes and gear that couldn't even come close to today's standards. Total madmen. Total visionaries.

In 2010, Brett, Richie, and Wade were inducted into the Mountain Bike

Hall of Fame for the incredible contributions they made to the sport. They helped launch a movement that keeps progressing — and they're all still at it today. Wade's running his eco-conscious bike care brand, Godfather's Garage, and still riding with Rocky Mountain's crew. Richie's hosting his "Schley Rides" podcast, still riding hard and staying active in the MTB industry and media. And Brett? He's still out there inspiring and pushing stoke in both snowboarding and mountain biking. An amazing set of OGs who helped shape the sport and continue to live it.

These days, Brett Tippie is still a huge presence in mountain biking — announcer, entertainer, host of The Brett Tippie Podcast, and full-time shredder. MTB is where his name carries the most weight today, but every winter he drops sweet tree-run powder clips from Canada that keep his snow roots alive. Beyond all the accomplishments, Tippie is just a genuinely rad dude. His journey hasn't always been easy. He's battled addiction and come out stronger, more grounded, and more inspiring than ever. He hasn't just left a mark on these sports — he's made a lasting impact on people.

I hit him up and sent him a message asking if he could help me get an e-bike through YT Industries, a brand he was riding for, representing, and had solid ties with. He knew about my background in the snowboard world and said he'd see what he could do.

Sure enough, he came through. Tippie hit up the marketing team at YT, and next thing I knew, he had a Decoy e-bike lined up with a 25% discount. That was during the peak of COVID, when inventory was locked down and getting a new bike was nearly impossible. When I showed up at YT to pick it up, some of the employees were tripping out. They couldn't believe I scored a Decoy — some of them had been trying for months to get their hands on one since there was no new inventory available at that time.

I guess it pays to have a rockstar connection like Brett Tippie pulling some strings for you.

And that's how my e-bike journey really began. It leveled up my mountain biking experience. Twice the trails, twice the descents, and zero guilt about skipping the grinding uphill. Just pure stoke.

Meeting Tippie — online and later in person — weren't just cool moments. They were full-circle experiences where two different chapters of life — snowboarding and mountain biking — collided in the coolest way. I'm still grateful for that hookup, but more than that, I'm stoked to call Brett a friend. He's a legend, an inspiration, and a solid dude.

E-Bikes: A Whole New World

When e-bikes first started showing up in the mountain biking scene, everything changed. Suddenly, riders could go so much farther, pedal up hills faster, and avoid getting maxed out with spiked heart rates and drained leg strength during those brutal, steep climb sections.

It opened up an entirely new way to experience the trails — twice the distance, double the laps, and still energy left in the tank by the end of the day. That kind of upgrade quickly proved hard to beat.

Even though e-biking might seem easier at first glance, when you ride at a fast pace, it can actually be a better workout than riding an analog bike. Mark Hill, who runs The Segment Channel, did an in-depth study comparing the two, and here's what he found in a 60-minute ride test on the same trails:

E-Bike vs. Analog Bike – Real Ride Stats, Up and Down the Same Trails
Calories burned:

E-Bike: 1,014

Analog: 922

(Measured using a chest strap heart rate monitor)
Peak heart rate:

E-Bike: 182 bpm

Analog: 180 bpm

Average heart rate:

E-Bike: 155 bpm

Analog: 152 bpm

Distance covered:

    E-Bike: 12 miles

    Analog: 6.7 miles

Elevation gained:

    E-Bike: 1,740 ft

    Analog: 1,000 ft

Analog   E-bike

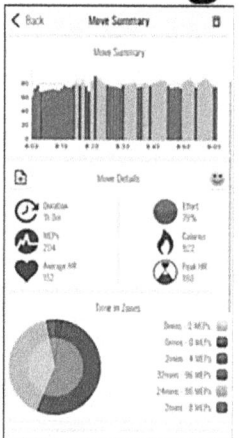 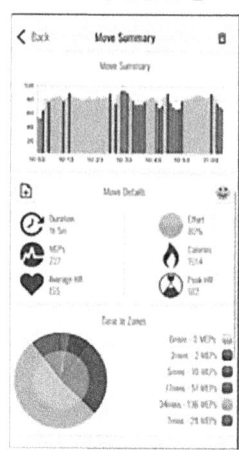

YT Jeffsy   YT Decoy

Of course, not everyone was quick to accept the shift. Some of the old-school purists saw e-biking as cheating or claimed it wasn't "real" mountain biking. But for those chasing adrenaline, flow, and the rush of downhill trails, the climb up was never the goal — it was just the price of admission. With full-suspension e-bikes, it became possible to get in double the runs in the same amount of time. What's not to love about that?

The Forest Service and trail rangers didn't love it either — not at first. To them, e-bikes were just motorized machines breaking the rules. But what they didn't understand is that e-bikes aren't tearing up trails like a Sur-Ron or electric dirt bike — they're just making it easier for riders who don't have pro-level lungs and legs to climb hills and enjoy the same epic terrain. They don't cause any more wear than a regular mountain bike, and they've opened up the outdoors for a whole new crew of passionate riders.

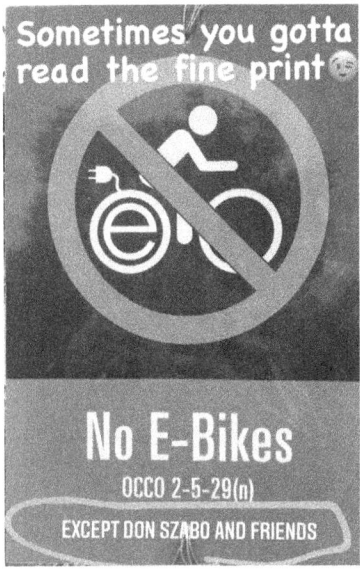

This sign says it all

I've been riding e-bikes on these trails for over five years now, long before the rules started to soften. Sure, technically, it wasn't allowed — but like a lot of things in life, there's a right way to bend the rules if you're smart about it. These days, many rangers have eased up on enforcing that outdated no e-bike rule, thanks to riders who've explained how power-assist pedaling really works, pitched in on trail maintenance, and shown we're not here to destroy — we're here to ride, respect, and rebuild. So when you see that "No E-Bikes" sign out there, make sure to read the fine print. It clearly says: Except Don Szabo and friends.

Before long, a whole community started forming around this new way of riding. Riders with that same mindset — chasing more laps, more fun, and more smiles — started finding each other. E-bikes became the ultimate tool for expanding the mountain biking adventure beyond the old-school analog approach. Forget shaving grams off components — something traditional bike riders often obsess over, spending big bucks on lightweight parts just to make their bikes a little lighter and maybe climb a bit easier. E-biking was about unlocking more possibilities: riding farther, climbing easier, going uphill faster — without all the hassle and cost.

That's when a Riverside crew came into the picture. I had to drive about an hour to meet up with them in their local riding zone, but it was worth it — those inland trails offered a solid change from my usual spots. It's a tight group of like-minded e-bikers who truly understand the mission. At the center of it all is Orven Zaragoza — an ex-pro rider with deep technical knowledge of bikes and a crazy-good memory for trails. He can piece together great rides from memory at whatever location we're riding, recalling tiny details like which tree, bush, or rock marked a key turnoff to the next great trail.

With Orven leading the charge, every ride feels like a proper adventure. Midweek meetups with them are serious business. Everyone shows up on time, dialed in, ready to hit the trail at true e-bike pace — fast, focused, and efficient. No messing around. Hit the ride, knock out the laps, get back to the vehicles, and slide right back into the demands of everyday life. Done deal. Simple as that.

In contrast, some of my Laguna Bike Shed crew rolls in late, talks some smack, and laughs their way into the ride once everyone is finally ready. It's less of a scheduled mission and more of a party on wheels. Although some serious riding still goes down, the riding is partly an excuse to hang out, crack jokes, and maybe have a post-ride drink or two. It's definitely a much looser crew.

Different crews, different tempos — but at the end of the day, it's all love for the ride that keeps us rolling.

Orven's riding style always stands out — just a half-shell helmet and no knee pads. No joke. For him, it's all part of keeping things mellow and controlled. He believes that riding light — without a full-face helmet or knee pads — keeps him from pushing too hard. And oddly enough, for him, it works. He rides great and rarely crashes. For other riders, that wouldn't work.

Crashes can come out of nowhere — even on the simplest sections — and some people are just magnets for disaster no matter what.

Weekend trips with that crew are next-level. But one ride stands out above the rest: the Palm Canyon Epic, or PCE. It kicked off with a 3 AM wake-up at home and an early meet-up in Palm Springs, followed by a shuttle way up into the mountains, deep in the pines. (A shuttle is a private or paid vehicle that brings people and their mountain bikes to a higher elevation and a distant starting point — well above where they'll finish the ride.) The trail started 26 miles out from the desert floor, winding its way all the way back down to Palm Springs.

Even with the benefit of the shuttle, most of the e-bike battery still got used up on the ride. There's a long, punishing sand wash toward the end that drains both legs and battery fast. Serious respect goes out to those who ride this — and other punishing climbs and trails — without any electric assist. That takes a whole different level of strength and endurance. For some, that's the path. For others, it's about maximizing the fun and covering more ground in less time.

And then there was the rainbow — out there in the distance, guiding our way the entire ride. The rain the night before had also left behind perfect hero dirt, the kind that locks tires in and makes every turn feel just right. The first mile of trail had a set of optional jumps, and most of them I sent blind — just trusting the flow or following someone who knew the speed and lines. A few of the more technical jumps definitely required some knowledge of the terrain to make happen, but they got done after riding that fun jump section a few times at the start of the long, epic ride.

The rest of the ride was great — nonstop flow, fun terrain, and endless good vibes. That 26-mile ride, with a rainbow leading the charge, hero dirt under the tires, and a dialed-in crew, stands out as one of the most beautiful and memorable rides ever. Every part of it — from the terrain to the scenery to the people — was truly special. That's what e-bikes unlock: more moments like that, in all kinds of places, with different crews of cool people. Much longer, more fun rides. Total game-changer.

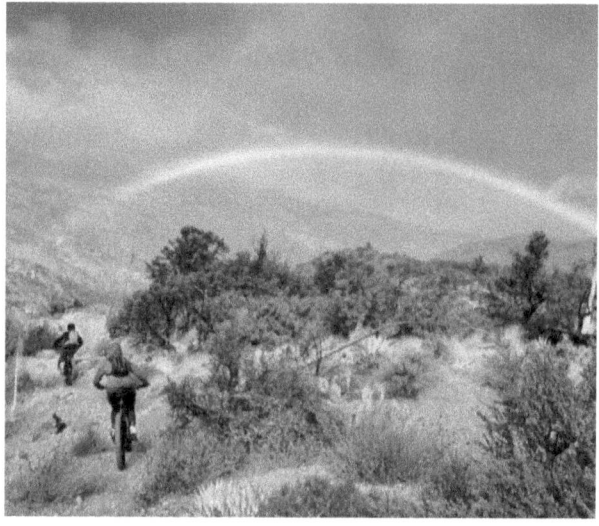

26 miles, chasing the rainbow — epic day

Whistler Bike Park
Trail Tow-ins & Big Mountain Sends

I caught wind that Calvin Yu and a crew of some guys I knew and rode with (and some I didn't know yet) were headed to Whistler, up in Canada. I'd been hearing for years that it was one of the most legendary bike parks on the planet, and there was no way I was gonna miss out on this great place I'd heard so much about. With only two weeks left before the trip, I had to hustle to get things ready. I managed to line up a bike bag for travel from a friend and, between juggling the chaos of life, the next thing I knew — I was on a flight headed to British Columbia.

I reached out to Pascal Gallant — Martin Gallant's brother — who I'd crossed paths with a few times on snowboards back in the '90s. Pascal had gotten deep into mountain biking, and when I hit him up, he didn't hesitate: "Come on up — we'll meet at the lifts and ride the mountain." That's all I needed to hear.

We linked up with Pascal on our first day after warming up with a few runs through Whistler's massive playground of trails. When we met at the bottom lift, he asked, "You guys been down *A-Line* yet?" referring to one of the park's most famous jump lines. I told him no, and then asked him the critical question: "Do you know the speed for all the hits?"

Without missing a beat, he grinned and said, "I know it like the back of my hand."

That was what I needed to hear. We took the lifts up the mountain, *dropped into A-Line*, and I locked in behind him, matching his moves. This kind of riding is what we call getting "towed in." It doesn't involve a rope or any actual towing — it's all about following someone who knows the trail. You match their speed, follow their lines, and use their experience to help you clear each jump and flow through the section like you've done it before. It's one of the best ways to learn a new zone, especially a trail as fast and flowing as A-Line.

And wow — A-Line was a full-on adrenaline rush. I didn't have to overthink it. I just trusted Pascal's pace, mimicked his body positioning, and followed his rhythm through the flowy rollers and massive tabletops. It instantly reminded me of motocross. Back in the day, my moto buddies would tow me into big jumps or through a new track the same way — leading the way so I could lock in and learn. The feeling was similar. The jumps on A-Line might've been half the size of what I was launching back in the moto days, but now I was riding at twice the age I was then — so the math kind of balanced out.

Downhill mountain biking is powered by gravity, whereas motocross, you have a throttle. But once you're in the zone — especially on a new trail — it's all about trusting the ground, trusting your guide, and trusting yourself. If you've got a rider in front who knows the terrain, you can lock into their lines and get pulled right into the flow. That's exactly how it went on A-Line — full send on a 1.8-mile trail with around 30 jumps, clean hits all the way down, and the kind of run that makes you want to turn right back around and do it again.

And when we did go again, there is a jump called the "Moon Booter" that became even more fun each time. This beast sits about halfway down the trail, kicking off with a very high-banked right-hand berm that rolls you into a long, fast downhill stretch for at least a couple hundred feet. It swoops into a 20-foot-tall jump — or "booter" — built for liftoff. Hit it with the right speed and you're flying 30 to 50 feet through the air, grinning the whole way. The landing? Butter-smooth, long, and forgiving — designed for serious airtime. Easily one of the best hits on A-Line. Pure fun, every single time.

After that, Pascal turned to us and said, "Wanna go hit *Dirt Merchant*?" I was like, "Let's go — I'll follow your line."

Dirt Merchant was next-level. Bigger hits, *hips*, step-downs, step-ups, and features that had me grinning ear to ear. Following Pascal's lead made it feel like a slingshot ride through a dream trail. Many of the jumps pushed 20 to 30 feet, and the hips meant you had to throw the bike sideways in the air and land angled into the next section. He knew all the lines and how to move through them, and I just mirrored his flow — staying loose and letting the trail pull us along like we were strapped into a roller coaster. But this time, we were the ones in control.

One standout feature halfway down the trail was a *bridge drop* — you had to launch about 15 feet down and 15 feet out. You had to land it smooth and keep your momentum. Not long after that drop came a good-sized step-up jump. You'd land from the previous drop, roll through around a hundred feet of swooping trail, keeping your speed up, and then launch nearly 30 feet out — gaining 10 vertical feet of airtime onto a landing that was at least 20 feet higher than the very bottom of the swooping trail. I don't know if my measurements are correct, but it doesn't matter — I just know the rush was real. I had no idea that step-down and step-up even existed. I wasn't one of those guys who studies videos or obsesses over trail previews. I just rolled in blind behind Pascal and trusted his *tow-in* to take me where I needed to go. It was wild — the kind of thrill you don't plan for. You just trust, commit, and send it.

The trail twisted, dropped, carved, and flowed like a wild roller coaster. Banks, berms, and jumps led from one feature to the next. The rush was real — and it's etched in my mind like a signature line and a really good time. Following someone down an exciting trail for the first time like this is a rush that can't be explained by words alone.

We ended up hitting A-Line and Dirt Merchant multiple times, mixing in some other solid trails that Pascal knew well — he knows Whistler Bike Park like the back of his hand. We were lucky to have him as a guide, especially when you're dropping into jump lines and technical sections blind. Tow-ins from someone who knows the flow make all the difference. Riding with an old friend like that, after not seeing each other for decades, made it even more special.

And this wasn't just a one-time trip — it happened a few times on other visits to Canada, including the first time I met back up with Sean Johnson in over 25 years a few months later. We talked about those car-hood-sliding days in Japan and caught up on all kinds of things in life and had a blast riding together. It was amazing to see him in a whole new chapter. From his wild, drunken Whiskey video days to now — married, with a kid, living on Vancouver Island and running his own company, Storm Saunas. The craftsmanship and design of the saunas he builds are incredible. He's proof that people can change direction, learn new skills, and create something positive and meaningful with their lives. Seeing that kind of transformation firsthand just reminded me how powerful growth can be — at any stage in life.

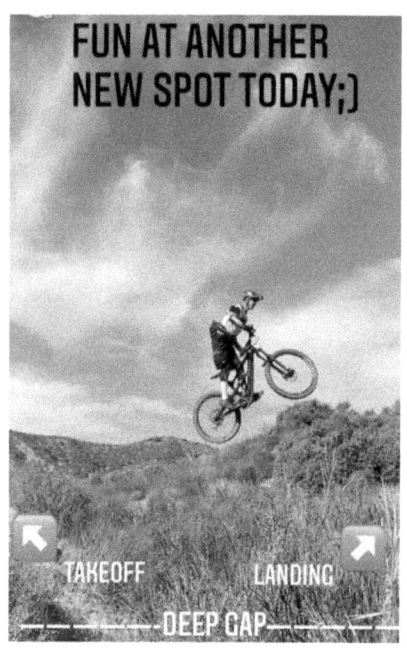

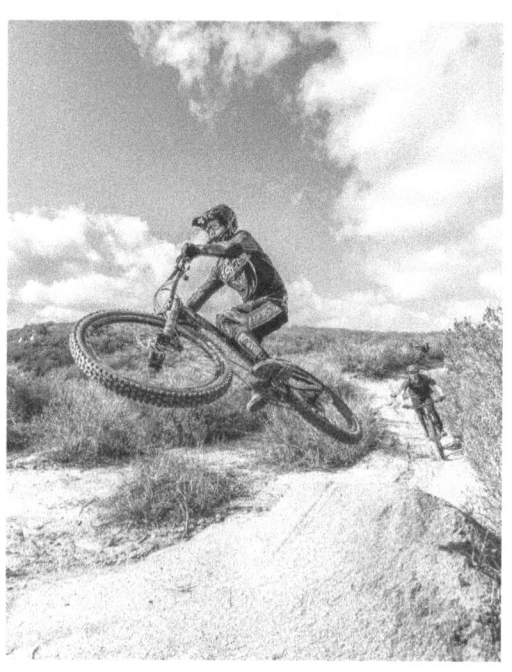

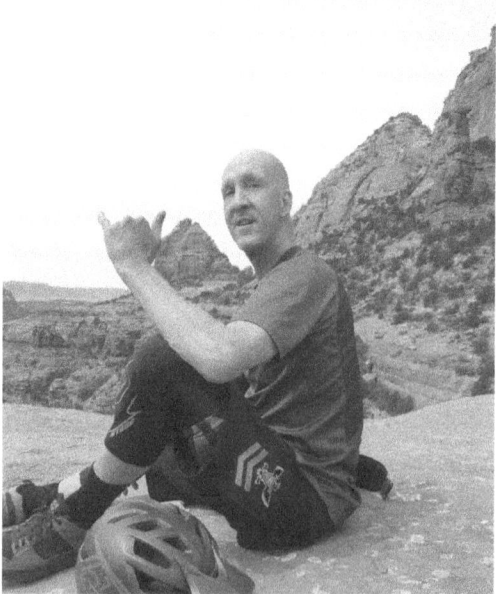

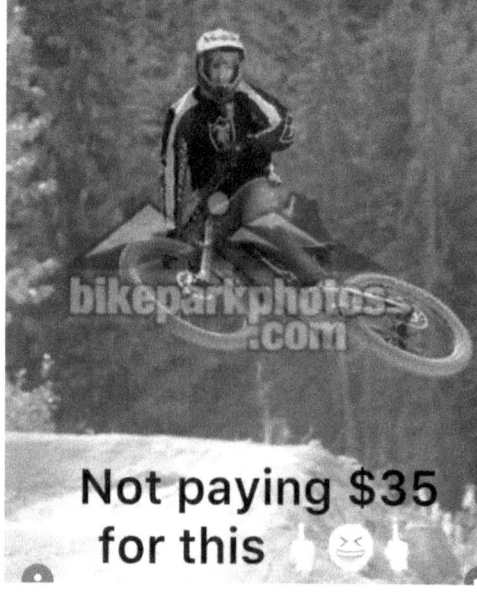

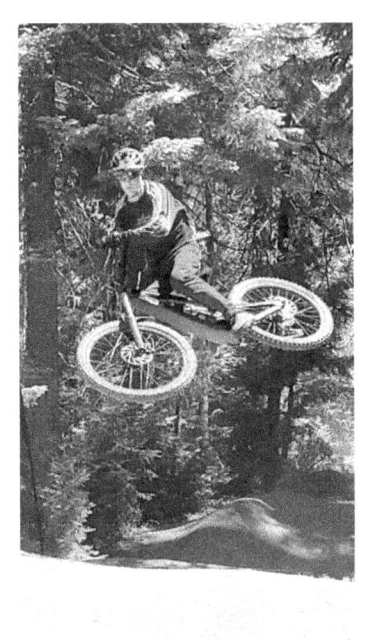

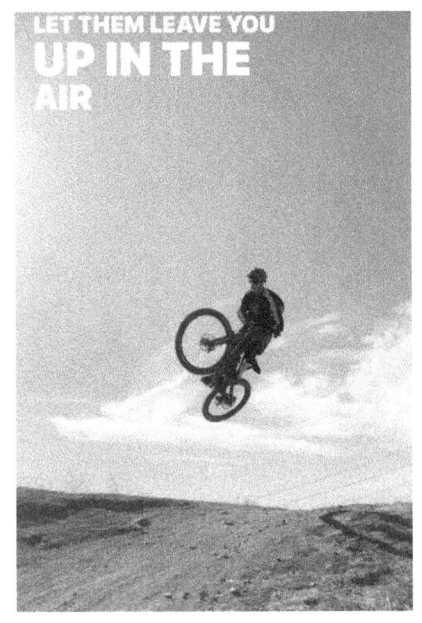

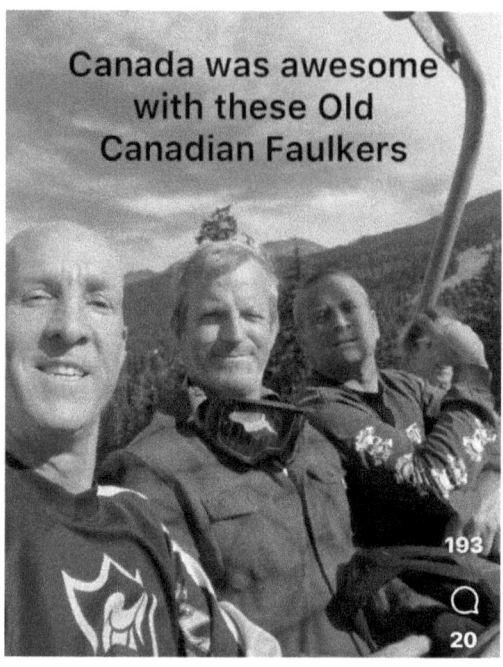

From snow in the 90's to MTB in '22. Me, Sean Johnson and Pascal Gallant

Crabapple Hits — Big Jumps

Toward the end of the week, we made our way over to the Crabapple jump line. Word was — it was on another level.

When we got there, the jump line was empty. It was intimidating just standing at the top. A straight-up *progression line*: 10-footer, 20-footer, 30-footer, 50-footer...and a 65-foot gap toward the end. No joke. The kind of jumps that separate the senders from the spectators.

The local wisdom was this — if you hit the 30-footer clean and stayed off the brakes, you'd have the speed to hit the 50 and then the 65-foot gap just right. First run through, I hit the 10, 20, and 30-footer, but came up a little short and *clipped the knuckle* of the landing on the 30, so I grabbed brake and played it safe. No sense sending the next two if the speed wasn't there.

But I wasn't done. I went back up to the top of the line, reset, and knew exactly what I had to do — get a bit more speed into the 30 and then just let it fly for the next two jumps. The crew waited at the bottom, watching. They weren't feeling like sending it that day, so it was all on me.

Drop in — 10-footer, clean. 20-footer, smooth. 30-footer, perfect landing. I stayed off the brakes and let the bike fly into the 50-footer — clean jump. Then came the 65-footer.

I came into the dip before the takeoff with solid speed, feeling locked in. I launched, giving it just a little *whip* for style — meaning I threw the bike sideways, kicked the back end out just enough, not too wild. A whip is all about that flair — that little signature midair. It can also help you stay more comfortable while jumping if you know how to use it to your advantage.

The best riders in the world throw their bikes so far sideways — or even upside down — you wonder how they bring it back around. I've seen riders throw the rear wheel past the front wheel midair and still stick the landing. Next-level talent for sure.

I'm not throwing world-class whips like that, but I added just enough flair to make it mine — and it helped me feel comfortable in the air over the jump. My buddy Henry was posted up by the 65-footer with his phone rolling video and got a great clip. I heard him yell out, "Yeah, Szab!" as I floated through the air, spotted my landing, brought the bike back straight, and landed the jump clean.

It was one of those personal milestones that just hit different. Vision, confidence, and skill all lined up — and it went smooth. I was riding a trail bike with just 150mm of travel — not even a full-on downhill rig like most of the other riders, who were on 180-to-200mm suspension bikes built for this stuff. They thought I was crazy sending Crabapple on my trail bike setup, but hey — I made it work. Because that's what you gotta do. You don't always need the perfect gear. Sometimes, you just need the mindset — the knowledge that you've got the skill, and the confidence to send it and make it happen.

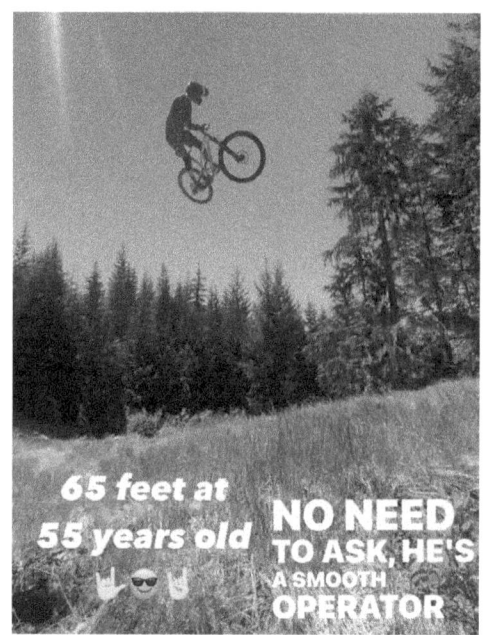

Crabapple hits on the trail bike

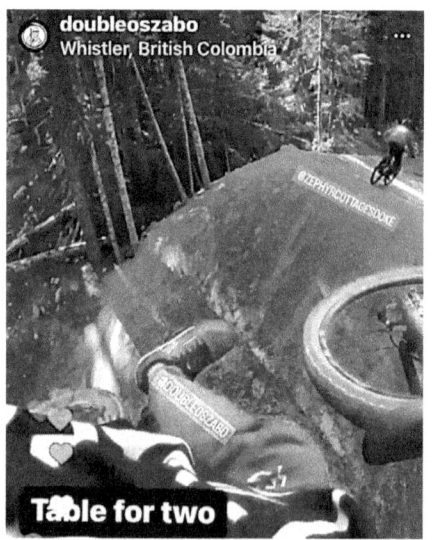

It's hard to get your bike completely flat in the air

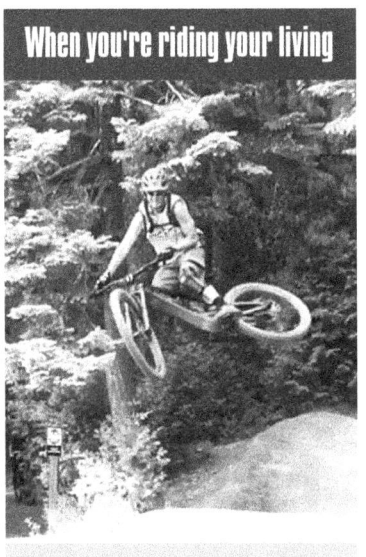

When you're riding your living

Everything else is just waiting

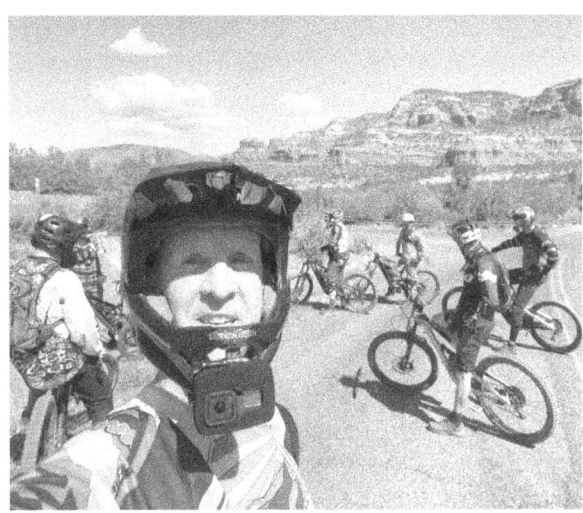

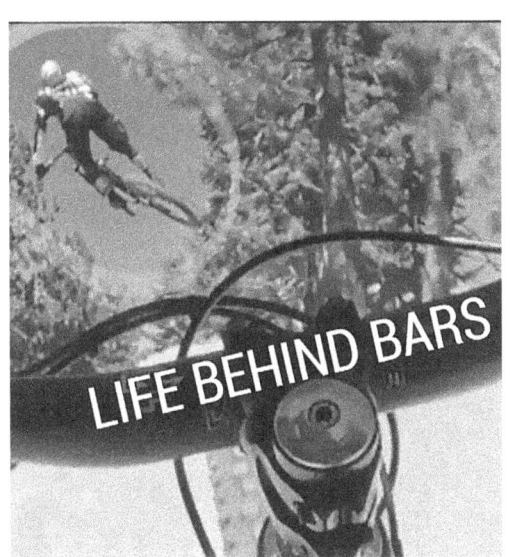

LIFE BEHIND BARS

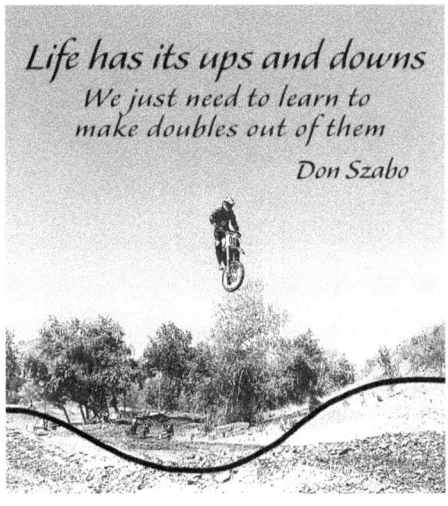

Life has its ups and downs
We just need to learn to
make doubles out of them

Don Szabo

Old Friends, New Night-Riding

That afternoon, Whistler took on a whole new vibe. Ken Achenbach rolled into Whistler Bike Park to meet up — his name carries weight, not just as a pioneer in snowboarding, but as a longtime friend from the old snowboard days. Ken, now a savvy realtor with a past full of groundbreaking snowboarding innovation, has a legacy too long to get into here. He also launched the Camp of Champions in Whistler, which gave generations of skiers and snowboarders the chance to train, have fun, and level up for over 25 years. Ken always had that drive and big ideas to build the sport from the ground up.

Alongside him was Don Schwartz, a guy whose resilience after a brutal helicopter crash made him an icon of survival and grit in extreme sports. Since then, Don's gone on to write a book, Beating the Impossible, and his story was featured in the documentary In the Blink of an Eye. He's stayed active in the mountains, proving that mindset and grit can carry you through just about anything.

I won't get into the full backstories — they're legendary in our circles — but seeing them again reminded me of reconnecting with the younger, wilder versions of ourselves that we used to be, back when we all rode snowboards together in the late 80's through the late 90's.

Later, Ken picked me up in his truck with his e-bike, and we set out to meet Brett Tippie for a night ride. Brett — a bundle of energy with his dad jokes, witty humor, and contagious laugh — had an e-bike ready for me and all the lights we'd need for riding in the dark.

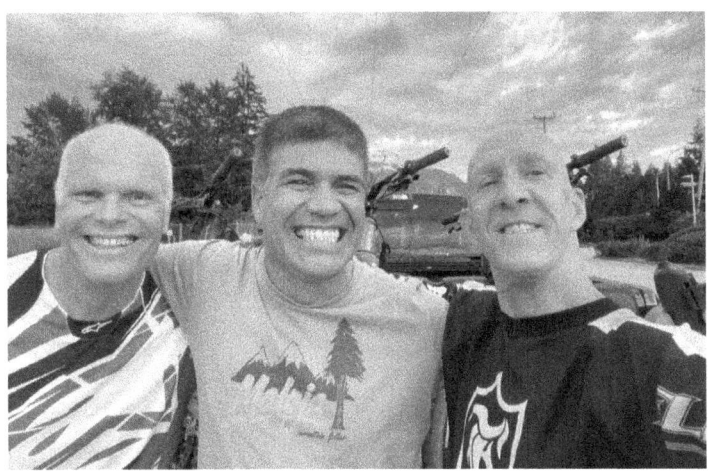

Pre-night ride with Ken Ach and Brett Tippie

Night riding is a whole other beast — it transforms the trails into shadowy adventures where every turn feels brand new, which it was for me. With the crisp glow of our bike lights and Tippie guiding us, we tore through trails, laughing, riding, and having a blast with every turn of the handlebars.

After the ride, Tippie welcomed me to his home. I crashed in a makeshift spot in the basement — classic road-trip vibes. The next morning, I met his amazing family and rolled out with him to his local Harley-Davidson dealership. Tippie's a local hero up there. The dealership said, "Take whatever rental Harley you want — for the week. It's on us."

Of course, he hit the guy with a classic dad joke, then rode off on a Harley while I followed behind him in his truck. That drive back was nothing short of stunning. Canada has some seriously beautiful terrain — and great trails if you know where to go around Vancouver and Squamish. Amazing hills, deep forests, and wide-open skies. Just one of those views you want to bottle up and keep forever.

I didn't ride Whistler that day. I'd been pushing it at Whistler all week and got this day to chill. So it turned into a cruiser hangout day with Tippie — laid back but still full of energy.

Back at the bike park, the crew returned to the Crabapple jump line with the 65-footer.

I heard our friend Albert gave it a go — and that's when things went south. He got the wrong trajectory off the jump takeoff, went over the bars, and on the landing, slammed hard.

The diagnosis: he fractured his neck in three places. It was serious, but luckily, it wasn't worse. No paralysis, no displaced bones — just fracture cracks. Still, it shook all of us. That's the kind of fall that makes you pause.

He stayed up in Canada a little longer to recover while the majority of the crew flew home to the States. And for a while, he talked about walking away from mountain biking.

That was such a bummer to hear — but understandable. He's got two young kids and a family to take care of. That crash rattled him — and all of us. But in true Albert style, the mountain bike passion eventually came back. A few months later, he was back on the trails. You can't keep a good man like him down.

Now he's still the same Albert — happy, full of energy, cracking jokes, laughing, and sharing his infectious stoke on the trail.

That kind of spirit is contagious. It's what brings people together again and again. Injuries may knock us down, but it's that inner fire that keeps us rolling. And Albert — he's the perfect example. He's back on the bike, ripping the trails just as hard as ever, laughing, and bringing the good vibes like he never missed a beat. He's got the right mindset to keep the good times rolling — and when you've got that kind of energy flowing, it pulls everyone along for the ride.

Virgin, Utah

One of the most unforgettable mountain bike trips I've taken was to Virgin, Utah. This area is known for its rugged and dramatic landscapes, featuring expansive mesas, steep canyons, and iconic red rock formations. The terrain offers a mix of rugged, rocky sections, technical descents, and sculptable dirt that holds well to carve while still breaking free to be molded into whatever riders can envision — a natural playground to test their skills and creativity. The natural beauty is breathtaking, with panoramic views that make every ride a visual feast.

It's also home to the Red Bull Rampage — the most insane freeride mountain bike event on the planet. Unlike traditional races, Rampage isn't judged by speed. It's about style, difficulty, creativity, and landing the kind of jumps and lines that seem impossible to the average rider. These guys hand-build their own routes down towering cliffs, sending massive drops and tackling technical features that blur the line between riding and flying. It's raw, powerful, and demands absolute commitment and respect.

Now, I'm the first to admit — I don't have anywhere near the skill or the balls to do what those Rampage riders pull off. But just being out there, surrounded by the same terrain they've made legendary, is amazing. There's something sacred about Virgin. The red rock cliffs stretch endlessly in every direction, and the silence of the desert is only broken by the sound of tires gripping dirt, rocks, your own breath echoing inside your helmet, and the stoke you share riding this place with others.

I was riding with my friend Kyle Lecocq, who knows this area well. He took me out on the Flying Monkey Trail, which winds its way past the infamous King Kong trail. Just being close to that kind of legendary ground lit a fire inside me. Flying Monkey was no joke — tight lines, sketchy sections, and enough exposure to keep your focus razor-sharp. It was an adrenaline-filled trail that was amazing to ride down.

The next day, after another awesome night camping under the stars with friends, we hit the Grafton Trail — another beast of a downhill run. It was also fast in spots and technical in others, with just enough rocks and sudden drops to keep you on your toes all the way down. We were laughing, breathing hard, and riding right on the edge of control — and that's exactly what made it so damn fun.

When we reached the bottom, Kyle casually pointed toward a gap and said, "That's the Grafton Gap."

I followed his gaze and saw it — this massive dirt-to-dirt jump spanning a significant gap between two ridgelines. Before I could say anything, Kyle looked at me and grinned. "Think you can hit it?"

I took a minute to soak it in. It was huge — about two stories high and just as wide. But something in me clicked. Maybe it was the adrenaline still surging from the trail, or maybe it was the energy of the place. I nodded and said, "Yeah…I can do it."

Before I knew it, his friend was pulling a vehicle up and parking it right under the gap. Apparently, this wasn't going to be just any jump — I was about to clear a car. That raised the stakes fast. I hiked my bike up above the lip of the jump, heart pounding, trying to block out everything but the line. I stood at the roll-in, eyes scanning from the takeoff to the landing.

The gap wasn't really visible from up there, but I knew what I had to do. The desert air was still, the horizon wide open. I visualized the motion — lifting off, floating across, landing clean.

Then I dropped in.

As I hit the takeoff, I committed. I launched into the air, fully locked in, watching that landing zone like a hawk. I cleared the car nicely. The tires reconnected with dirt, and for a moment, I was riding that high…until I realized something.

I should've immediately been on my brakes.

I hadn't really looked at the runout after the jump. I'd just focused on what I had to do to clear it. In the distance in front of me, the trail dropped off into a massive twenty-foot-deep wash. I didn't realize it was there. It came up fast, and now I was quickly approaching the edge — even though I was already on the brakes trying to stop.

Then, at the last second, I spotted it — a steep, rutted chute carved into the dirt wall going into the wash. It wasn't vertical, maybe 70 or 80 degrees, and it looked just barely rideable.

As I skidded to the edge, I made the decision: I'm going to ride down it.

I leaned my weight back, dropped in, and surfed that nasty chute all the way to the bottom of the wash, making the tires navigate through the ruts.

What started as a big jump turned into a full-on survival mission. First, soaring over a car. Then, navigating a steep descent into an unexpected wash. It gave me one of the biggest adrenaline spikes I've had in a while — even though this entire place had already been providing plenty of thrills. I came out the other side laughing and feeling absolutely alive. It was awesome.

That's Virgin, Utah, for you. It's rugged, raw, and beautiful in a way that makes you feel small — but it also invites you to go big. That place has a soul. For a few days, a few runs, and that wild section, I felt like I was a part of it.

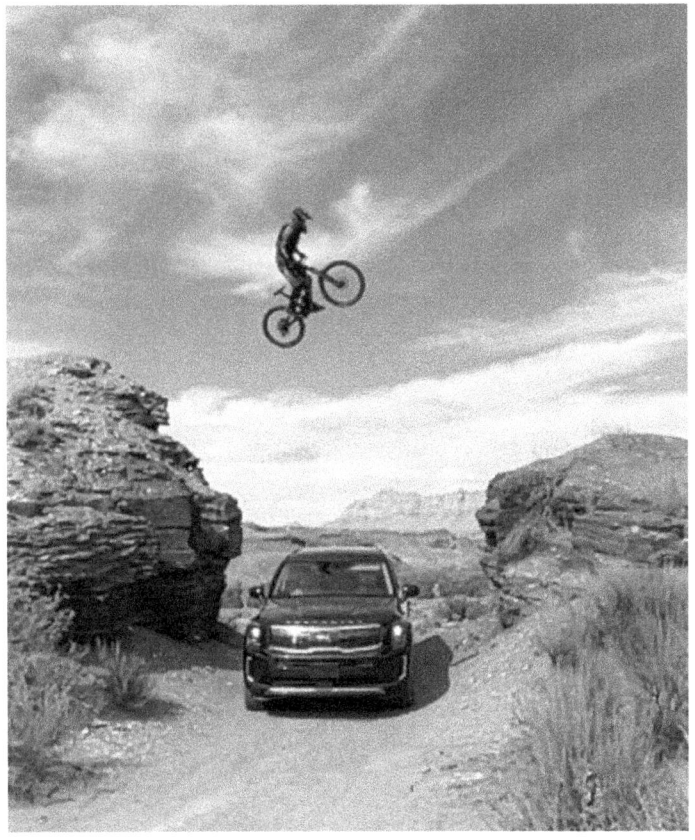

Grafton Gap — friend parked his car, I jumped it

-Chapter 17-
Asia Rocks

In late 2022, my hard-working sister, an engineer who had dedicated nearly 25 years to her company, found herself at a crossroads. Her company relocated its headquarters to Texas, leaving her with a tough decision: uproot her life or stay in California and take a new path. She chose to stay, though the transition left her in a strange limbo, consulting here and there as she navigated her next steps in her work life.

During one of our conversations, she expressed a desire to travel while she had the rare opportunity — before diving back into another engineering position. Thailand had caught her interest, and I suggested she make it happen. At the same time, I felt a strong pull to return to Japan — a place that had been such a huge part of my life from the late '80s through the late '90s. I wanted to reconnect with my old friend Sohn, who had been my Japanese snowboard distributor and partner in countless adventures that started over 35 years ago. The thought of catching up after all these years was too good to pass up.

As we talked, we realized we both wanted to go to Asia, and the idea of traveling together started to take shape. Neither of us knew how it would go. Would we have a great time together, or end up driving each other crazy? There was only one way to find out. So, with two weeks in Japan and two weeks in Thailand planned, my sister and I dove into the adventure.

Around this time, my growing interest in revisiting Japan connected in a unique way with a surprising friendship I'd developed through Instagram.

Algorithms on social media are a strange thing, and Instagram — now my preferred platform — played an unexpected role in shaping this part of the journey.

I've been on Facebook for years and still use it here and there, but when I'm not outside in nature or living real life, Instagram is the online zone I like to visit most to connect with friends or the mountain bike community and build relationships that matter. One of those connections began in 2020 and, three years later, led me to meet her halfway across the world in 2023.

One evening, while scrolling Instagram, I came across a post that was part of the Women Supporting Women Challenge. Her image was captivating, and the words she wrote struck a chord. It was written by Rynn Kawahara, a woman living in Japan, offering words of encouragement and support to other women. I clicked on her profile — a rare occurrence for me. She was a singer, and I was drawn into her world through her photos and energy. I liked a few of her posts and moved on, but the connection didn't end there.

Rynn visited my page to see who I was — a stranger taking interest in a few of her posts. What she found surprised her. She saw my world of action sports, then discovered deep ties to Japan, and posts about losing my wife and mother to cancer struck a chord with her. She reacted to many of my posts, seeing shared values and a unique window into my life. Cancer was something close to her heart, and she appreciated my love for Japanese culture. Despite our very different lives, we discovered surprising commonalities and began communicating regularly.

Rynn and I formed a modern online friendship built on curiosity and mutual respect, with many conversations that crossed continents and time zones. She stays up into the late hours, and we'd chat often as I was waking up. We developed a bond that felt real, even if it was only rooted in electronic communication, pictures, and videos. It's remarkable how technology can bring people together in such unexpected ways.

When I told Rynn that Karen and I were planning a trip to Japan, she didn't just offer to meet up — she offered to show us around Tokyo and arranged for us to stay with her friend Rieko. Her enthusiasm to help us made the trip feel even more exciting. For me, this wasn't just a chance to visit a place I loved, but also to connect with someone I had developed a friendship with.

Our plan for Japan was now taking shape. The first leg of the trip would be spent in Tokyo, where Rynn would show us around and Rieko would host us at her apartment overlooking the city. After a week in Tokyo, we would travel to Kyoto, a city I'd never explored before, to reconnect with Sohn, my old snowboarding distributor and friend. In the past, my trips to Japan had always taken me north, chasing the best snow all the way to the north island of Hokkaido. But this time, we'd head west — to Kyoto's rich cultural history and the chance to see Sohn, which made it the perfect destination.

With everything coming together, it felt like the right balance of reconnecting with the past and embracing new friendships. First up, our time in Tokyo with Rynn.

Exploring Tokyo with Rynn

We kicked off our trip in Tokyo, staying with Rieko, a friend of Rynn's that she had lined up for us. Her apartment was perched on the 14th floor with stunning views over the skyline — a perfect welcome to the week ahead. That first night, Rynn brought an amazing spread of sushi and traditional Japanese dishes, setting the tone for what would be a fantastic adventure.

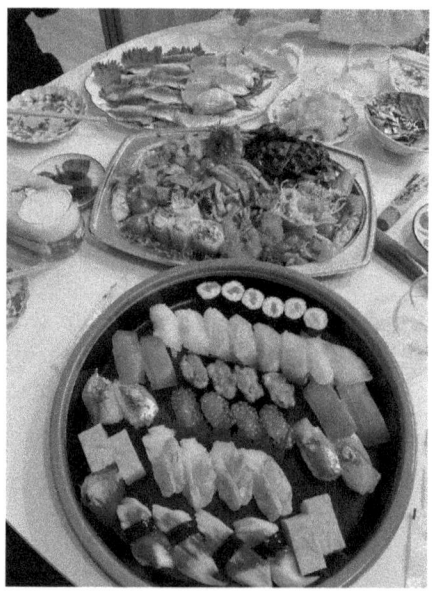

Tokyo night #1 — Rynn brought the sushi goods

Rieko was a wonderful host, warmly welcoming us and showing us around their city in a way we never could have discovered on our own — giving us a true local's perspective on the heartbeat of the city.

Rynn turned out to be the ultimate tour guide. She took us to temples like the Meiji Shrine, rich with history and tradition. We checked out cultural experiences like Kabuki theater, and she gave us fascinating insights into Japanese customs and daily life. There's nothing quite like exploring a place with someone who knows it inside and out, and her enthusiasm for sharing her world made everything that much more special.

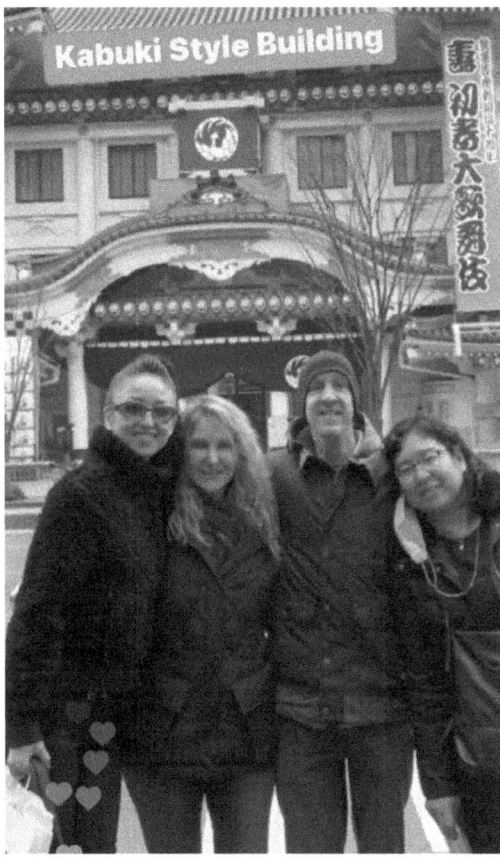

Kabuki style with the crew

The Rhythm of Japan

One thing that really stood out was the efficiency of Japan's public transportation. The trains and buses weren't just reliable — they were precise, arriving exactly on time and making it effortless to get wherever we wanted to go. It was a stark contrast to the sometimes-chaotic, clunky systems back in the U.S. where most people don't even consider using public transportation because it's so inefficient. While I love the freedom and openness of America, I couldn't help but admire Japan's commitment to organization and functionality — not just in transportation, but in other areas of life, like the cleanliness everywhere.

One particularly memorable stop was a visit to the area where Rynn had went to college in Aoyama. While wandering the streets, we stumbled upon a Vans skateboard shoe store with a massive photo of my old friend Steve Caballero doing a boneless skateboard trick. I couldn't resist taking a shot of me holding up one of his signature shoes in front of the display — creating a layered moment where past and present collided in the coolest way, in a completely different world than the one I'd grown used to living in back in the U.S.

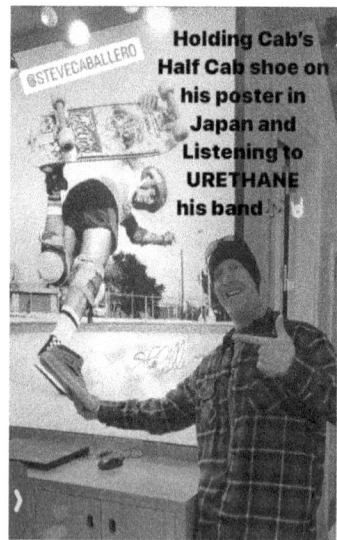

.Holding Cab's shoe model in front of his poster in Japan

During our time in Tokyo, we visited the grounds of the Imperial Palace — one of the Japanese emperor's residences, and a place sacred to anyone living in Japan. For the Japanese people, seeing the Emperor is a deeply meaningful experience, something etched into the memory of anyone lucky enough to witness it. As we stood near the palace, we actually saw the Emperor himself, waving from the window of his open limo to a small crowd of people gathered to take in the beauty and history of the grounds.

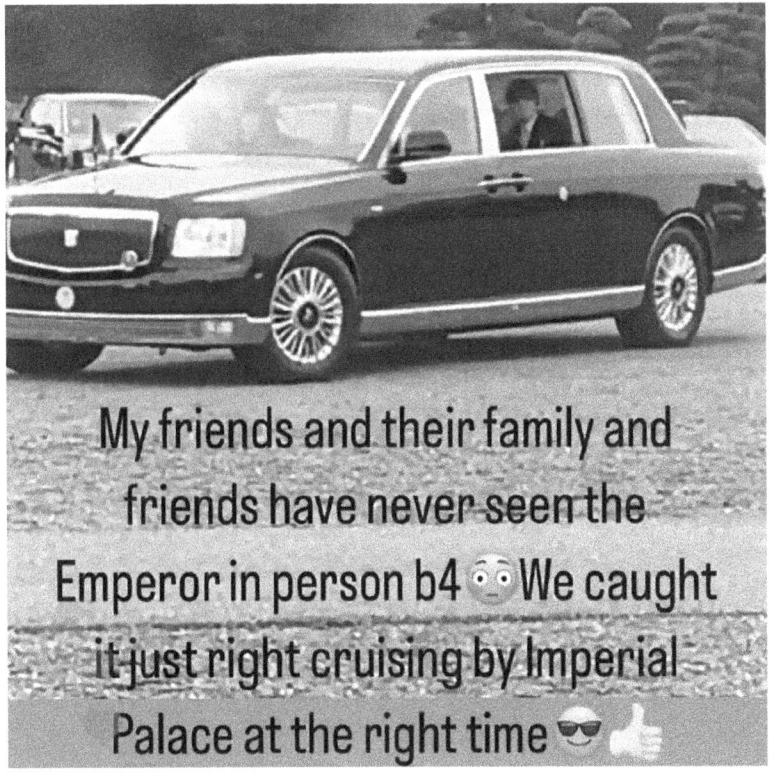

My friends and their family and friends have never seen the Emperor in person b4 👀 We caught it just right cruising by Imperial Palace at the right time 😎 👍

When Double O Szabo calls — even the Emperor listens

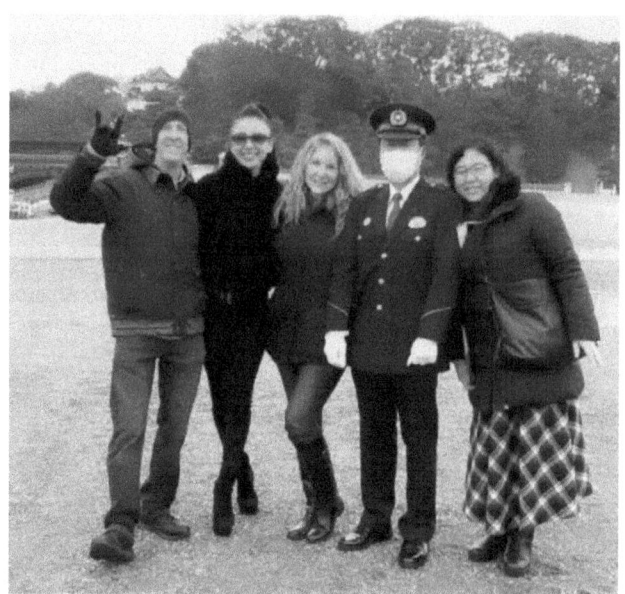
Got the guard to drop his guard and snap a pic with us

Rynn couldn't believe it. Even her mom and sister had never seen the Emperor in person before — neither has most of Japan's population. Watching her light up with excitement, and later hearing her tell her mom and friends what she had seen, made the moment even more special.

Rynn's Musical World

For Karen and me, the most unforgettable experience of the trip so far happened when we watched Rynn perform at the music studio with Shinji on guitar.

She pours her passion and energy into their music project, grinnBos, with a strong sense of mission and purpose. She dedicates herself to studio work, crafting their unique sound and style to deliver positive messages through their music.

The reserved, soft-spoken woman we had spent the week with — the one I had come to know online and now in person — suddenly became a commanding presence. The stage brought out a version of her that was vibrant, powerful, and magnetic. Her voice was strong and brimming with emotion, and the way she moved, performed, and sang drew us in completely. Shinji kept the rhythm stylishly steady on an acoustic guitar, adding his own flair and providing a sound that balanced beautifully with hers, creating a rich tone between the two of them.

Even though I couldn't understand most of the lyrics — aside from the songs she sang in English, which is impressive on its own — I still felt the power in her performance. I recognized some of the songs from what she had shared with me in the past through her Instagram music page. We had also done a few collaboration videos, combining her beautiful, rockin' music with my mountain biking footage — blending her world and mine in a unique cultural mix we both posted on Instagram. Seeing her come alive in her element was inspiring — an amazing transformation my sister and I will never forget.

Our time in Tokyo was filled with meaningful connections and cultural experiences that gave my sister and I a deeper appreciation for Japan, beyond the snowboarding days I'd experienced decades ago. But this was just the beginning. The second week in Japan would take us beyond Tokyo, as I reunited with Sohn and reflected on our adventures that started over 35 years ago. We also made new memories that will last well into the future.

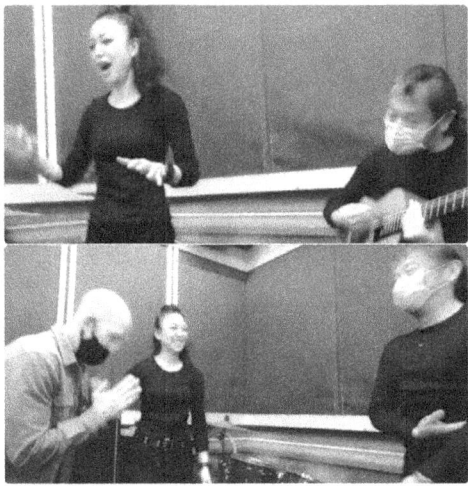

Rynn and Shinji rockin' the studio

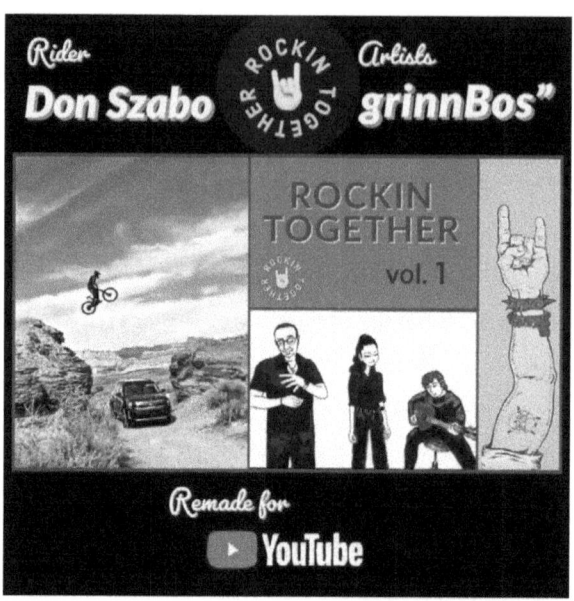

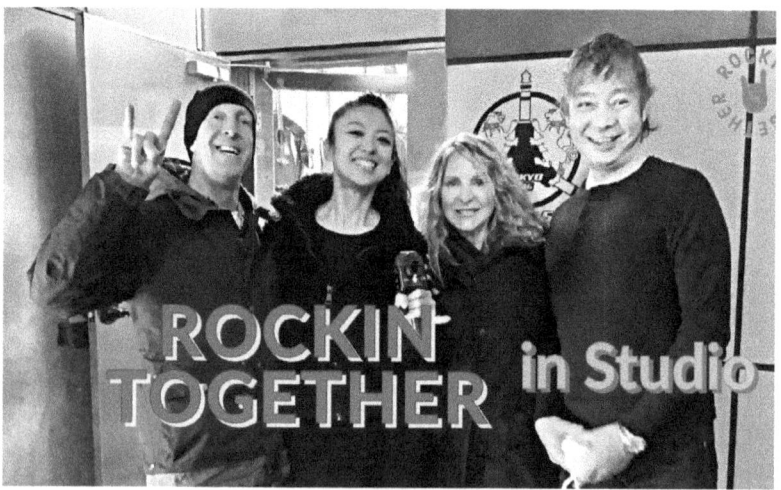

Rockin' together, in the studio and online

Kyoto Bound

So far our Asia trip was a journey of connection, beauty, and unforgettable moments. After exploring Tokyo with Rynn and watching her incredible transformation on stage, Karen and I boarded a bullet train west to Kyoto. Meeting up with Sohn there felt like revisiting an old chapter of my life — reconnecting not just with a longtime friend, but with someone who had played a pivotal role in my early snowboarding career.

From 1988 through 1991, Sohn was my Japanese distributor for Nectar Snowboards and a good friend. He was instrumental in promoting my pro models, and together, we traveled across Japan for a few years, visiting snowboard shops, organizing on-snow demos, and building excitement around the sport. But what set Sohn apart wasn't just his business sense — it was his ability to make things happen. He had the connections, the vision, and the follow-through to turn ideas into reality. He knew how to work with shops, generate buzz, and bring fans to the mountains where we would ride with locals and showcase the energy of snowboarding firsthand to those checking it out.

Sohn even lined up TV coverage, helping introduce the sport to a broader audience in Japan at a time when snowboarding was still carving out its place on the slopes. His drive and strategic thinking played a huge role in making those years so memorable for me. Seeing him now — a highly successful businessman with ventures in multiple industries, including his involvement in the golfing world — was both inspiring and a reminder of how far he's come since those early days. He also has a place on Oahu in Hawaii and we keep in touch online, sharing glimpses of our lives. Some of the people we interact with there are old friends; others are digital acquaintances we may never meet in person, but there's still a connection.

Looking back, those years traveling Japan with Sohn weren't just about promoting my snowboard model — they were about experiencing a culture that left a lasting impact on me. The excitement of those shop tours, the energy of the on-snow demos, and the friendships forged along the way have stayed with me ever since.

Kyoto's timeless beauty provided the perfect setting for our reunion. The

Golden Temple shimmered like something out of a dream, its reflection in the still waters creating a sense of surreal perfection. This trip was especially unique because the temple was dusted with snow — a rare sight in Kyoto. The snow accentuated the temple's beauty, with the golden roof and intricate details glowing against the white backdrop. The structure, adorned with real gold, was breathtaking. Its monetary, cultural, and spiritual value added to its awe-inspiring presence, especially for those familiar with its history.

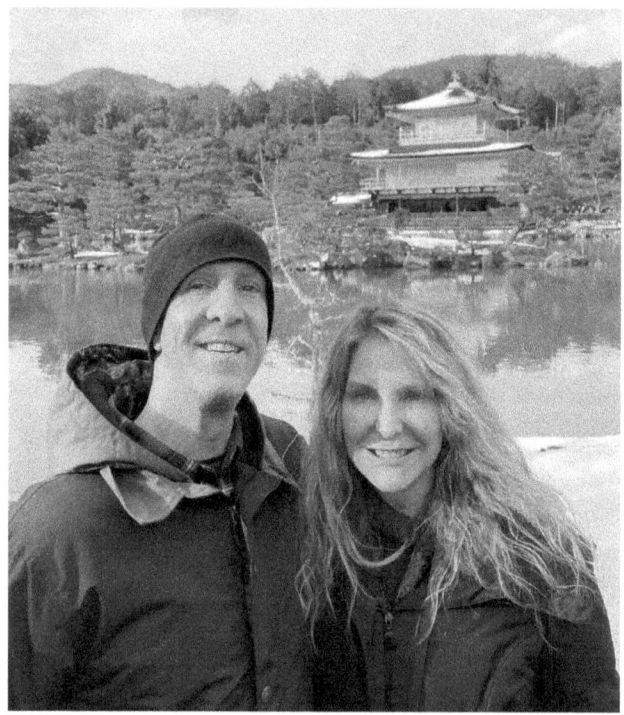

Golden Temple. Real gold. That's mental

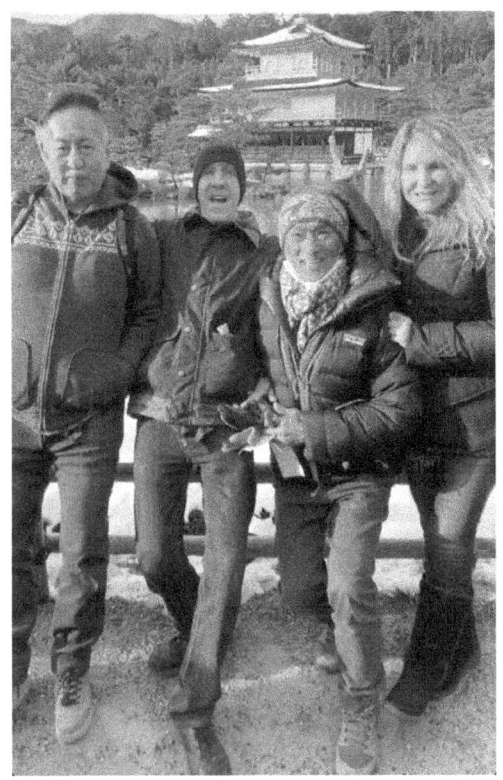

Crew in the front, gold in the back

Another day, we walked through the towering bamboo forest — a place that felt almost spiritual. The calm energy of the swaying bamboo invited reflection, blending nature's beauty with ancient history. As we walked, the forest seemed to echo quietly and our conversations turned to the years we had spent apart. Sohn fondly reminisced about meeting my dad and how vital and full of life he was back then in the late 1980s. It was a heartfelt moment as we reflected on those early days.

Sharing these moments with Karen and Sohn felt like bridging the past and present, grounding us in the richness of the moment.

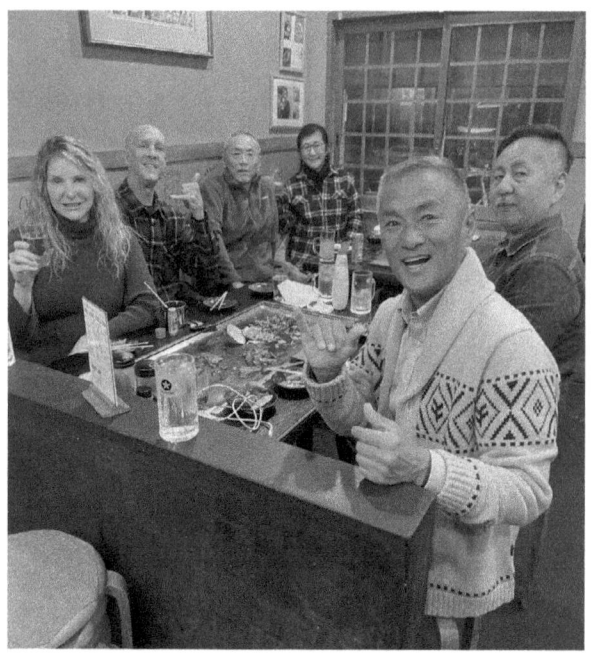

Sohn's secret restaurant did not disappoint

One evening, Sohn took us to a hidden, unmarked restaurant that felt like stepping into another world. The eight-course meal was amazing, but what came after was unforgettable. The owner shared his collection of ancient Japanese artifacts: delicate plates, ornate cups, and a sword — all at least a century old. These weren't just objects — they were pieces of history, carrying the weight of craftsmanship and tradition.

Holding these treasures, I reflected on the concept of value. It's not just about the physical rarity of an item, but the stories and meaning it carries over time. Whether it's artifacts, shared memories, or relationships, the things we value most are those that are irreplaceable.

Reflecting on my time with Sohn, I couldn't help but feel a deep sense of gratitude and pride. What began as a business partnership over 35 years ago has grown into a lifelong friendship. Seeing how far he's come is nothing short of inspiring. Back in the late 1980s, I knew he had potential. He had an eye for business and a determination that was hard to miss. But to witness his transformation into a highly successful businessman across multiple industries is truly impressive.

Sohn's achievements go far beyond what I could have imagined back then. Owning a second home in Hawaii and spending a good portion of his time there, living his best life, is proof of the incredible journey he's had. I'm proud of him — not just for his success, but for the person he is and has become. Our friendship, which started with a handshake and a business deal, has become a bond I'll always treasure.

As we said our goodbyes, I reflected on how rare it is to find a connection that withstands the test of time and distance. Knowing that we've stayed in touch and shared laughs all these years is something I'll always be grateful for. Leaving Sohn, I carried a renewed sense of appreciation for the paths our lives had taken — and the intersections that brought us back together.

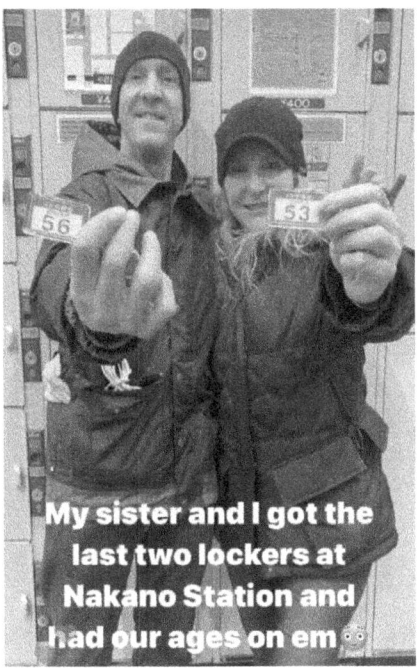

My sister and I got the last two lockers at Nakano Station and had our ages on em

Coincidence? Or cosmic alignment?

Tropical Thailand

From Japan, Karen and I left all of our winter clothing in lockers at Nakano Station and flew to Thailand, trading Kyoto's quiet elegance for the tropical vibrance of Southeast Asia. The humid heat hit us immediately, and Thailand's lush landscapes unfolded like a vibrant, living postcard. Without local guides this time, Karen and I relied on her resourcefulness to plan our adventures. Using an app called Viator, she uncovered some incredible tours that made our time in Thailand unforgettable.

We zipped through bustling streets in Tuk Tuks — quirky open-air vehicles pedaled by drivers that let us take in the sights during the journey. We also went on a restaurant Tuk Tuk tour around town that combined delicious food with the thrill of exploration at six different restaurants, one of them even being a Michelin-starred spot known for its exceptional quality. We also went to a Muay Thai fight, where almost every fight ended in a knockout. The crowd's energy was electric, and the raw intensity of the matches was an authentic taste of Thailand's passion for adrenaline-fueled competition.

One of the highlights was the trip to James Bond Island, made famous by the 1974 film "The Man with the Golden Gun". We boarded a long motorized boat with a few dozen other people and skimmed across the warm tropical waters toward the dramatic limestone spires that jutted out of the sea like something out of a movie — which, of course, they literally were. It felt like the perfect setting for Double O Szabo and his sister Karen to strike a serious back-to-back pose, pretending to hold up guns like we were on assignment.

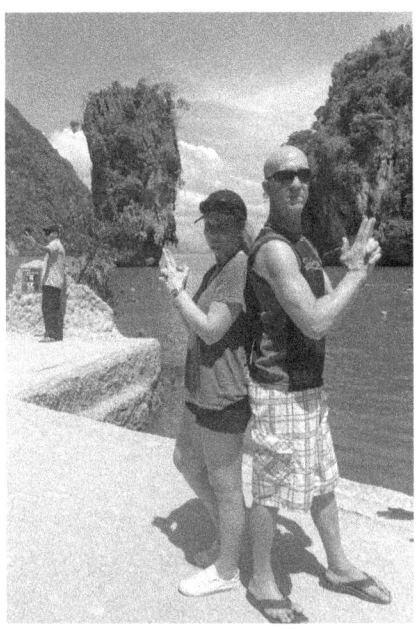

James Bond Island, gun pose with Karen

Another day was a long, beautiful kayak tour. We boarded a different large motorized canoe that took dozens of passengers past jagged limestone cliffs, lush island greenery, and emerald waters to a stunning island. Once there, we switched to smaller kayaks and paddled through caves and hidden lagoons. We also explored another island, walking its shores and soaking in its natural beauty. On another day, we ventured through tight jungle channels in single canoes, surrounded by dense greenery. And on yet another, we tore through the jungle on quads — riding four-wheelers through thick, tropical terrain and kicking up dirt and sand the whole way.

Thailand's natural beauty was intoxicating — a feast for the senses that left us in awe.

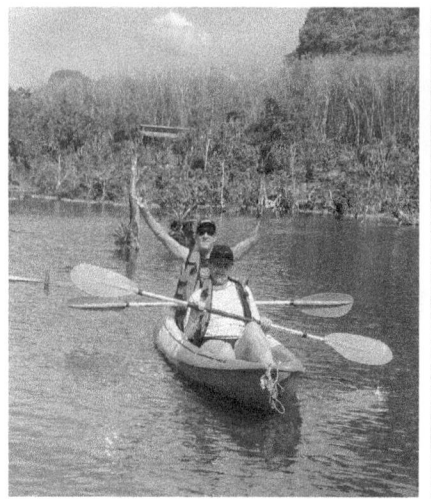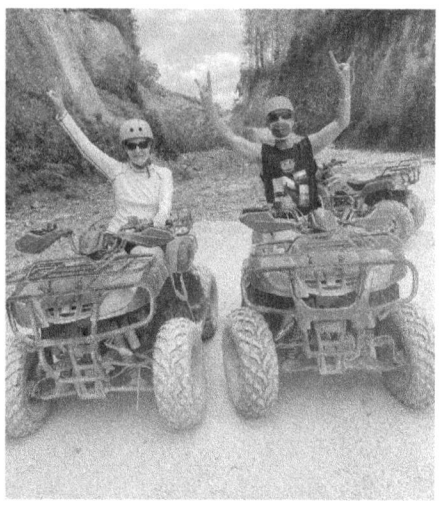

Canoes and quads in Thailand — good times

The he-she cabaret was perhaps the most unexpected and intriguing part of our trip. We knew going in that the performers were transformed from men into elegant and, at times, questionably beautiful women. The show itself was dazzling, blending choreographed routines with humor and a touch of glamour.

After the show, we met the performers, whose variety added to the intrigue. Some were petite and delicate, while others — like the two towering figures I ended up taking a picture with — were well over six feet tall. Their height and look were their strange contribution to the mix of characters on stage, creating a sense of awe and fascination among the intrigued spectators. The photo we captured that night shows a smirk on my face, a joking gesture, but we were full of a mix of amusement and wonder. It's a moment I won't forget — capturing the wild, unpredictable magic of Thailand and reminding us that things are not always what they seem to be.

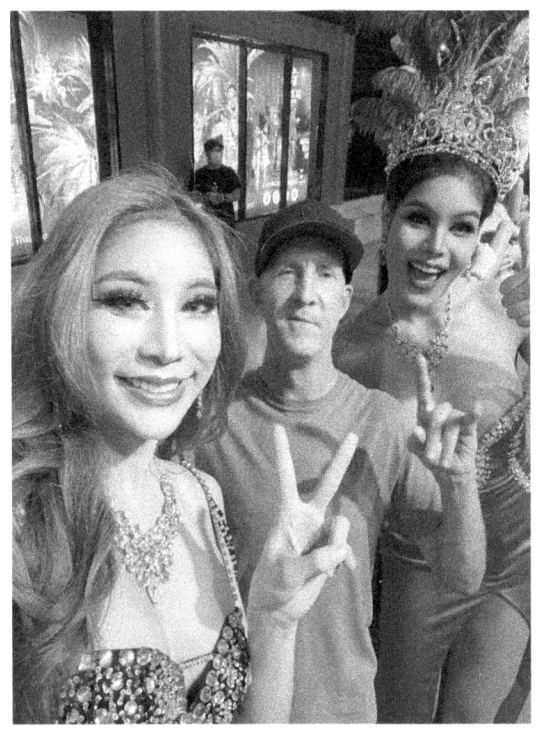

A He-She x 2 + me = 3

As Karen and I packed up to leave, I couldn't help but reflect on how this trip had been about so much more than sightseeing. From Rynn's thoughtful guidance and magic in Tokyo, to reconnecting with Sohn in Kyoto and seeing my same old friend — now an accomplished businessman — to experiencing the vibrant energy of Thailand, the adventure reminded me of life's contrasts and the beauty of embracing them all as we go through life's amazing journey.

-Chapter 18-
Mindset Matters

Mindset is a word that gets thrown around a lot — and yeah, I've used it plenty. Not because I think I'm an expert, but because I've seen firsthand how much of a difference it can make. Especially when life hits hard and things get tough.

Mindset isn't just about getting through the hard stuff — it's also about getting better, stronger, and more intentional in everyday life. You can use it to improve any area you choose to focus on. Whether it's your health, relationships, career, or even just your daily attitude, mindset is a tool that can help you level up any part of life you want to make better.

Mindset isn't something most people are taught growing up. It's usually learned through experience — often the hard way from trial and error and a deep need to do life differently. It's something that can quietly shape everything — how we show up, how we recover, and how we grow.

The cool thing about mindset is how far-reaching it is and how it cuts through every part of your life. The right mindset doesn't guarantee that life gets easier, but it changes how you face what's in front of you.

There are countless tools out there for building a stronger mindset, but here are a few foundational ones that can make a real difference, especially during challenging times:

• Gratitude – Focusing on what's still good, even in the middle of pain, can shift everything. It's easy to get stuck on what's missing. But being thankful for what you have — even the small things — can bring surprising strength and clarity.

• Reframing Challenges – Setbacks happen to everyone. But they don't have to be dead ends. With the right perspective, even painful moments can become powerful turning points. Asking, "What can I learn from this?" is a mindset shift that brings growth instead of bitterness.

• Present Focus – Getting stuck in the past or worrying about the future pulls energy away from what really matters: the now. Staying present in the moment — this breath, this choice, this step — helps keep things grounded and manageable.

• Positive Self-Talk – The way we speak to ourselves matters. Negative thoughts will always show up, but they don't have to stay. Replacing them with encouragement, honesty, and strength is a habit that builds inner confidence and resilience.

• Self-Compassion – Everyone struggles. Everyone messes up. The difference comes in how we respond to ourselves afterward. Showing some grace instead of criticism can help create the space to heal, rebuild, and keep moving forward.

• Small wins matter. Progress doesn't have to be huge to make a difference. Choosing a better meal, getting out for a walk, a bike ride, hitting the gym, or checking something off your to-do list — it all adds up. These little actions build momentum. And when confidence is low, stacking small victories and actually acknowledging them can help rebuild it from the ground up.

Every morning, before even getting out of bed, I run through a simple practice I call my mindset mantra: I'm grateful for the roof over my head, the food in the fridge, and that my body still works well enough to do the things I love — and the things I need to do. I thank the Lord for another day, for the love I share with the people still in my life, and I take a moment to send love to the ones who've passed on. That's how the day starts. From there, I try to notice the good stuff as the hours unfold — even the small things. And when that feeling locks in — not just in my mind but in my heart — everything shifts. Gratitude becomes less of a reaction and more of a way of life.

These are just a few starting points. There's a whole world of books, videos, and voices out there that offer powerful tools to go deeper. A few worth checking out:

• Tony Robbins – A pioneer in the space of personal growth. His approach blends mindset, energy, and real-world action to help people make big changes from the inside out.

• Rob Dial – Host of The Mindset Mentor, he delivers short, focused podcast episodes and videos packed with insight — great for anyone looking for bite-sized but powerful mindset tools.

• Adam Mock – A smart and solid mind in this space who I met through mountain biking. He wrote a great book called Rescue Your Dreams, packed with practical info, prompts, tasks, and journaling exercises to help you level up your life and reconnect with the dreams you left behind. A great book from a great friend and well worth checking out.

• Michael Bernoff – A master of communication and mindset. I've done multiple live events, phone, and online trainings with him, and his work is practical and instantly usable. He focuses on small, intentional shifts that lead to big personal change. He teaches you how to communicate better — both with yourself and others — and helps you create real, lasting progress in your life.

The truth is, there's no one-size-fits-all formula. The key is to find what resonates with you and keep showing up. Mindset isn't a one-time fix. It's a practice. A commitment. A way of life.

Start small. Stay open. Keep growing. No matter where you're at, change is possible.

Heather, Mindset Reflection

In life, we often find ourselves at a crossroads, faced with the choice to either stay stuck in old patterns or embrace the possibility of change. For me, that pivotal moment came just two weeks after my wife Heather passed away. Her death marked the end of a long, painful journey with cancer — a journey that tested every ounce of my resilience. In her absence, I was grief-stricken and directionless, unsure of how to move forward in life after losing my partner of 15 years.

Two weeks later, I found myself in Scottsdale, Arizona, attending my first

Core Strength Experience with Michael Bernoff. I was raw, emotionally spent, and desperate for a way to rebuild — not just my life, but my mindset. What I found there changed everything.

In those final months of Heather's life, what tore me apart most was knowing the fate of the woman I loved. Death was closing in, and I was powerless to stop it. Every glance at her reminded me of what I was about to lose, and no strength I had could change where it was headed. On top of that heartbreak were the relentless challenges of being her caregiver — watching her body weaken day by day, carrying the weight of trying to ease her pain while quietly breaking inside myself.

I stayed home to be by her side, to take care of her, and to let her rest. Sometimes when I needed a break from the weight of it all, I turned to the internet. That's where I stumbled across Tony Robbins, whose messages about mental strength and the power of gratitude resonated deeply with me. He said something that stuck: "When you're thinking of what you're grateful for, you can't focus on the negatives." It was simple yet powerful, and I began weaving gratitude into my daily routine.

Not long after, I discovered Michael Bernoff, another powerful voice in the mindset space who had also learned from the legendary Jim Rohn. Michael's energy and approach to personal development were magnetic. He spoke about rewiring your brain, creating new thought patterns, and breaking free from the habits that hold you back. I was intrigued and decided to try his five-day phone course, Call to Action. It was a small commitment — just a couple of hours each day — but the impact was undeniable.

When I later learned about his live event, Core Strength Experience in Scottsdale, Arizona, I knew I had to go. I arranged everything — Heather's care, my sister's support, and even help from the neighbors with our daughters — to make sure I could attend. The timing was surreal. Heather passed away just weeks before the event, but I still felt compelled to go.

The Core Strength Experience

Walking into that event was like stepping into a different world. The room was alive with energy — people from all walks of life, all seeking something greater for themselves. At the start of the event, you're paired with an accountability partner through an amazing process, setting the tone for the three-day immersion. For nearly 12 hours each day, Michael guided us through exercises, discussions, and activities that pushed us to confront our deepest fears and desires. I learned so much through the different processes he put us through — it was amazing.

One moment stands out vividly. Michael asked a question to the audience, and though it wasn't directed at me, I felt like I should raise my hand. He called me up on stage, where we talked about where I was mentally after Heather's passing. Standing in front of 300 people, I laid it all out there: "For the past year, my head has been in the dirt, dying alongside my wife. I thought my life was heading downhill — straight to hell — and now that she's gone, it might be."

But Michael didn't let me stay in that dark place. Through his guidance, I began to see that my story wasn't over. He helped me reframe my thoughts, teaching me that mindset isn't just about thinking positively — it's about reshaping how you see the world and your place in it. By the end of that weekend, I felt something I hadn't felt in a long time: hope.

After that first Core Strength Experience, I was on fire. I felt alive again, filled with energy and purpose. That summer, I reconnected with friends in Oregon and lived in a high state of mind, enjoying life in a way I hadn't in ages — and glad that Heather was no longer suffering. But as the months passed and the reality of her being gone set in, I fell back into old thought patterns. I hadn't fully locked the mindset into myself yet.

One dark night, those thoughts almost consumed me — but fate had other plans. Even in my lowest moment, something inside me — a spark of what I had learned — pulled me back. I knew I had to re-engage with the tools Michael had given me. I returned to Core Live (formerly Core Strength Experience) four more times — in 2017, 2019, 2024 after Covid, and again in 2025 — each time gaining clarity and power in my mindset.

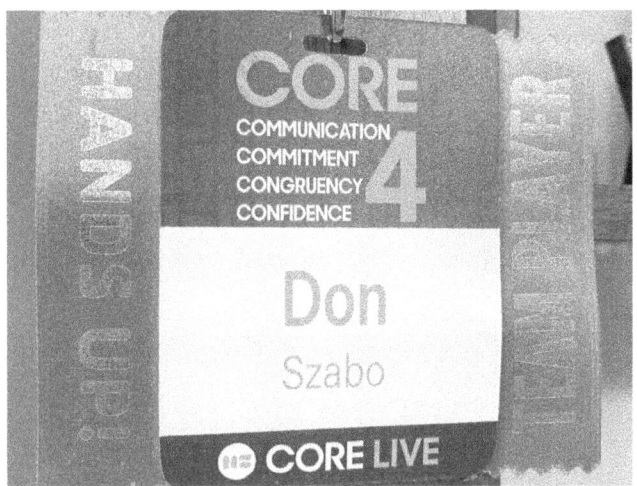

CSE is now CoreLive. New name — same powerful experience

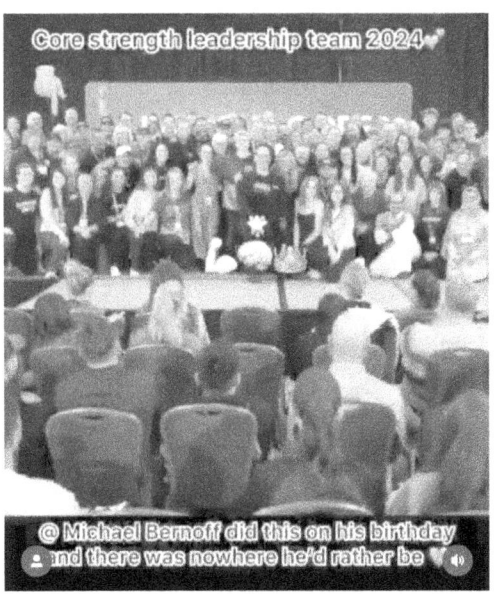

Nowhere I'd rather be too

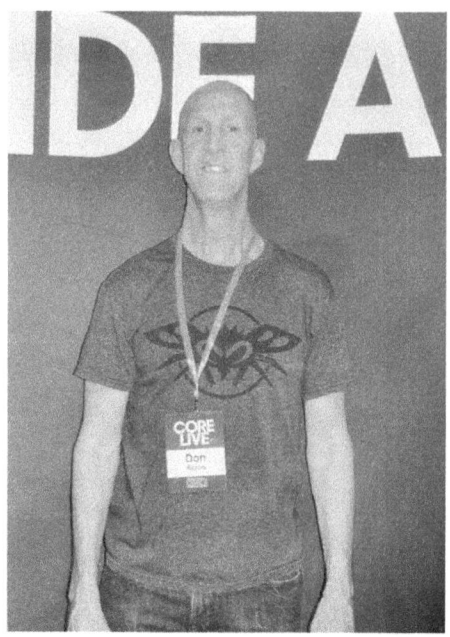
Just before a few powerful days

Three Stools and a Breakthrough

One of the most powerful moments I've ever witnessed took place live on stage at one of Michael Bernoff's Core Strength events. It was raw, real, and absolutely mind-melting — not just for me, but for all 300 of us in that room who sat frozen, wide-eyed, watching something unbelievable unfold right in front of us.

Michael called a woman up from the audience — someone brave enough to share that she'd been carrying deep trauma from her past. You could feel the weight of it the second she started talking. It was still living inside her — not just in the way she moved, but in the way her voice trembled. You didn't have to see her up close to know it was real — you could hear it and feel it.

Michael asked her to also share something she was proud of. Then he asked about a time in her life when she felt pure happiness. She spoke, and her energy shifted. There was a light in her voice when she talked about those better times. It was a genuine, open conversation that set the tone for what was about to happen next.

Then Michael walked over, and an assistant had placed three stools on the stage.

He turned to her and said, "This one represents your trauma."

He pointed to the next: "This is the moment you're proud of."

And the third: "This is your happiness moment."

He told her to begin moving from stool to stool — starting with the trauma. She sat down and began describing what had happened to her. But before she could finish her story, Michael told her to switch — to the proud stool. She had to instantly shift her thoughts and talk about that moment instead. Then again — switch to happiness. Then back to trauma. Then proud. Then happy again.

It picked up more and more speed. The order changed. The switches got faster. She wasn't allowed to finish any story — just fragments, bouncing between pain, pride, and joy. Her mind was forced out of old patterns, constantly rerouted, unable to settle into the groove that trauma had carved over the years.

And then — on what must've been the tenth or twelfth switch — she went to step toward the trauma stool again…and Michael kicked it down.

Hard. Flat to the floor.

Boom. Gone.

He looked her in the eyes and said, "I know you're proud. I know you're happy. So…what's the problem?"

She stood there for a second. Looked down at the space where that trauma stool used to be. Looked back up.

And softly, but with total sincerity, she said, "I don't know."

And then…she smiled.

The room went wild. Cheers, applause, people on their feet. I guarantee some people had goosebumps. You could hear the shift in her voice. The pain was gone. The weight that had been crushing her for years had lifted — right there in front of all of us. She walked back to her seat smiling. Proud. Happy. Whatever used to hold her down no longer had a grip on her life.

It was unreal. This wasn't a trick. It wasn't just a clever stage moment. It was a real transformation. Her brain had been rewired in minutes — and we all saw it happen with our own eyes.

Michael Bernoff is not a motivational speaker. That's usually a rookie term — anyone who's a master at their craft is much more than that. His work is rooted in the principles of neuro-linguistic programming (NLP) and his own invention, Human Interaction Technology (HIT). He understands how the brain works and how to create lasting change, helping people break free from trauma, fear, and limiting beliefs. I've seen him do what seems like magic — helping people overcome PTSD, heal from abuse, and find clarity in their lives.

But what makes Michael truly unique is his ability to connect. His events are about transforming how you see yourself and the world. Through exercises and group activities, he teaches you to communicate better — both internally and externally. It's about rewiring your brain to move forward in life with purpose and confidence.

Michael's work is life-changing. His ability to help people rewire their thoughts, break free from negativity, and move toward their goals is unparalleled. He's not just teaching mindset — he's teaching a way of life.

I've learned that the mind is the most powerful tool we have. It can either trap us in a cycle of pain and doubt or propel us toward greatness. The choice is yours.

This chapter isn't just about Michael Bernoff or the Core Strength Experience — it's about what those moments taught me: that no matter how far you've fallen, you can always climb back up. Mindset matters. It always has, and it always will.

The Power of Mindset

It's easy to look at someone else's life — especially those who seem to have it all — and think, They must be so happy. They must have it all figured out. But time and again, we're reminded that external success doesn't guarantee internal peace. Robin Williams, Kurt Cobain, Chris Cornell, Anthony

Bourdain—the list goes on. These were people who inspired millions, whose talents and achievements made them seem untouchable. Yet behind the curtain, they were struggling.

Their stories are a stark reminder that no amount of fame, money, or recognition can save you if your mindset isn't in the right place. They let their demons and their negative thought patterns take them down paths they couldn't escape. They are tragic examples of what happens when we neglect our mental health — when we let the darkness overpower the light.

I've come to believe that mindset is one of the most valuable tools we have. It's not something you achieve once and then forget about — it's something you have to nurture and work on constantly. Just like you need to eat, sleep, and exercise to maintain your physical health, you need to actively cultivate a positive and resilient mindset to stay mentally strong. There is no finish line in this work. You're either growing, or you're stagnating. And stagnation, in its own way, is a kind of death.

Living Fully

We're all dying, one day at a time. That's the reality of life. From the moment we're born, the clock starts ticking. But instead of letting that reality weigh you down, choose to embrace it. Life is finite, which means every moment matters.

I've never been the type to grit my teeth and endure life, hoping for some mythical reward at the end of the road. I've always believed in enjoying the journey as much as possible. Yes, there are responsibilities, and yes, there are moments when life demands sacrifice. But those moments shouldn't define the whole of our existence.

This mindset has meant living passionately and fully — even when it's cost me. It's meant chasing the adrenaline that comes with action sports — from skateboarding and snowboarding in my youth, moto in the middle, surfing sprinkled across the years, to mountain biking today. It's meant making decisions that others might call reckless, but that I know have made my life richer and more fulfilling. One of my favorite quotes is, "When you're riding, you're living — and everything else is just waiting." Classic quote that resonates with me deeply.

Lessons from the Edge

Looking back, I can see how mindset has shaped every part of my life. It's been the difference between seeing injuries as setbacks or badges of honor, between seeing life's detours as failures or new opportunities. And it's what's kept me going, even in my darkest moments.

If there's one thing I've learned, it's that we all have the power to shape our reality. Mindset isn't just about thinking positively — it's about reframing how we see the world and our place in it. It's about choosing to see challenges as lessons, pain as growth, and life as a journey worth taking head on — and making it the best it can be by being intentional.

This doesn't mean life will always be easy. There will always be struggles, setbacks, and moments of doubt. But if we can keep working on our mindset — if we can keep striving to see the beauty in the chaos — then we can live lives that are not only meaningful, but truly our own.

Chapter 19

Love Life and Rock On 🤘😎🤘

The Highs and Lows of Adrenaline

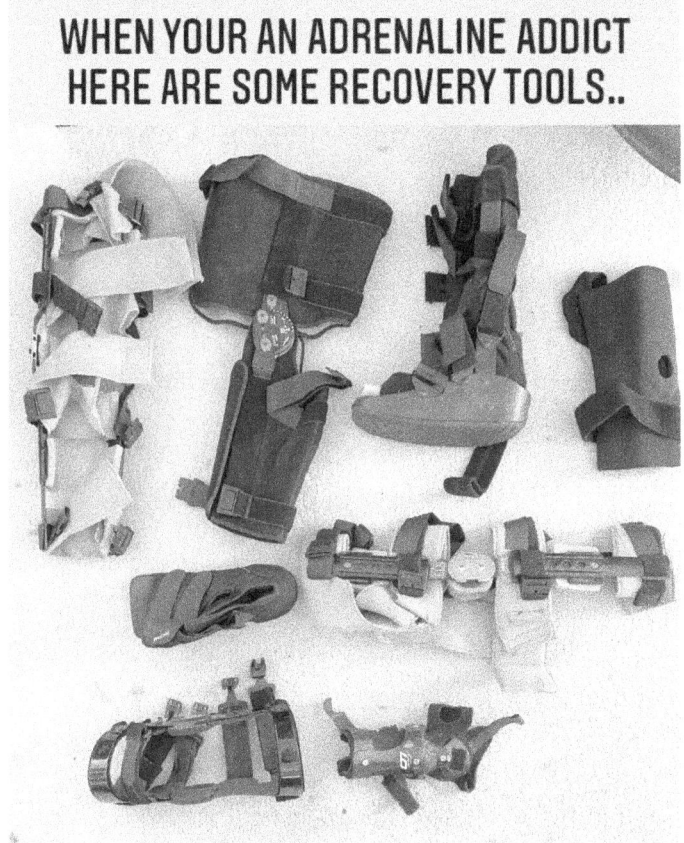

WHEN YOUR AN ADRENALINE ADDICT
HERE ARE SOME RECOVERY TOOLS..

My addiction has never been to substances or vices that traditionally consume people. My addiction has always been adrenaline — the rush of pushing boundaries, the thrill of conquering risk, and the feeling of being fully alive in those high-intensity moments. It's an addiction that's left its mark on me, both physically and mentally. Ten action sports surgeries and more injuries than I can count are just part of the toll from decades spent chasing that rush.

Like I said, some might call it foolish, especially as I've gotten older. They see all the scars, the damage — a torn bicep, tweaked fingers and toes — and think it's time to stop. But it's part of who I am. To me, these aren't just injuries. They're proof I lived with everything I had. They're the cost of embracing life with open arms.

Sure, there are times I wonder if I could've been smarter, maybe a little more careful. But the truth is, I believed I could pull off what I was doing — and sometimes, things just happen at the speed, height, or difficulty of what we're doing. It's not a matter of if you're going to crash — it's *when*. That's just an accepted fact.

I'm a donor, but let's be honest — when they get my body when it's over, they might just throw it in the trash. Too many broken parts, too much wear and tear. But that's the point. I used it. And I think a life well lived leaves some scars behind. I'm going to try to be a bit more careful, but like I said, things happen.

Because for me, life has never been about playing it safe. The choices we make are what shape the ride. And while I might not have mastered the art of caution, I've learned to respect the game — to see the beauty in every scar, injury, story, and every moment — for better or worse — no matter what happens, for the love of what we do.

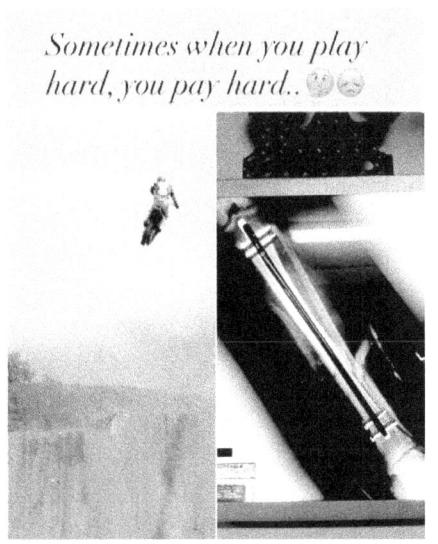

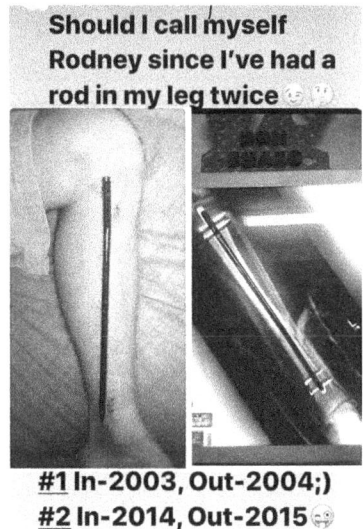

Lower left tibia, repeat offender

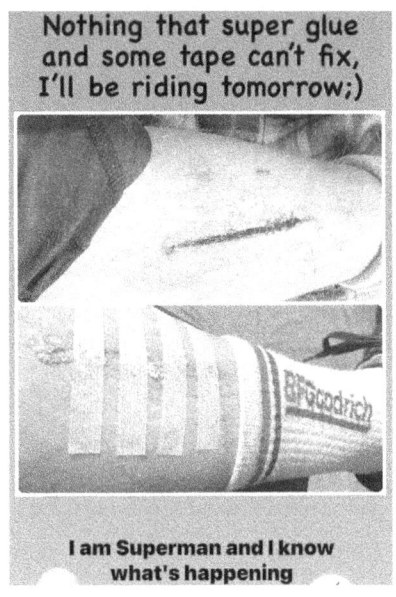

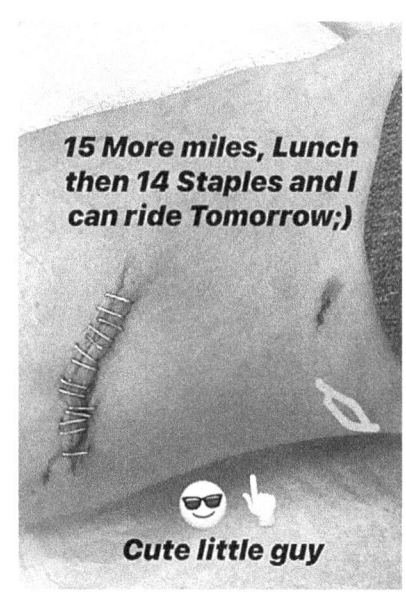

My leg modeling career is over

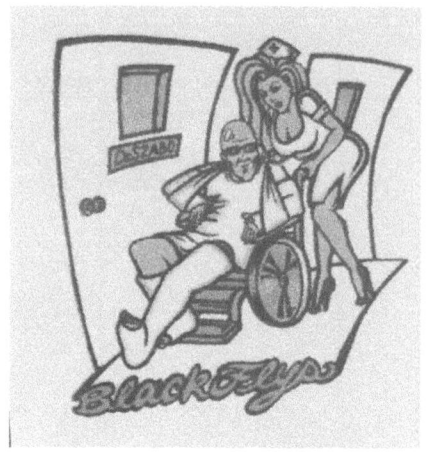
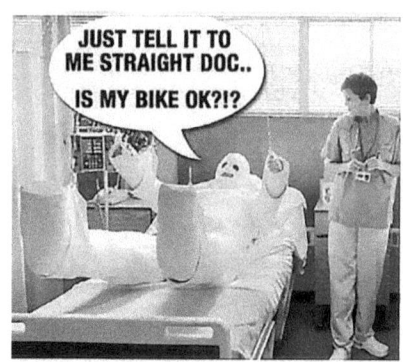

Szabo Injury Cartoon (L), is my bike OK image (R)

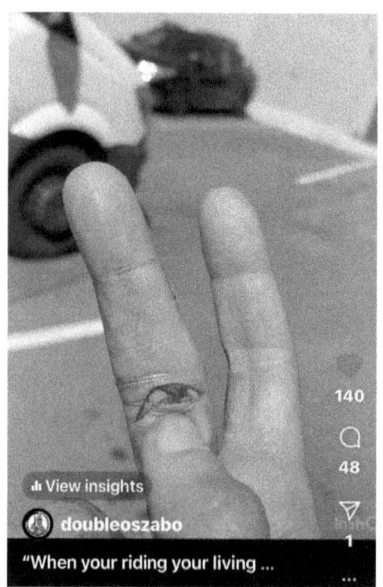
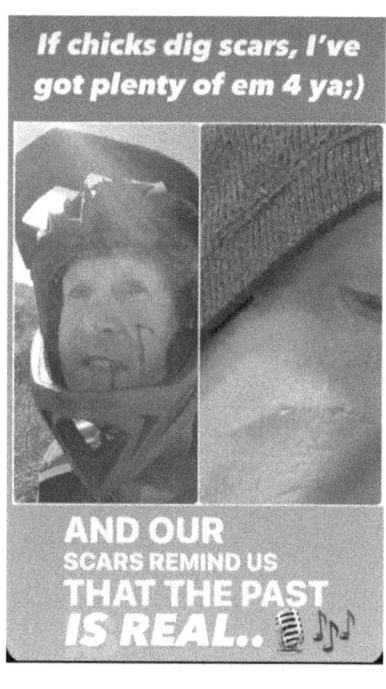

Finger split Peace Sign-ish (L), My "Chicks dig scars" pic (R)

Stacked 2023 Setbacks

After an awesome month long trip to Asia filled with good vibes and reconnections, I came back home ready to get back into my regular rhythm. For me, part of that meant mountain biking. I was stoked to hit the dirt again and picked up right where I left off, heading out with a friend to a jump trail spot I didn't know very well called Area 51.

We hit all the big lines, including a 30-foot road gap and a 40-foot double — the kind of hits that make your heart race and remind you why you love this sport.

But on the last run toward the end of the day — well, it's always the last run, right? Never say "last run" out loud. That's the unwritten rule. The second you call it, you jinx it. It's like tempting fate, and more often than not, something goes sideways. Just say, "one more," or "another run," and keep the universe calm.

Anyway, I lost sight of him in front of me on the trail. Instead of backing off — which is what I should've done, since I was basically riding blind at that point — I foolishly tried to keep pace and catch up, since he knew the trails well. I came out of a corner and saw a jump I thought was straight on. Without hesitation, I sent it. But the trail had other plans — it hooked left, and I didn't. I landed off the trail and rode straight into a big rock, cartwheeling in the air before slamming hard into the ground.

Result? A fractured hip and femur.

Next thing I knew, I was in a hospital bed. After a few days of recovery there, I still wasn't in shape to go home — mainly because I didn't have anyone who could care for me. So they moved me into a nursing center for a few more days to help with some basic necessities.

While lying there recovering, frustrated and off my feet, I started thinking about something I've struggled with my whole life — my weight. I've never been able to gain any, so I got what I thought was a bright idea. Since I wasn't exercising during this downtime, I figured it was the perfect opportunity to try to pack on some pounds since I wouldn't be burning off the calories out biking or doing much of anything. Bad call.

Instead of clean calories, I went all in on unhealthy heavy food. I loaded up on eggs, bacon, unhealthy meals — every week I was eating In-N-Out 4x4 burgers, four patties stacked high with fries on the side. I ate like that for months, thinking I was doing my body a favor to gain weight. But all I was really doing was setting the stage for disaster.

Just as I started bouncing back from the hip and femur fractures, something even worse hit me. Out of nowhere, my wrist and an old dislocated finger flared up with a kind of pain I'd never experienced before. It was excruciating — way worse than when my tib/fib broke and the bone was sticking out of my lower leg. That was visual, gnarly, and painful — but this? This was a deep, hot, sharp internal pain that screamed from the inside out and made my hand completely nonfunctional and in constant pain.

It turned out to be a full-blown arthritis flare-up attack — similar to gout.

It may have been caused by the opioids I took during the initial pain from the fractured hip and femur. It was never really clear what it was, but I can tell you that it hurt like hell and it took me out for quite a while. For the next two months, I had to deal with this new wave of agony on top of the physical recovery I was already going through. The worst of the pain eased after a few weeks, but gripping anything — especially handlebars — was impossible. After a few weeks, I honestly started to wonder if the pain would ever go away.

Once the pain in my hand started to settle down a few weeks later when not using it, I gave riding a shot — but it still hurt a lot. It felt like my wrist bones were bouncing off each other while riding. Still, I kept testing it. A few times a week, I'd try again and again, and little by little, the pain faded until it was finally gone after a couple of months.

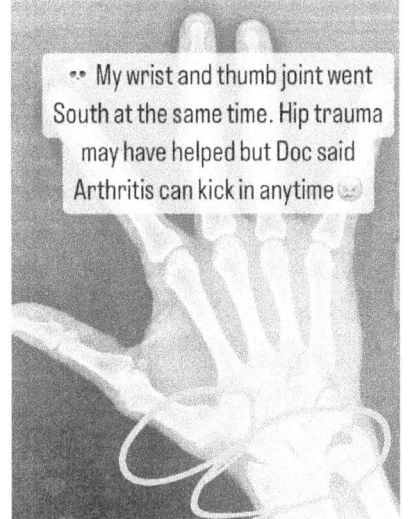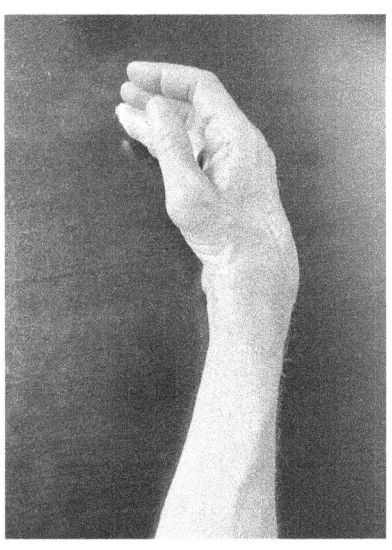

Four brutal blows — hip and femur fractures, and a freak arthritis hand attack.

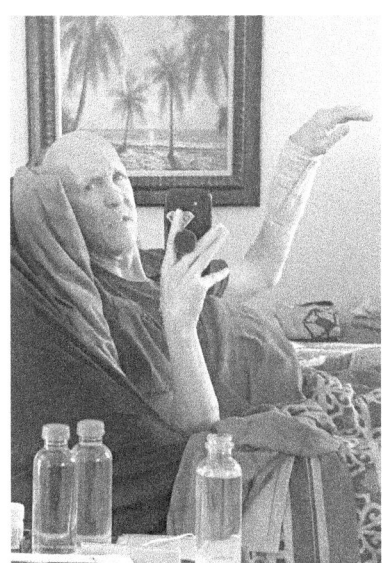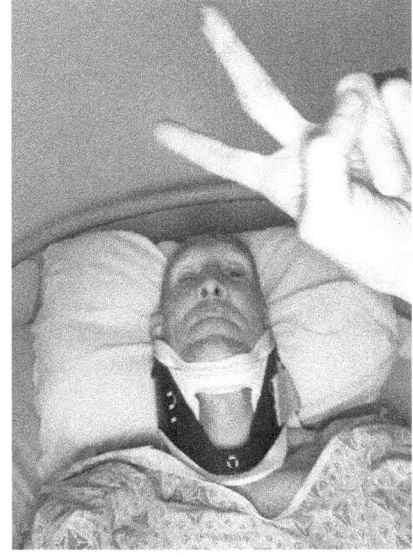

Heart attack and broken ribs. 2023 tried to break me, but I'm still standing.

But then came the biggest hit of all.

Four months of eating all that heavy junky food — with zero cardio — was like a ticking time bomb. One night, after yet another heavy meal, I felt something I'd never felt before. It was like an elephant was standing on my chest. Not just pressure — this was crushing. The weight wouldn't let up. I waited for it to pass, but 30 minutes went by and it only got worse.

I had a friend drive me to the hospital, and as soon as they hooked me up to the heart monitor, things escalated fast. The machine lit up with warning signs, and within moments, they were giving me nitroglycerin. I only remembered that word from old cartoons I watched in the '70s — it always caused explosions and chaos. But in real life, it's no joke. Turns out nitroglycerin is one of the first things they use to manage the symptoms of a heart attack — not to cause an explosion, but to stop one from happening inside your chest by relaxing blood vessels and improving blood flow to the heart.

And that's exactly what was happening. I was having a heart attack.

They ran a camera through my heart arteries and found one that was severely blocked — they said it was 98% closed off. The doctor placed a stent in that artery to open it up, and two more stents in other narrowed heart artery areas. He told me I was lucky. If I had waited any longer, it could've been a full blockage. And that would've been it. Lights out. I would've been gone.

That's when it finally hit me. My mom had suffered a stroke. Cardiovascular disease runs in my family, and I had inherited that risk — and this was almost the last nail in the coffin. I just hadn't connected the dots until I was lying in a hospital bed, wondering if that elephant standing on my chest was about to crush me for good.

Another two months of rehab followed — this time for my heart. I slowly worked my way back into shape with steady cardio until I was keeping my heart rate high for half an hour, five days a week, just like the doctor asked. I was simply grateful to be upright, breathing, and still here. A few friends and people I know weren't so lucky — now, unfortunately, they're on the other side of the dirt.

Eventually, I started easing back into mountain biking on my own. Shorter, safer rides near home just to rebuild my flow, confidence, stamina, and fitness. Then I got a message from Mark Hill, who runs The Segment Channel. He invited me out to Greer Ranch. Compared to the solo recovery rides I'd been doing at home, it sounded like fun.

We had a blast riding, and he got some great clips. I hit a jump I'd done dozens of times before. But this time, I hadn't adjusted my suspension for more aggressive riding, since I'd just been solo cruising until that day. Big mistake. I got bucked forward, nose-wheelied into a tight turn, almost saved it — but went over the handlebars and slammed into the catch berm. That's a built-up corner of the trail. It's a shaped dirt berm designed to hold your speed after a jump, but instead of flowing through it, I landed hard right into it, flat on my back.

Pretty sure I cracked or broke a couple of ribs on that one. There's not much you can do unless they're badly displaced, so it was just another six weeks of downtime and gritting it out. The clicking and sharp pain kept getting better until I was riding again around a month and a half later.

The only upside? I was eating clean by then and had learned some lessons the hard way. But man — 2023 came for me like a freight train, stacking test after test, daring me to break. It took me down for about eight of the 12 months that year. Between the hip and femur fractures, the freak arthritis attack, the heart attack, and then the busted ribs, it was one of the roughest physical years I've ever faced — one setback after another.

But here I am — still riding, still breathing. And still choosing to fight.

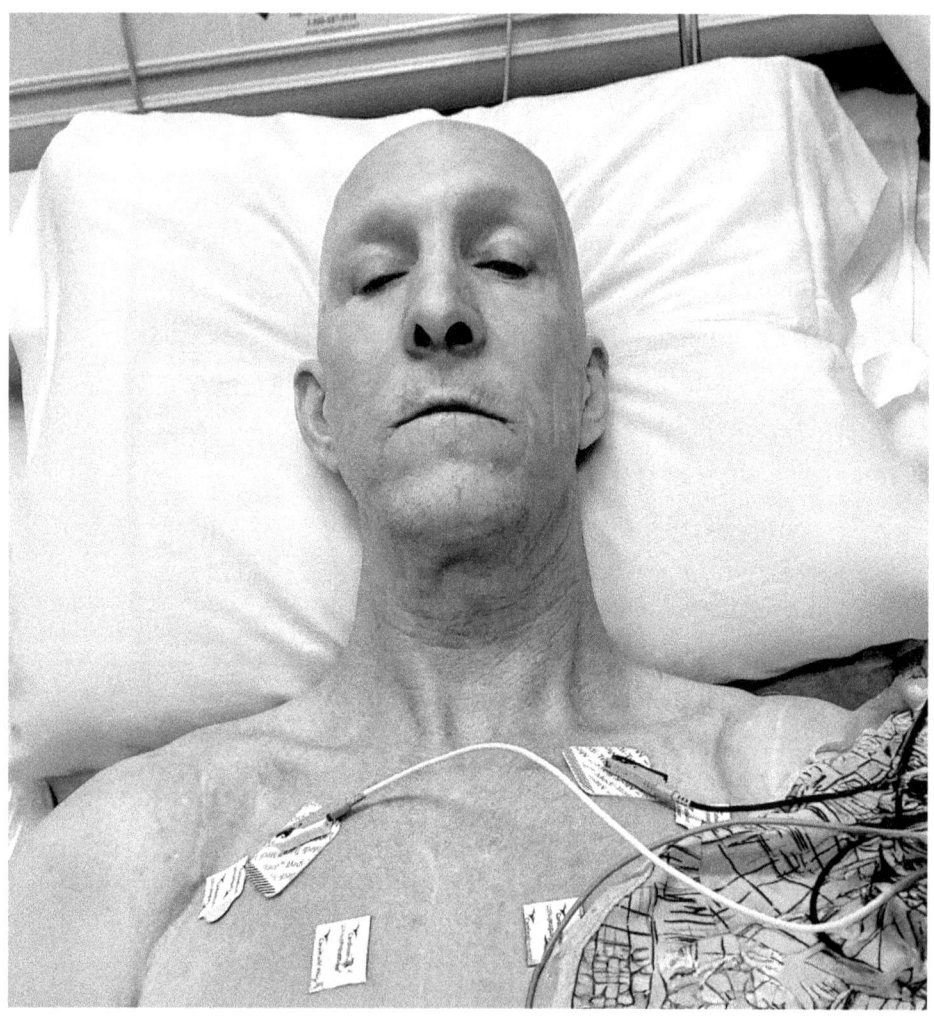

A heart attack with 98% blockage — I should be dead, but it wasn't my time ...

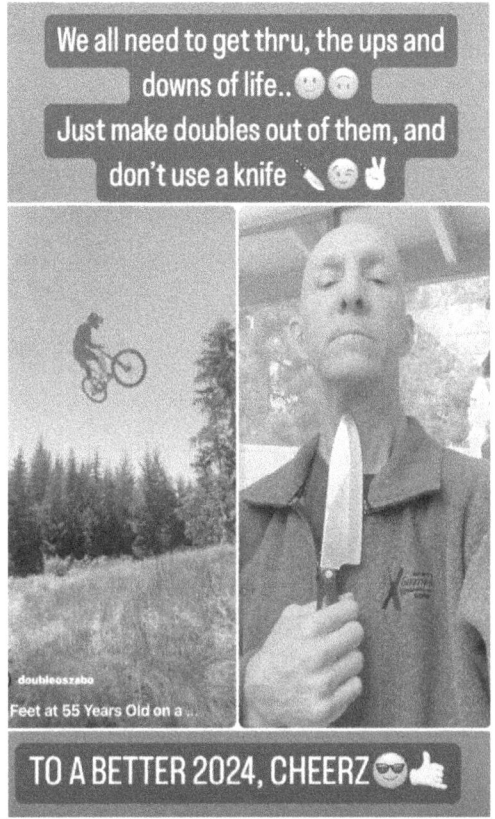

Health is Wealth

There's no replacement body. No spare parts waiting in the garage. Once things start to break down, the choice becomes clear: rebuild — or let it all fall apart. Fighting for health isn't about perfection. It's about staying in the game.

There's so much advice out there about diets, supplements, training routines. But underneath all of it, there are a few core principles that can help keep the engine running better — no matter the mileage.

Food matters. It fuels energy, recovery, and mental clarity. Before the heart attack in 2023, as you know, I had gone off the rails — trying to gain weight by eating heavy meals, loading up on fat and red meat, and barely moving, thanks to the femur and hip fractures and the arthritis flare-up. It was a slow-motion disaster. Cardiovascular disease had been building for years without me knowing, and that lifestyle choice poured gasoline on the fire. That brush with death forced a hard reset.

Eating clean isn't about trends or extremes — it's about being intentional. Real food. Heart-healthy choices. Less garbage. More fuel. It's a mindset shift as much as a dietary one. Eat to support the mission. Eat to stay strong — not to escape emotions or dull pain and not just for flavor.. That change alone can help keep a person alive and thriving.

New health tools are coming fast — and they're not gimmicks. These are real breakthroughs. I've already dabbled in stem cells and peptides, but there's a whole new wave on the rise.

One of the biggest breakthroughs right now is full-body MRI scans — changing the game in early detection. In a single scan, with no radiation, doctors can detect tumors, aneurysms, heart disease, and even early-stage cancers that haven't shown symptoms yet. They can also spot liver issues, prostate problems, spinal compression, or hidden inflammation in your organs before things go off the rails. It's proactive instead of reactive — and that shift alone can save lives. Early detection and personalized treatment are no longer a dream; they're becoming real.

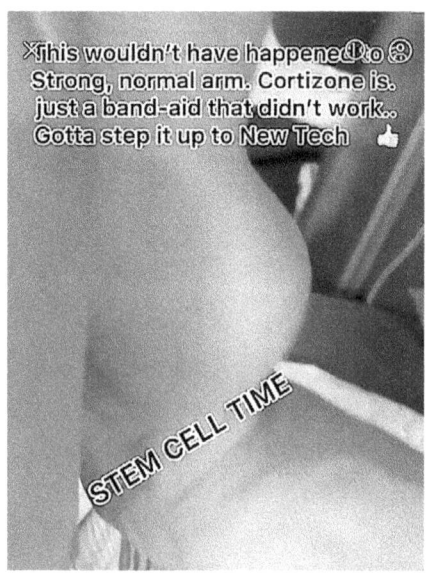

I've dabbled in stem-cell
and peptide treatment

Beyond imaging, new devices are making it possible to track health in ways that used to sound like science fiction. Imagine wearing a patch that quietly runs the kinds of blood tests you'd normally need needles and lab visits for. These "lab-on-a-patch" sensors are being developed to monitor inflammation, heart stress, or even drug levels — all continuously, all without the hassle. That constant feedback could mean catching problems in their earliest stages, when treatment is most effective.

Diagnostics are also becoming faster and sharper. There's already an AI-powered stethoscope that can detect heart disease in just 15 seconds, picking up subtle patterns no human ear could hear. It can flag valve disease, arrhythmias, or early heart failure before symptoms even appear. For many, that speed could be the difference between a silent, life-threatening condition and one that gets treated in time.

Brain health is seeing breakthroughs as well. The FDA has approved a simple blood test that can spot Alzheimer's-related changes with accuracy once only possible through costly scans or invasive spinal taps. For families facing the uncertainty of memory loss, that kind of early clarity can open doors to planning, treatment, and hope.

Even our gut — the so-called "second brain" — is being unlocked in new ways. A swallowable capsule, no bigger than a vitamin, can now travel through the digestive tract, recording real-time data about pH, metabolites, and even neurotransmitters like dopamine. That kind of insight could lead to person-alized nutrition and treatment plans that stop problems before they start.

Taken together, these advances signal a powerful shift. We are moving from waiting for illness to strike toward a future where medicine can predict, prevent, and personalize care. This isn't far-off speculation — it's unfolding now.

I know I need to carve out time to dive deeper, because this isn't science fiction anymore. It's happening. And if we pay attention, we might just get ahead of things — before bad things get ahead of us.

The future of health is arriving, and it's giving us tools we've never had before. The message is clear: stay curious, stay moving, and stay open to the new. Because with these advances, we're not just adding years to our lives — we're adding life to our years.

Movement is still life, and the basics remain the same: get the heart rate up, five days a week, for at least thirty minutes. Not for vanity — for survival. Cardio. Strength training. Show up. Lift. Move. Sweat. Ride. Rebuild. When the body is under load, the mind sharpens. When the muscles fire, so does discipline. Strength carries into every other part of life.

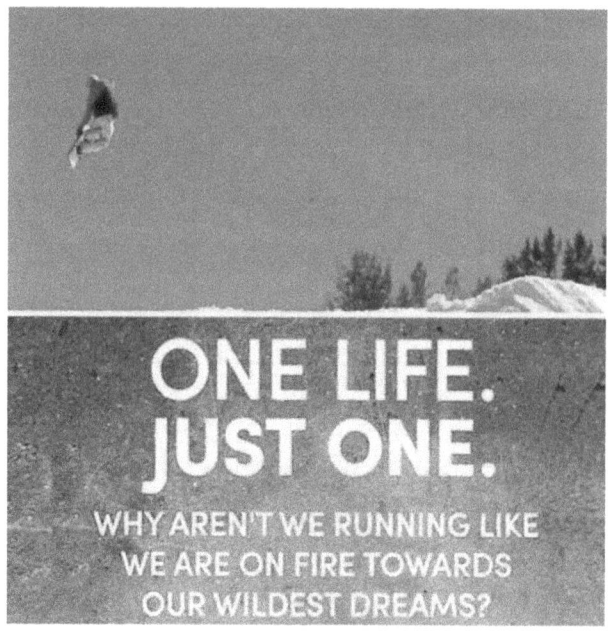

Yoga & the Breath

Stretching and yoga? Total game changers. Flexibility might've felt optional once, but not anymore. Stretching keeps things moving, reduces injury, and helps with recovery. And yoga? That's more than just movement. It teaches presence. Control. Breath. Balance — not just on the mat, but in life. It builds a different kind of strength. Quiet. Centered. Focused. It helps shut out the noise and reconnect with what matters.

When you breathe in, think: peace, love, and happiness. That's what one of my instructors, Zahir, always says — and it stuck with me. On the exhale, you let go of the stress, the heaviness, the mental noise. It's not just a breathing rhythm — it's a mindset reset. And the crazy part? It works.

My other instructors Kim, Suzanne and Jer emphasize the breath during yoga. A lot of teachers say it's the most important part of the practice. I used to think that just meant breathing through tough poses. But now I know it's way deeper than that. The inhale is your invite — to calm, strength, focus, or whatever you need. The exhale is your release — letting go of tension, anger, pain, or whatever's been weighing you down. Somewhere in between the two is where the real magic is. That's presence.

You don't need to be in a yoga studio to feel it. This kind of intentional breathwork — taking in the good and letting go of the bad — can be used anytime, anywhere. It's like gratitude. A simple tool, but powerful when you actually use it. And the best part? You don't have to be anywhere in particular — just present.

You can walk into a yoga class angry, anxious, or totally drained — and walk out lighter, clearer, and more connected. The poses open the body, but it's the breath that opens the mind. For me, yoga has become mindset training in motion.

Every inhale is a chance to shift your state — toward peace, clarity, or strength.

Every exhale is a release — a letting go of tension, noise, or anything weighing you down.

And sometimes, just repeating Zahir's words — peace, love, and happiness — can bring you right back to center.

Part of taking care of your health isn't about staying young — it's about staying alive. Really alive. Choosing to participate. To play. To be able to chase sunsets and *singletrack* for longer — and actually feel good while doing it. To have more time for the things and people you love. To be present and ready for whatever comes next in your life.

Wherever someone is on their path — whether starting over, pushing through setbacks, or just staying consistent day by day — there's no better time than now to take your health seriously. Train the mind like a muscle. Be intentional. Keep the engine running the best you can. Because when health and mindset line up, everything else starts to follow. Life doesn't just go on — it gets better.

Enjoy the Ride — Make It Great

Go out and live your life. Chase your dreams. Make things happen. Don't wait around for the perfect moment or for retirement to finally bring happiness — because that day might never show up. Plan for the future, sure, but don't sacrifice your joy today thinking you'll start living "later." Some people live that way and never even make it to that "later." Life is short. Live now. They say 85% of the things we worry about never even happen — and the ones that do? We handle them better than we expected, and we learn something from it. Things work out. Don't waste your energy stuck in fear. Life moves way too fast. Enjoy the ride while you've got the chance.

It's been a gift to share my story and some of the lessons I've picked up through the highs, the lows, and everything in between. If any of it helps someone else live better, love harder, or get through their own rough patch, that means everything to me. I truly wish you the best life — one filled with purpose, passion, and peace.

Back in the '90s, I traveled the world without a cell phone. It was a simpler time — free in so many ways. You'd walk up to people, ask for directions, figure things out face to face. No GPS, no apps, no "likes" — just real life unfolding, moment by moment in front of you. Those days were awesome.

Looking back, I feel like I grew up at the perfect time for me. I got to ride the wave of action sports before it went mainstream and the world got consumed by tech. Skateboarding all over Southern California by word of mouth, snowboarding different resorts around the country and globe — we found creative ways to chase what we loved, even when we were broke. We hustled. Sometimes we'd walk into a ski resort's marketing office and tell them we were shooting photos for a brand or magazine, asking for a few lift tickets in exchange for giving their mountain credit. Sometimes they got something out of the deal, sometimes they didn't — but we always had a blast. It was a wild, free, incredible time to be alive. Those years taught us how to hustle with heart, and how to turn passion into opportunity. Thousands of hours. Thousands of memories. Truly some of the best years of my life.

Of course, life hasn't always been smooth. I've had moments that felt like the end of the world. Times so dark, I questioned whether I even wanted to be in this world anymore. The mind can twist things so badly, I started to believe everyone would be better off without me. But mindset is everything. It's like a muscle. You have to train it, strengthen it, protect it — because it carries you when nothing else will.

Now I look at my beautiful daughters and hope they'll feel the same way about their own time growing up. The world they're stepping into will be almost unimaginable compared to what we've known. Robots cooking meals. Smart tech running the house. Self-driving cars. It's already happening — and it's just the beginning. Breakthroughs in AI, healthcare, and technology are moving forward all at once, feeding off each other and accelerating faster than we ever thought possible. The future is coming fast — and it's beyond anything we've seen before.

And they'll also remember their mom — my amazing wife, Heather — who left this world way too soon. One day, cancer will be a curable disease. I truly believe that will happen in their lifetime. People won't have to feel the kind of pain, fear, and loss that we've experienced. It breaks my heart that Heather missed that future. But I believe she's needed up there now, just like we needed her here. They say the good ones are taken first. Miss you babe…♡

I don't know what the future holds. But I'm beyond grateful for the life I've been given, and the era I grew up in. I wouldn't trade it for any other. I wasn't meant for candles and horse-drawn wagons — I was meant for this time. For boards, bikes, chaos, curveballs, love, and freedom. And for all the madness? It's been one hell of a ride.

To my daughters, my future grandkids, and anyone who reads this: Enjoy the ride. Live fully. Love fiercely. Don't wait. No matter where you are in life, it's still a beautiful world and an amazing journey — for those willing to stay present, keep progressing, and live fully every day.

Even with all the twists and turns, it's been a great life. A powerful one. And the best part? The story's not over. At 59, I know there are still more passions and more gears to go through in the years ahead. At least I hope so. You never really know — so live now.

Whatever your story is, make it great.

I've known people who seem to have everything but are miserable — or no longer here. And I've seen others who have nothing but are the happiest people you'll ever meet. The difference? It's mindset. The choice is yours.

What we all need to do is…

Love Life and Rock On.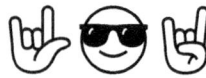

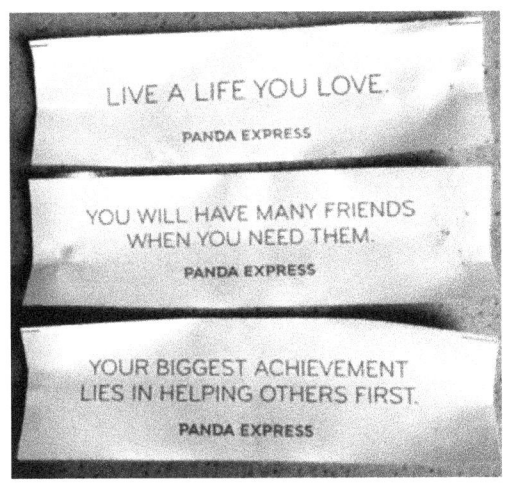

Kaylee and Ashlyn are the sweetest fortune cookies life gave me

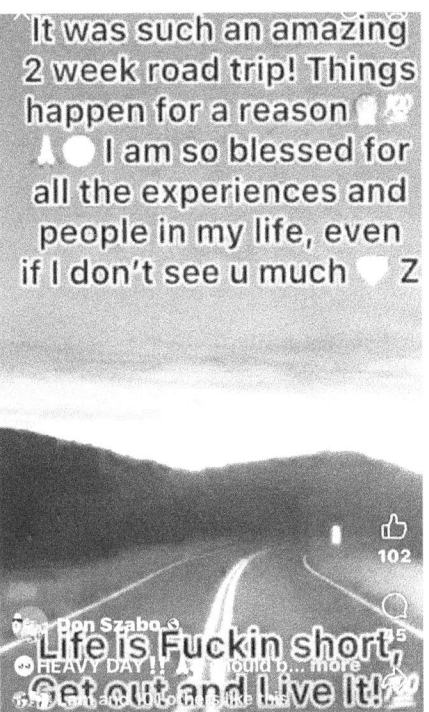

Life is Fuckin short! Get out and Live It!

Glossary Of Terms

- **A-Line** = trail name of a famous jumpline at Whistler Bikepark, BC, Canada.

- **Action Sports** = Extreme Sports, just a cooler way to say it, and referring to the core sports like skateboarding, surfing, snowboarding, moto, and MTB.

- **Blind Drop** = usually jumping downward, you can't see where you are landing. Quite often the feature is looked at first, remembered what to do and then go do it with the vision of what to do in your mind.

- **Boardercross** = a multi person snowboard race thru a course with jumps, turns and obstacles to the finish line.

- **Bridge Drop** = wooden structure to ride across / drop off of.

- **Bulletproof Terrain** = very icy snow.

- **Bumps into Doubles** = bumps into jumps.

- **Charging Chutes** = aggressively riding down skinny steep areas, requiring skill and control going down a difficult thin run.

- **Cliff Jump** = jumping your snowboard, mountain bike, or moto off a Cliff with the intention of landing and riding away.

- **Clipped the Knuckle** = came up a little bit short of the landing but rode it out ok.

- **Corked spin trick** = an off axis ariel, usually involving a spin and a flip at the same time while in the air doing the trick.

- **Dirt Merchant** = trail name of famous bigger jumpline at Whistler Bikepart, BC, Canada.

- **Double** = a jump over a gap between two dirt mounds.

- **Double Overhead** = a wave that is twice as high as you are.

- **Double Step-down** = jumping down a cliff, to a landing, and then jumping down to a further landing to finish this performance.

- **Drop** = whether dropping into a wave ramp or trail. Also a single physical drop on whatever you're riding (bike / board).

- **Foam Pit** = a soft landing area made of foam blocks. People learn tricks into soft foam before landing the trick on ground.

- **Full Send** = maximizing the jump.

- **Gaps** = a jump from take off to landing that doesn't have an area to ride in between. You gotta jump to the landing between the takeoff jump.

- **Halfpipe** = basic shape originally built for skateboarding, You go up transitions on both sides, turn 180 degrees to ride to the other side. Tricks add difficulty when maneuvering on each side.

- **Hips** = jumps that you land in a sideways direction from the direction started.

- **Inverted Aerials** = going upside down while doing an aerial and land back right side up how you started the aerial.

- **Jump Lines** = trails that are made with multiple jumps down the trail to ride.

- **Line** = an exact path that a person is taking in whatever sport they are doing.

- **Masonite** = a hardboard, usually in a 4' x 8' master sheet to use as is or cut down to needed size. Usually for a smooth nice, good wheel grip skateboard ramp surface to ride.

- **MTB Scene** = mountain bike scene.

- **No Footed Trick** = adding difficulty by taking your feet off whenever you're riding, usually while in the air and putting them back in place for the trick landing.

- **Over The Falls** = getting thrown forward by a wave and crashing in front of it.

- **Progression Line** = getting bigger and bigger jumps as you move along the trail.

- **Quads** = a four wheel off-road vehicle you sit on top of and ride like a dirt bike, it has handlebars to steer and control it.

- **Ramp** = a usually wooden built structure to skateboard up transitions to do tricks on. Quite often in a half pipe formation.

- **Resi-Mat** = soft rideable surface put on the landing of a jump. If you fall, this soft surface will help you not get hurt.

- **Sharp Intricate Lines** = technical line, not a wide open line/path.

- **Shredding** = riding really well at whatever sport a person is doing.

- **Shuttle** = a vehicle, paid or private, that transports mountain bikers and their bikes to a high point for a downhill ride.

- **Singletrack** = A narrow dirt trail for one mountain bike or motorcycle rider.

- **Skid Plate** = dirt bike engine protector on the bottom of motorcycle.

- **Slashing Turns** = turning abruptly to show or do your quick turn abilities.

- **Step Up** = you leave jump and land on a higher landing.

- **Stoked** = strong set of emotions, creating happiness and joy for yourself or with others, all being happy together.

- **Thread through** = going through a tight area.

- **Toy Hauler** =Trailer with a fold-down ramp that carries dirt bikes and/ or quads and doubles as living space anywhere you park.

- **Tow-In** = following a riders moves in front of you. Mimicking their speed and Lines usually over jumps or difficult terrain.

- **Triple Overhead** = a wave that is three times higher than you.

- **Whip** = MTB or Moto trick of putting the bike sideways and/or tipped over while in the air, bringing it back straight and landing back on your wheels at the end.

Back-Words

I probably created this book backwards. I'm not a trained writer, and I'm not much of a reader either. Most of the content I take in is by listening — sometimes while hiking or walking. That's exactly how this book came to life. I spoke most of it into my phone while walking 10–20k steps a day. Sometimes through neighborhoods, sometimes out on a trail, always enjoying the view and letting my heart pour out through my words into my phone.

Later, I tuned up the words and listened back to the chapters during food prep, bike prep, workouts, mellow rides, driving, and more. Anytime something didn't sound right, I'd fix that section on the spot — or try to make a note to revisit it later. I never read a guide or followed a format. I just told my truth — my stories — and how it all felt, in my own words. Like Frank Sinatra — and later, the Sex Pistols — sang, "I DID IT MY WAY."

I want to thank Adam Mock for bringing his creative vision to the covers and so much more. He's a brilliant friend who's given unwavering, thoughtful advice. His book Rescue Your Dreams is a powerful and well-articulated journey to reclaim the life people forgot they wanted — truly inspiring, with an incredible process built around prompts, journaling, and reflection.

Rynn Kawahara — thank you for being a great friend and for your awesome help with the artwork on the book covers and so much more. Thanks for tirelessly working via three-way text with me and the artist, Amadeus Tafoya, who brought the vision to life. You've got a sharp eye for design. I'm sure being a creative music artist in Japan helps, and you also have a heart of gold. I'm truly blessed that the algorithms brought us together 5 years ago. Keep rockin' girl.

A big thanks to my lifelong friend Vince Kitchen — for putting out his book Normally Unusual first and telling me it was time to do mine. Funny enough, it all came together while I was at one of Michael Bernoff's Mindset events. I thank him as well for helping guide my Mindset journey over the past 10 years and counting. He's an amazing man with so much knowledge and insight in that space — it's truly incredible what he does, as you have seen and this is only a glimpse of what he is truly capable of.

To all my Action Sports friends who endorsed this book —
So many people look up to you, and I'm proud to call you my friends. It's been awesome to ride, skate, snowboard, and push limits with you over the years. I've bounced between sports my whole life, chasing the next rush and enjoying every Action Sports discipline that I wanted to do. Many of you are multitalented and thrive in more than just sports — some through art, music, or giving back in powerful ways — but each of you chose one sport to focus on, committed to it, excelled at it, and became masters over the years — and it shows. The level you've reached is nothing short of inspiring. You are true legends in the eyes of the world, and that's something to be proud of. Much respect.

I'm grateful to each of you for having my back on this book journey. It truly means a lot to me, and you've all lived such amazing lives. You should write a book — I'll endorse it, ha ha.

Dave England's path has been a bit different. We started skateboarding together back in the '80s, and in the '90s we also surfed, rode snowboards, and pushed our limits — he always charged harder than most. At one point, he even rode snowboards at a local pro level. But what really made him famous wasn't Action Sports — it was becoming a legend of chaos and comedy through the Jackass series and now the movies. So no, he's not a career athlete like the rest — but he's a true original, and I'm proud to call him a friend...even if he is a Jackass.

To my mom, dad, and Heather ♡. You're no longer on this side of the dirt, but I feel you with me. I see your hands in so many of the good things that have lined up in my life, even when I don't fully understand the reasons. I still wrestle with God's plan when it comes to losing Heather — but I've learned to keep showing up and to find joy in what remains. It's a beautiful life, and I'll continue to be grateful for it every day. Love you forever.

Thanks to my sister, the rock of common sense in my life when I needed it most. I'm glad we got to take that month-long trip to Asia together when you were in between your 25-year engineering career and the amazing work you do now. I'm stoked I got to document some of that trip here with words and a few pics. You definitely got the brains out of the deal. I just "send it" in sports and in life and hope to stick the landing. Love you sis...♡

To my amazing daughters — thank you for giving me purpose when everything else felt lost. Watching you grow into strong, thoughtful, beautiful young women — pursuing your own paths in college and in life — it blows my mind. You're growing up so fast, and I know it will only continue. I can't wait to see each new chapter unfold. The future is yours, and I hope I get to see as much of it as possible. I love you with all of my heart. I have so many great memories with you, and can't wait to make more of them...♡

And to you — thanks for walking through "The Life of Z" with me. If something in here reminded you that you can take a hit, face the unexpected, and still keep pushing forward...then you get it. Because that's the point. Sometimes, the mess becomes the message. Things go sideways. Dreams change. People we love get taken from us. But that doesn't mean we're done — it just means we've gotta adjust. Sometimes, what looks like the end is just a different road we didn't see coming. And if you stuck with me through the life stories, the highs and lows, the crazy stunts, the crashes, the injuries, the heartbreak, and the mindset shifts needed to deal with it all — and you felt any of it — then you were in it with me. And that means more than you know. We don't get to choose what happens to us. But we do get to choose what we do next. Even when the world feels upside down, there's still a road forward. We can't always see it, but it's there. Whatever's ahead for you, I hope you grab it with both hands and make it count. You've got this — with the right mindset, you can make it happen.

Life's not about perfection. It's about pushing forward, adapting, and living with purpose — and enjoying the ride.

Stay strong, stay wild, and live your story to the fullest.

CheerZ 🤘😎🤘

I'd also like to thank Dave from Bluejay Ink for arranging my words and photos for the book production. A lot goes into making a book and I'd highly recommend giving it a shot if it's something you're passionate about. For me, it's been a mind-expanding, heartfelt journey and I'm so thankful I was able to do it. It's not easy — and there are a lot of moving parts — even though books themselves stand still in time…

About the Author

Don "Double O" Szabo is a lifelong adrenaline junkie who's spent nearly 50 years pushing the limits of what the human body and spirit can endure. He came up through the legendary Southern California Action Sports scene, rising as a top-tier sponsored skateboarder with his sights set on going pro — until the mountains pulled him in a new direction. Don transitioned into professional snowboarding for over 10 years, traveling the world and being featured in some of the most iconic videos and magazines of the late '80s through the late '90s. He's lived life airborne, sideways, and full-throttle ever since.

His snowboard career ended early after a motocross injury that required multiple surgeries forced him to stop — but his passion for adrenaline never left. Don kept chasing the edge, riding moto for a total of 20 years — pushing big jumps, doing wild stunts, and racking up injuries that came with living wide open. These days, it's mountain biking that fuels him most. The speed, the flow, the risk — it's the perfect mix of freedom and challenge that keeps him going, and he still can't get enough.

He's survived many crashes, multiple concussions, a coma, and a heart attack — and has the scars and ten Action Sports surgeries to prove it. Off the bike and board, he's a father, health-conscious adventurer, storyteller, and a survivor of things that others didn't walk away from. He's lost his mom, dad, and the love of his life to cancer, battled through grief, and somehow kept finding reasons to get back up and ride again. He's known both the highest highs and the lowest lows, and keeps choosing to show up with a smile.

With a voice forged through pain, passion, and perspective, Don shares raw, unfiltered stories from the front lines of Extreme Sports and life itself. His memoir is more than a highlight reel — it's a testament to resilience, mindset, and purpose. Riding has become more than just an adrenaline rush; it's also a way to reconnect, reset, and keep moving forward.

When he's not inspiring others, he's staying active in the gym, doing yoga, cooking, hiking, biking, and soaking in the natural beauty around him — whether near home or traveling. Still riding, still breathing, still chasing the next thrill, but also embracing the next chapter of life with passion, purpose, and gratitude for the ride through this beautiful world.

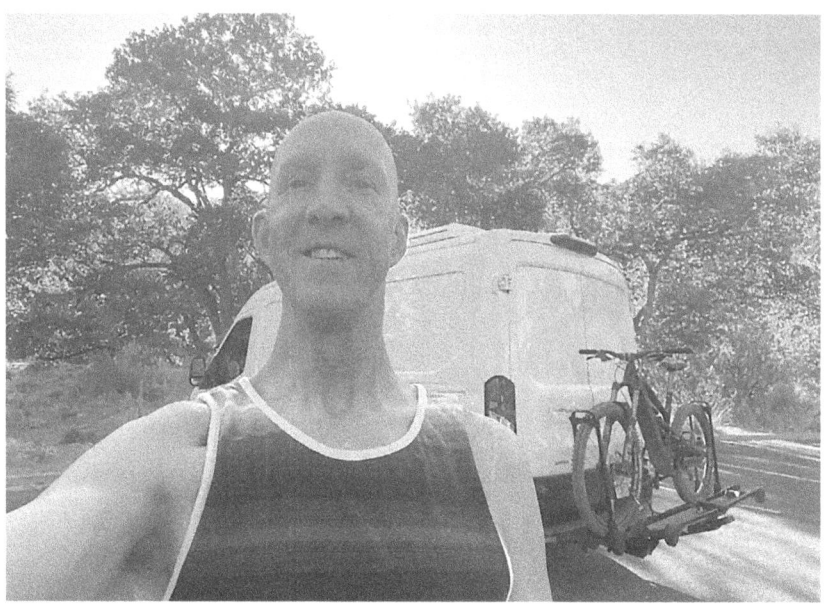